Drugs of Addiction

and Non-Addiction

Drugs of Addiction
and Non-Addiction
Their Use and Abuse

A Comprehensive Bibliography
1960–1969

⌐⸴⌐⸴⌐⸴

by
Joseph Menditto

The Whitston Publishing Company
Incorporated
Troy, New York
1970

3/1971

(given)

© 1970 by
Joseph Menditto

Library of Congress Catalog Card Number: 79-116588

Printed in the United States of America

To my wife Vinnie
and our four children,
Connie, Marcus, Eva and Joey,

& HINDU LOBBI.

PREFACE

The present compilation contains about six thousand entries
for works published between 1960-1969, and is designed to provide users with a convenient and comprehensive guide to the
research material in the field of addiction. Few bibliogra-
phies on the subject exist. The most significant difference
between this work and others lies in the purpose of the project. Some have preferred to cover a longer period, requiring
selectivity, others have chosen to deal with a specific subject within the subject. It seemed to me that there was a
need for a work which would survey extensively the literature
of the last decade, almost entirely omitted from other works
of the same nature. Thus the effort has been made, and I hope
it will prove worthwhile.

The form of bibliographical arrangement follows the pattern
mostly familiar to the users. Thus under each subject, the
listing is the following: Books and Essays; Doctoral Dissertations; Periodical Literature. The first two are arranged by
author, the last is alphabetical by title. An author index
is provided.

To the users I must further explain that the subdivision
within the periodical literature in "General" and "Scientific"
is purely arbitrary. This special effort was made on the
grounds that such division would facilitate the research according to the special interest of the individual. By all
means errors and misjudgments in each category will and do
exist. I apologize for the inevitable errors.

This bibliography owes a main debt to Stephen H. Goode,
Director of Russell Sage College libraries, whose advice and
encouragment were an essential element and a firm support
from beginning to end; also I should like to express my ap-
preciation to my colleagues and the library staff, in parti-
cular Annette Daley, for their patience, tolerance and help-
ful assistance. I suspect that they will be as relieved as
I by the end of such effort. At last I am indebted to my
wife and our children for the help received and for allowing
me a freedom from family obligations while compiling the present bibliography.

CONTENTS

AMPHETAMINES AND STIMULANTS: Books and Essays

Beckman, Harry. DILEMMAS IN DRUG THERAPY. Philadelphia:
    Saunders, 1967.
Blum, Richard H. "A history of stimulants," SOCIETY AND
    DRUGS. San Francisco: Jossey-Bass, 1969, pp. 99-114.
Brow, Thorvald T. THE ENIGMA OF DRUG ADDICTION. Spring-
    field, Illinois: C.C. Thomas, 1961.
Burn, Harold. DRUGS, MEDICINES AND MAN. New York: Scrib-
    ner, 1962.
Dureman, Ingmar. DRUGS AND AUTONOMIC CONDITIONING; the
    effects of amphetamine and chlorpromazine on the simul-
    taneous conditioning of pupillary and electrodermal re-
    sponse elements. Stockholm: Almquist and Wiksell, 1960.
Evans, Wayne O. THE SYNERGISM OF AUTONOMIC DRUGS ON OPIATE
    OR OPIOID-INDUCED ANALGESIA: a discussion of its poten-
    tial utility and an annotated bibliography. U.S.A. Med-
    ical Research Laboratory Report, no. 554, 1962.
Geller, Allen, and Boas, Maxwell. DRUG BEAT; a complete
    survey of the history, distribution, uses and abuses of
    marijuana, LSD, and amphetamines. New York: Cowles Book
    Company, 1969.
Hoffer, A., and Osmond, H. THE HALLUCINOGENS. New York:
    Academic Press, 1967.
Hyde, Margaret O. MIND DRUGS. New York: McGraw-Hill, 1968.
International Narcotic Enforcement Officers Association.
    NON-NARCOTIC DRUG ABUSE. 5th annual conference, 1964,
    sponsored by Smith, Kline & French laboratories. Phila-
    delphia, 1965
Isbell, Harris. "Dependence on Central Stimulants," CECIL
    AND LOEB TEXTBOOK OF MEDICINE, ed. Beeson and McDermott,
    12th edition. Philadelphia: Saunders, 1967, p. 1504.
Kalant, Oriana Josseau. THE AMPHETAMINES: toxicity and
    addiction. Springfield, Illinois: C.C. Thomas, 1966.
Mario Negri Institute of Pharmacological Research, Sympos-
    ium, Milan. INTERNATIONAL SYMPOSIUM ON AMPHETAMINES
    AND RELATED COMPOUNDS. 8 sessions. no. 1. Structure-
    activity relationships of amphetamines and halogenated
    amphetamines; no. 2, Distribution and metabolism of am-
    phetamines; no. 3, Interaction of amphetamines with
    biogenic amines; no. 4, Physiological significance of
    the interaction of amphetamines on the cardiovascular
    system; no. 5, o.p.; no. 6, Effects of amphetamines on
    food intake and lipid metabolism; no. 7, Effects of am-
    phetamines on the central nervous system: experimental;
    no. 8, Effects of amphetamines on the central nervous
    system: clinical, ed. S. Garattini and E. Costa. New
    York: Raven Press, 1969.

Russo, J. Robert, ed. AMPHETAMINE ABUSE. Springfield, Illinois: C.C. Thomas, 1969

Smith, Kline & French Laboratories, Philadelphia. HANDBOOK ON DEXEDRINE, BRAND OF DEXTROAMPHETAMINE SULFATE, ESKATROL DEXAMYL. Reference manual. 7th ed. [Philadelphia, c1966].

U.S. Congress. Senate. Committee on Labor and Public Welfare. CONTROL OF PSYCHOTOXIC DRUGS. Hearing before the Subcommittee on Health of the Committee on Labor and Public Welfare, U.S. Senate, 88th Congress, 2d session, on S. 2628, a bill to protect the public health by amending the Federal food, drug, and cosmetic act to regulate the manufacture, compounding, processing, distribution, delivery, and possession of psychotoxic drugs, Aug. 3, 1964. Washington: U.S. Govt. Print. Off., 1964.

U.S. Congress. Senate. Committee on Labor and Public Welfare. PSYCHOTOXIC DRUG CONTROL ACT OF 1964; report to accompany S. 2628. Washington: U.S. Govt. Print. Off., 1964.

AMPHETAMINES AND STIMULANTS: Doctoral Dissertations

Atkinson, Bobby L. "The effect of amphetamine on a simple and complex paired-associates" (Thesis, unpublished, University of Houston). DISSERTATION ABSTRACTS. 28 (3-B): 1154, 1967.

Cleeland, Charles S. "The effects of amphetamine and chlorpromazine on a fixated response" (Thesis, unpublished, Washington University). DISSERTATION ABSTRACTS. 27(6-B): 2156, 1966.

Cole, Sherwood O. "The hypothalamic regulation of eating behavior and amphetamine-induced anorexia" (Thesis, unpublished, Claremont Graduate School and University Center). DISSERTATION ABSTRACTS. 28(10-B): 4280-4281, 1968.

Cone, Allie L. Jr. "Effects of ambient sensory input and d-amphetamine upon roughness discrimination in the rhesus macaque" (Thesis, unpublished, Emory University). DISSERTATION ABSTRACTS. 28(5-B): 2155, 1967.

Denber, Herman C. "Intracellular localization of psychomimetic and psychotropic drugs" (Thesis, unpublished, New York University). DISSERTATION ABSTRACTS. 28(11-B), 4410, 1968.

Elfner, Lloyd Francis. "Systematic shifts in the subjective octaves of high frequencies produced by cross-ear stimulation, sleep loss, and d-amphetamine" (Thesis, unpublished, University of Wisconsin). DISSERTATION ABSTRACTS. 23(4): 1421, 1962.

Kistner, Joseph M. "Effects of chlorpromazine and d-amphetamine on sequential stereotypy of avoidance responses" (Thesis, unpublished, University of Pittsburgh). DISSERTATION ABSTRACTS. 28(10-B): 4717, 1968

Lovingood, Billy Wade. "The effects of dextro-amphetamine sulfate and caffeine on selected psychomotor, strength, and intellectual performance tasks and physiological parameters of young white men exposed to a restricted environment" (Thesis, unpublished, University of North Carolina). DISSERTATION ABSTRACTS. 24(9): 3625, 1964.

Luther, Baldev R. "A comparative study of some arousal-related measures in psychiatric patients and surgical patients" (Thesis, unpublished, University of Minnesota). DISSERTATION ABSTRACTS. 27(6-B): 2140, 1966.

McGuire, Louis C., Jr. "Reinforcing effects of intravenously infused morphine and L-amphetamine" (Thesis, unpublished, University of Mississippi). DISSERTATION ABSTRACTS. 27(11-B): 4146, 1967.

McKearney, James W. "The relative effects of d-amphetamine, imipramine and harmaline of tetrabenazine suppression of several operant behaviors" (Thesis, unpublished, University of Pittsburgh). DISSERTATION ABSTRACTS. 28(4): 1712. 1967.

Peterson, Ernest. "The effect of four psychotropic drugs on sensitivity to electrically induced pain" (Thesis, unpublished, Princeton University). DISSERTATION ABSTRACTS. 23(8): 2994-2995, 1963.

Pickens, Roy W. "Conditioning of locomotor effects of d-amphetamine" (Thesis, unpublished, University of Mississippi). DISSERTATION ABSTRACTS. 26(9): 5565, 1966.

Thurmond, John B. "A study of the effects of amphetamine and broadband noise on the Macaca mulatta's absolute visual threshold" (Thesis, unpublished, Emory University). DISSERTATION ABSTRACTS. 25(9): 5411-5412, 1965.

Weiner, H. "The effects of "unwanted" signals and detro-amphetamine sulfate on observer responses" (Thesis, unpublished, University of Maryland). DISSERTATION ABSTRACTS. 21: 685, 1960.

Weitzner, Martin. "The relationship of M.A.S. score and amphetamine to verbal and motor tasks" (Thesis, unpublished, Boston University). DISSERTATION ABSTRACTS. 24(4): 1716-1717, 1963.

Worrall, Norman. "A special case of semantic conditioning and some effects of d-amphetamine" (Thesis, unpublished, Indiana University). DISSERTATION ABSTRACTS. 28(1-B), 1967.

AMPHETAMINES AND STIMULANTS: Periodical Literature

General Publications

"Abuse of amphetamines," by Edison, C.R. J.A.M.A. 205: 882-883, Sept. 16, 1968.

"Abuse of amphetamines in dangerous area" (editorial). NEW YORK J. MED., 64:2634, 1964.

"Abuse of barbiturates and amphetamines," by Seevers, M.H. POSTGRADUATE MEDICINE. 37: 45-51, Jan., 1965.
"Abuse of barbiturates, stimulants, LSD, as great a danger as illegal narcotics," by Braude, A. AMERICAN ASSOCIA- TION OF INDUSTRIAL NURSES JOURNAL. 15: 40-41, Jan., 1967.
"Abuse of methylamphetamine." LANCET. 2:818, Oct. 12, 1968.
"Abuse of methylamphetamine," by Glatt, M.M. LANCET. 2:215- 216, July 27, 1968.
"Addicted! addiction to diet pills." GOOD HOUSEKEEPING. 164: 12 passim, May, 1967.
"Addiction to amphetamines." BRITISH MEDICAL JOURNAL. 5354:339-400, 1963.
"Addiction to amphetamines," by Brandon, S. BRITISH MED- ICAL JOURNAL. 5366:1204, 1963.
"Addiction to amphetamine," by Myers, W.H., and Law, E. BRITISH MEDICAL JOURNAL. 5371:1536, 1963.
"Addiction to stimulants," by Bell, D.S. MEDICAL JOURNAL OF AUSTRALIA. 1:41-45, Jan. 14, 1967 (46 ref.).
"Alcoholism compounded; addiction to tranquilizers and stimulants." SCIENCE NEWS. 94:338-339, Oct. 5, 1968.
"Amphetamine." LANCET. 1:1374-1375, 1965.
"Amphetamine," by Nachshen, D.S. LANCET. 2:289, 1965.
"Amphetamine," by Roberts, H.J. LANCET. 2:909-910, 1965.
"Amphetamine," by Wilson, C.W. LANCET. 2:496-497, 1965.
"Amphetamine abuse." MEDICAL LETTER ON DRUGS AND THERA- PEUTICS. 10:63-64, Aug. 9, 1968.
"Amphetamine abuse. Pattern and effects of high doses taken intravenously," by Kramer, J.C., et al. JOURNAL OF THE AMERICAN MEDICAL ASSOCIATION. 201:305-309, Jul. 31, 1967.
"Amphetamine abuse by hospitalized chronic schizophrenic patients," by Rockwell, D.A. BRITISH JOURNAL OF PSY- CHIATRY. 114:239-240, Feb., 1968.
"Amphetamine abuse in the United Kingdom." BULLETIN ON NARCOTICS. 20(2):56, April-June, 1968.
"Amphetamine addiction," by Bell, D.S., and Trethowan, W.H. JOURNAL OF NERVOUS AND MENTAL DISEASES. 133:489-496, 1961.
"Amphetamine addiction," by Durrant, B.W. PRACTITIONER. 194:649-651, 1965.
"Amphetamine and barbiturate abuse," by Mansfield, N.J.H. CANADA'S MENTAL HEALTH. 17:2-5, Sept.-Oct., 1969.
"Amphetamine and delinquency," by Scott, P.D. LANCET. 2:534-535, 1964.
"Amphetamine and phenmetrazine addiction. Physiological abnormalities in the abstinence syndrome," by Oswald, I., and Thacore, V.R. BRITISH MEDICAL JOURNAL. 5354:427- 431, 1963.
"Amphetamine, barbiturates, and accommodation-convergence," by Westheimer, G. AMERICAN MEDICAL ASSOCIATION ARCHIVES OF OPHTHAMOLOGY. 70:830-836, 1963.
"Amphetamine consumption in Northern Ireland," by Moorehead, N.C. JOURNAL OF THE IRISH MEDICAL ASSOCIATION. 61:80- 84, March, 1968.

"Amphetamine dependence," by Connell, P.H. PROCEEDINGS OF
THE ROYAL SOCIETY OF MEDICINE. 61:178-181, Feb., 1968.
"Amphetamine dependence in Dublin," by Walsh, D. JOURNAL
OF THE IRISH MEDICAL ASSOCIATION. 58:161-163, 1966.
"Amphetamine drugs," by Flemming, A.S. PUBLIC HEALTH RE-
PORTS. 75:49-50, 1960.
"Amphetamine intoxication and dependence in admission to
a psychiatric unit," by Johnson, J., et al. BRITISH
JOURNAL OF PSYCHIATRY. 112:617-619, Jun., 1966.
"Amphetamine misuse," by Connell, P.H. BRITISH JOURNAL OF
ADDICTION. 60:9-27, 1964.
"Amphetamine prescribing," by Reed, F.S. BRITISH MEDICAL
JOURNAL. 2:108, Apr. 8, 1967.
"Amphetamine psychosis: I. Description of the individuals
and process," by Ellinwood, E.H.,Jr. JOURNAL OF NERVOUS
AND MENTAL DISEASES. 144(4):273-283, 1967.
"Amphetamine toxicity, population density, and behavior,"
by Thiessen, D.D. PSYCHOLOGICAL BULLETIN. 62(6):401-410,
1964.
"Amphetamine usage by medical students," by Smith, Stanley,
and Blachly, Paul H. JOURNAL OF MEDICAL EDUCATION.
41:167-170, Feb., 1966.
"Amphetamine use and abuse in psychiatric patients," by
Rockwell, Don A., and Ostwald, Peter. ARCHIVES OF GEN-
ERAL PSYCHIATRY. 18(5):612-616, 1968.
"Amphetamines and barbiturates." BULLETIN ON NARCOTICS.
21(3):43-46, July-Sept., 1969.
"Amphetamines and barbiturates; the up and down drugs."
TODAY'S EDUCATION. 58:42-44, March, 1969.
"Amphetamines and driving." BULLETIN ON NARCOTICS. 21(1):
46, Jan.-March, 1969.
"Amphetamines in general practice," by Brandon, S., and
Smith, D. JOURNAL OF THE COLLEGE OF GENERAL PRACTITION-
ERS. 5:603-606, 1962.
"Amphetamines: in the arm." OIL, PAINT AND DRUG REPORT.
192:3 passim, July 31, 1967.
"Amphetamines: up, up and away." THE ATTACK ON NARCOTIC
ADDICTION AND DRUG ABUSE. 3:3, Summer, 1969.
"Appetite-suppressing drugs as an etiologic factor and
mental illness," by Breitner, C. PSYCHOSOMATICS. 4:
327-333, 1963.
"Barbiturate curbs to go into effect; producers and dis-
tributors of barbiturates, amphetamines and drugs must
keep records." OIL, PAINT AND DRUG REPORT. 188:7 passim, Dec. 27, 1965.
"Barbiturates and amphetamines bill; do not overlook the
competitors." OIL, PAINT AND DRUG REPORT. 187:4 passim, Feb. 8, 1965.
"Barbiturates and amphetamines bill; House leadership clears
decks." OIL, PAINT AND DRUG REPORT. 187:5, March 8,
1965.
"Behavioral variables affecting the development of amphetamine tolerance," by Schuster, C., et al. PSYCHOPHARMA-
COLOGIA: 9:170-182, 1966.

5

"Blame pep pills for murder." CHRISTIAN CENTURY. 82:199, Feb. 17, 1965.

"Changes proposed to curb glue sniffing fad." THE HAWAII HEALTH MESSENGER (Hawaii Department of Health, Health Education Office). 14:1, 1963.

"Clinical manifestations and treatment of amphetamine type of dependence," by Connell, P.H. JOURNAL OF THE AMERICAN MEDICAL ASSOCIATION. 196:718-723, 1966.

"Cruel chemical world of speed; methedrine," by Shepherd, J. LOOK. 32:53-59, Mar. 5, 1968.

"Danger! A new kids' fad: gluesniffing," by David, L. THIS WEEK MAGAZINE. p. 4 passim, 1963.

"The danger of amphetamine dependency," by Lemere, F. AMERICAN JOURNAL OF PSYCHIATRY. 123:569-572, Nov., 1966.

"Delinquency and the amphetamines," by Scott, P.D. and Willcox, D.R.C. BRITISH JOURNAL OF PSYCHIATRY. 111 (478):865-876, 1965.

"Dependence on amphetamines and other stimulant drugs." JOURNAL OF THE AMERICAN MEDICAL ASSOCIATION. 197(12), Sept., 1966.

"Diagnosis of amphetamine addiction." BRITISH MEDICAL JOURNAL. 5434:589, 1965.

"Diagnosis of amphetamine addiction," by Beckett, A.H., et al. BRITISH MEDICAL JOURNAL. 5436:725, 1965.

"Diagnosis of amphetamine addiction," by Walker, P.G. BRITISH MEDICAL JOURNAL. 5431:384-385, 1965.

"Diagnosis of amphetamine addiction," by Wilson, C.W. BRITISH MEDICAL JOURNAL. 5435:659-660, 1965.

"D-men on the road; illegal peddling of amphetamine tablets." TIME. 89:69, May 5, 1967.

"Don't dodge the drug question; stimulants," by Hawkins, M.E. THE SCIENCE TEACHER. 33:33-34, Nov., 1966.

"Doping," by Mustala, O. DUODECIM. 80:132-138, 1964.

"Drugs that even scare hippies," by Rosenfeld, A. LIFE. 63:81-82, Oct. 27, 1967.

"The effects of amphetamine upon judgments and decisions," by Hurst, P.M., et al. PSYCHOPHARMACOLOGIA. 11(5): 397-404, 1967.

"Experimental effects of amphetamine: a review," by Cole, S.O. PSYCHOLOGICAL BULLETIN. 68(2):81-90, 1967.

"FDA sets date for speaking up by drug people (barbiturates and amphetamines involved)," OIL, PAINT AND DRUG REPORT. 189:4, Feb. 28, 1966.

"Fatal benzene exposure by glue-sniffing," by Wineck, C.L., et al. LANCET. 1:683, Mar. 25, 1967.

"Glue and gasoline 'sniffing,' the addiction of youth," by Bartlett, S., and Tapia, F. MISSOURI MEDICINE. 63:270-272, 1966.

"Glue sniffers," by Barker, G.H., and Adams, W.T. SOCIOLOGY AND SOCIAL RESEARCH. 47(3):298-310, 1963.

"Glue-sniffing," by Allen, S.M. INTERNATIONAL JOURNAL OF THE ADDICTIONS. 1(1):147-149, 1966.

"Glue sniffing," by Chapel, J.L., et al. MISSOURI MEDICINE. 65:288-292 passim, Apr., 1968.

"Glue sniffing," by Jacobziner, H. NEW YORK STATE JOURNAL OF MEDICINE. 63:2415-2418, Aug., 1963.
"Glue sniffing," by Sokol, J., and Robinson, J.L. WESTERN MEDICINE. 4:192, June, 1963.
"Glue-sniffing. II.," by Verhulst, H.L., and Crotty, J.J. NATIONAL CLEARING-HOUSE FOR POISON CONTROL CENTERS. 1964:1-8, 1964.
"Glue-sniffing; an adolescent craze." CONSUMER REPORT. 28:40, Jan., 1963.
"Glue sniffing among juveniles," by Sokol, L. AMERICAN JOURNAL OF CORRECTION. 27(6), 1965.
"Glue-sniffing among Winnipeg school children," by Gellman, Vera. CANADIAN MEDICAL ASSOCIATION JOURNAL. 98(8): 411-413, Feb. 24, 1968.
"Glue sniffing and heroin abuse," by Merry, J. BRITISH MEDICAL JOURNAL. 2:360, May 6, 1967.
"Glue sniffing - brief flight from reality," by Jackson, R., et al. JOURNAL OF LOUISIANA MEDICAL SOCIETY. 119: 451-454, Nov., 1967.
"Glue sniffing, a hazardous hobby," by Pierson, H.W., Jr. JOURNAL OF SCHOOL HEALTH. 34:252, 1964.
"Glue sniffing in children - deliberate inhalation of vaporized cements," by Glaser, Helen L. JOURNAL OF THE AMERICAN MEDICAL ASSOCIATION. 181:300, July 28, 1962.
"Glue sniffing: a new symptom of an old disease," by Shanholtz, M.I. VIRGINIA MEDICAL MONTHLY. 95:304-305, May, 1968.
"Glue-sniffing: a problem in Kansas?" NEWSLETTER (Kansas State Board of Health). 30(12):4-5, 1963.
"Habituation and addiction to amphetamines," by Kiloh, L.G., and Brandon, S. BRITISH MEDICAL JOURNAL. 11:#5295, pp. 40-43, 1962
"The hazard of amphetamine medication," by Breitner, C. PSYCHOSOMATICS. 6:217-219, 1965.
"The identification of amphetamine type drugs," by Clarke, E.G.C. JOURNAL OF THE FORENSIC SCIENCE SOCIETY. 7(1): 31-36, Jan., 1967.
"Identification of nasal inhaler fragments by gas chromatography," by Cromp, C.C. JOURNAL OF FORENSIC SCIENCES. 8:477-480, 1963.
"LSD and amphetamines." BULLETIN ON NARCOTICS. 20(3):17, July-Sept., 1968.
"Learning and drugs," by Bustamane, J.A., et al. PHYSIOLOGY AND BEHAVIOR. 3(4):553-555, 1968.
"Manifest anxiety, amphetamine, and performance," by Weitzner, M. JOURNAL OF PSYCHOLOGY. 60:71-79, 1965.
"A methylamphetamine epidemic?" by James, I.P. LANCET. 1:9;6, Apr. 27, 1968.
"Misuse of valuable therapeutic agents: barbiturates, tranquilizers, and amphetamine." BULLETIN OF THE NEW YORK ACADEMY OF MEDICINE. 40:972-979, 1964.
"Mixed toxicomania for amphetamines and oxazine derivatives in young patients," by Abély, P., et al. ANNALES MEDICO-PSYCHOLOGIQUES. 118:167-172, 1960.
"N-Alicyclic amphetamines," by Freifelder, M. JOURNAL OF

MEDICINAL CHEMISTRY. 6:813, 1963
"Narcotic and methamphetamine use during pregnancy: effect on newborn infants," by Sussman, S. AMERICAN JOURNAL OF DISEASES OF CHILDREN. 106:325-330, 1963.
"The naval medical officer as a psychiatric patient," by Arthur, Ransom J. AMERICAN JOURNAL OF PSYCHIATRY. 122(3):290-294, 1965.
"New kick: glue sniffing." TIME. 79:55, Feb. 16, 1962.
"Nonnarcotic addiction. Size and extent of the problem," by Sadusk, J.F., Jr. JOURNAL OF THE AMERICAN MEDICAL ASSOCIATION. 196:707, 1966.
"The occurrence of glue sniffing on a university campus," by Keeler, M.H., et al. JOURNAL OF THE AMERICAN COLLEGE HEALTH ASSOCIATION. 16:69-70, Oct., 1967.
"On 'doping'," by Silvestrini, B. BOLLETTINO CHIMICO-FARMACEUTICO. 103:541-544, 1964.
"Patterns and profiles of addiction and drug abuse," by Saker, Jordan. ARCHIVES OF GENERAL PSYCHIATRY. 15(5): 539-551, 1966.
"Pep pill menace." BRITISH MEDICAL JOURNAL. 5386:792, 1964.
"Pep pills act on brain like heat stroke." SCIENCE NEWS. 90:276, Oct. 8, 1966.
"Pills and Olympians." SCIENCE NEWS. 91:353, Apr. 15, 1967.
"Pills bill passes Senate, some ironing-out needed. (Controls over production and marketing of barbiturates, amphetamines, etc.)" OIL, PAINT AND DRUG REPORT. 187:3 passim, June 28, 1965.
"Pills measure moves to the half-way point. (Barbiturates and amphetamines)." OIL, PAINT AND DRUG REPORT. 187:5 passim, March 15, 1965.
"Pills traffic results in pelting for FDA." OIL, PAINT AND DRUG REPORT. 187:3 passim, Feb. 15, 1965.
"Potential impairment effects of amphetamine determined." JOURNAL OF THE AMERICAN MEDICAL ASSOCIATION. 189:35-36, 1964.
"Prevalence of habit forming drugs and smoking among the college students -- a survey," by Banerjee, R. INDIAN MEDICAL JOURNAL. 57:193-196, 1963.
"The problem of barbiturates and amphetamines," by Bordeleau, J. UNION MÉDICALE DU CANADA. 90:343-344, 1961.
"Problems in amphetamine usage," by Hart, R. BRITISH MEDICAL JOURNAL. 2:432, May 18, 1968.
"Psychological effects of amphetamines and barbiturates," by Nash, Harvey. JOURNAL OF NERVOUS AND MENTAL DISEASES. 134(3):203-217, 1962.
"Psychosis due to amphetamine consumption," by Beamish, P., and Kiloh, L.G. JOURNAL OF MENTAL SCIENCE. 106:337-343, 1960.
"Psychosis following the use of amphetamines," by Charalampous, K.D., and Hug, A. MEDICAL RECORD AND ANNALS (Houston). 56:31-32, 1963.
"Psychosis in a child associated with amphetamine administration," by Ney, Philip G. CANADIAN MEDICAL ASSOCIATION JOURNAL. 97(17):1026-1029, 1967.
"Purple hearts; the pep pill bill." ECONOMIST. 211:576,

8

May 9, 1964.
"Putting the brakes on speed; government to restrict the flow of illegal drugs." BUSINESS WEEK. p. 92 passim, Oct. 28, 1967.
"Reactions to use of amphetamines as observed in a psychiatric hospital," by Prout, C.T. NEW YORK JOURNAL OF MEDICINE. 64:1186-1192, 1964.
"Recent trends in substance abuse: glue-sniffing," by Allen, S.M. INTERNATIONAL JOURNAL OF THE ADDICTIONS. 1(1):147-149, 1966.
"Recognition of amphetamine addicts," by Ashcroft, G.W., et al. BRITISH MEDICAL JOURNAL. 5426:57, 1965.
"The relative value of self-report and objective tests in assessing the effects of amphetamine," by Agnew, Neil McK. JOURNAL OF PSYCHIATRIC RESEARCH. 2(2):85-100, 1964.
"A review of the evidence on glue-sniffing--a persistent problem," by Corliss, L.M. JOURNAL OF SCHOOL HEALTH. 35:442-449, Dec., 1965.
"A San Francisco bay area 'speed scene'," by Carey, James T., and Mandel, Jerry. JOURNAL OF HEALTH AND SOCIAL BEHAVIOR. 9:2, 164-174, 1968.
"Screening test for urinary amphetamine," by Eastham, R.D. BRITISH MEDICAL JOURNAL. 5439:925-935, 1965.
"Speed demons." TIME. 94:18, Oct. 31, 1969.
"The sniffing craze," by LaBenne, Wallace. PSYCHOLOGY. 5(4):14-16, 1968.
"Speed kills; Methedrine." NEWSWEEK. 70:87, Oct. 30, 1967.
"Speed: the use of amphetamines on the campus," by Burk, M.A. JOURNAL OF THE NATIONAL ASSOCIATION OF WOMEN DEANS AND COUNSELORS. 32:110-114, Sept., 1969.
"Stimulants and tranquilizers - their use and abuse," by Braceland, F.J. BULLETIN OF THE NEW YORK ACADEMY OF MEDICINE. 39(10):649-665, 1963.
"A study of illicit amphetamine drug traffic in Oklahoma City," by Griffith, John. AMERICAN JOURNAL OF PSYCHIATRY. 123(5):560-569, 1966.
"Successful treatment of amphetamine addiction in a schizophrenic woman," by Seelye, Edward E. AMERICAN JOURNAL OF PSYCHOTHERAPY. 21(2):295-301, 1967.
"A survey of the usage of amphetamines in parts of the Sydney community," by Briscoe, O.V., et al. MEDICAL JOURNAL OF AUSTRALIA. 1:480-485, March 23, 1968.
"A survey of the usage of amphetamines in parts of the Sydney community," by De Groot, J.C. MEDICAL JOURNAL OF AUSTRALIA. 1:826, May 11, 1968.
"A survey of the usage of amphetamines in parts of the Sydney community," by Kneebone, G.M. MEDICAL JOURNAL OF AUSTRALIA. 2:246, Aug. 3, 1968.
"Symposium: nonnarcotic addiction, clinical manifestations and treatment of amphetamine type of dependence," by Connell, Philip H. JOURNAL OF THE AMERICAN MEDICAL ASSOCIATION. 196(8):718-722, 1966.
"There's no hiding place down there," by Janowitz, Julian F. AMERICAN JOURNAL OF ORTHOPSYCHIATRY. 37(2): 296, 1967.

"Toulene fatality from glue sniffing," by Winek, C.L., et
al. PENNSYLVANIA MEDICINE. 71:81, Apr., 1968.
"Toxic reactions to amphetamines," by McCormick, T.C. Jr.
DISEASES OF THE NERVOUS SYSTEM. 23:219-224, Apr., 1962.
"Toxicomania caused by a psychostimulant drug," by Duarte,
A., and Maglio, M.A. SEMANA MEDICA (Buenos Aires).
121:1426, 1962.
"Toxicomanias caused by psychostimulating drugs," by Fer-
rero, R.G. SEMANA MEDICA (Buenos Aires). 117:1604-1605,
1960.
"Trace GSR conditioning with benzedrine in mentally defect-
ive and normal adults," by Lobb, H. AMERICAN JOURNAL
OF MENTAL DEFICIENCY. 73:239-246, Sept., 1968.
"Unsafe at any speed; Methedrine." TIME. 90:54 passim,
Oct. 27, 1967.
"The use and abuse of amphetamines," by Connell, P.H.
PRACTITIONER. 200:234-243, Feb., 1968.
"Use of amphetamines, marijauna, and LSD by students," by
Blachly, P. NEW PHYSICIAN. v.15, p.88-93, 1966.
"The uses and misuses of amphetamines," by Salsbury, C.A.,
and Wayland, R.B. MEDICO-LEGAL BULLETIN. 156:1-9, 1966.

AMPHETAMINES AND STIMULANTS: Scientific Publications

"Acute and chronic effects of glue sniffing," by Barman,
M.L., et al. CALIFORNIA MEDICINE. 100(1):19-22, 1964.
"Acute lethality of the amphetamines in dogs and its antag-
onism by curare," by Zalis, E.G., et al. PROCEEDINGS
OF THE SOCIETY OF EXPERIMENTAL BIOLOGY AND MEDICINE.
118:557-561, 1965.
"Acute poisonings by psychopharmacological agents in child-
hood," by Parada Bravo, R., et al. REVISTA CHILENA DE
PEDIATRIA. 35:314-323, 1964.
"Amentia with epilepsy-catatonia due to ES-amphetamine,"
by Vitelio, A. RIVISTA DI NEUROBIOLOGIA. 10:272-292,
1964.
"Amphetamine anorexia by direct action on the adrenergic
feeding system of rat hypothalamus," by Booth, D.A.
NATURE. 217(5131):869-870, 1968.
"Amphetamine, arousal and human vestibular nystagmus," by
Collins, W.E., and Poe, R.H. JOURNAL OF PHARMACOLOGY
AND EXPERIMENTAL THERAPEUTICS. 138:120-125, 1962.
Also: USA MEDICAL RESEARCH LABORATORIES REPORT. 1961,
no.526.
"Amphetamine effects on poor performance of rats in a shut-
tle-box," by Rich, Richard H. PSYCHOPHARMACOLOGIA.
9(2):110-117, 1966.
"Amphetamine psychosis. I. Description of the individuals
and process," by Ellinwood, E.H. Jr. JOURNAL OF NERVOUS
AND MENTAL DISEASE. 144:273-283, Apr.,1967.
"Amphetamine psychosis: theoretical implications," by

Ellinwood, E.H. INTERNATIONAL JOURNAL OF NEUROPSYCHIATRY. 4(1):45-54, 1968.

"An analysis of cat behavior using chlorpromazine and amphetamine," by Norton, Stata. INTERNATIONAL JOURNAL OF NEUROPHARMACOLOGY. 6(4):307-316, 1967.

"An analysis of urinary amine values on routine admissions to a mental hospital," by Abenson, M.H. ACTA PSYCHIATRICA SCANDINAVICA. 41:582-587, 1965.

"Antagonism of a behavioral effect of d-amphetamine by chlorpromazine in the pigeon," by Davis, Joel L. JOURNAL OF THE EXPERIMENTAL ANALYSIS OF BEHAVIOR. 8(5):325-327, 1965.

"Antagonism of reserpine behavioral depression by d-amphetamine," by Rich, R.H. JOURNAL OF PHARMACOLOGY AND EXPERIMENTAL THEARAPEUTICS. 146:367-369, 1964.

"Anxiety, meprobamate, d-amphetamine and the intra-subject variability of word associates," by Brody, Nathan, et al. PSYCHOLOGICAL REPORTS. 21(1):113-120, 1967.

"Aplastic anemia secondary to glue sniffing," by Powars, D. NEW ENGLAND JOURNAL OF MEDICINE. 273(13):700-702, 1965.

"Arousal and sensory change stimulation," by Jones, C. Dalton. CORNELL JOURNAL OF SOCIAL RELATIONS. 1(2):155-168, 1966.

"Behavior effects of caffeine, methamphetamine, and methylphenidate in the rat," by Mechner, Francis and Latranyi, Miklos. JOURNAL OF THE EXPERIMENTAL ANALYSIS OF BEHAVIOR. 6(3):331-342, 1963.

"Behavioral effects of interacting imipramine and other drugs with d-amphetamine, cocaine, and tetrabenazine, by Scheckel, C.L. and Boff, E. PSYCHOPHARMACOLOGIA. 5:198-208, 1964.

"Behavioral facilitation: the interaction of imipramine and desipramine with amphetamine, alpha-pipradrol, methylphenidate, and thozalinone," by Bernstein, B.M. and Latimer, C.N. PSYCHOPHARMACOLOGIA. 12(4):338-345, 1968.

"Behavioral variables affecting the development of amphetamine tolerance," by Schuster, C.R. et al. PSYCHOPHARMACOLOGIA. 9(2):170-182, 1966.

"Chemical interactions in methamphetamine reinforcement," by Pickins, Roy et al. PSYCHOLOGICAL REPORTS. 23(3, pt.2):1267-1270, 1968.

"Chlorpromazine and d-amphetamine in eyelid conditioning," by Ludvigson, H. Wayne. PSYCHOLOGICAL REPORTS. 14(2):402, 1964.

"Clinical manifestations and treatment of amphetamine type of dependence," by Connell, P.H. JOURNAL OF THE AMERICAN MEDICAL ASSOCIATION. 196:718-723, 1966.

"The combined effects of ethanol and amphetamine sulfate on performance of human subjects," by Wilson, L. CANADIAN MEDICAL ASSOCIATION JOURNAL. 94:478-484, 1966.

"Comments on the effect of amphetamine in avoidance conditioning," by Cole, Sherwood O. PSYCHOLOGICAL REPORTS. 19(1):41-42, 1966

"Comparative ability of normal and chronic schizophrenic

subjects to attend to competing voice messages: Effect of method of presentation, message load and drugs," by Rappaport, Maurice, et al. JOURNAL OF NERVOUS AND MENTAL DISEASES. 143(1):16-27, 1966.

"Comparison of amphetamine psychosis and schizophrenia," by Bell, D.S. BRITISH JOURNAL OF PSYCHIATRY. 111:701-707, 1965.

"Comparison of amphetamine sulphate and caffeine citrate in man, by Lader, M. PSYCHOPHARMACOLOGIA. 14(2):83-94, 1969.

"Comparison of drug effects on approach, avoidance and escape motivation," by Barry, Herbert and Miller, Neal E. JOURNAL OF COMPARATIVE AND PHYSIOLOGICAL PSYCHOLOGY. 59(1):18-24, 1965.

"Comparison of effects of dexamphetamine and LSD-25 on perceptual and autonomic function," by Claridge, G.S., and Hume, W.I. PERCEPTUAL AND MOTOR SKILLS. 23(2):456-458, 1966.

"A comparison of the analgetic potencies of morphine, pentazocine, and a mixture of methamphetamine and pentazocine in the rat. Rep. No. 602," by Evans, W.O. and Bergner, D.P. JOURNAL OF NEW DRUGS. 4(2): 82-85, 1964.

"A comparison of the cognitive functioning of glue-sniffers and nonsniffers," by Dodds, J., and Santostefano, S. JOURNAL OF PEDIATRICS. 64(4):565-570, 1964.

"A comparison of the effects of meprobamate, phenobarbital and d-amphetamine on two psychological tests," by Townsend, Arthur M. and Mirsky, Allen F. JOURNAL OF NERVOUS AND MENTAL DISEASES. 130:212-216, 1960.

"Complex response patterns during temporally spaced responding," by Hodos, William, et al. JOURNAL OF EXPERIMENTAL ANALYSIS OF BEHAVIOR. 5(4):473-479, 1962.

"Control of behavior by drug-produced internal stimuli," by Belleville, R. PSYCHOPHARMACOLOGIA. 5:95-105, 1964.

"D-Amphetamine-chlorpromazine antagonism in a food reinforced operant," by Brown, Hugh. JOURNAL OF EXPERIMENTAL ANALYSIS OF BEHAVIOR. 6(3):395-398, 1963.

"Decrement of avoidance conditioning performance in inbred mice subjected to prolonged sessions: Performance recovery after rest and amphetamine," by Bovet, Daniel, and Oliverio, Alberto. JOURNAL OF PSYCHOLOGY. 65(1):45-55, 1967.

"Decrements in avoidance behavior following mammillothalamic tractotomy in rats and subsequent recovery with d-amphetamine," by Krieckhaus, E.E. JOURNAL OF COMPARATIVE AND PHYSIOLOGICAL PSYCHOLOGY. 60(1):31-35, 1965.

"Deprivation and drug effects on prepyriform cortex electrical activity in rats," by Sutton, Dwight. PHYSIOLOGY AND BEHAVIOR. 2(2):139-144, 1967.

"Determinants of polydipsia: Effects of amphetamine and pintobarbital," by Segal, Evalyn F., et al. PSYCHONOMIC SCIENCE. 3(1):33-34, 1965.

"Determination and identification of amphetamine in urine," by Beckett, A.H., et al. JOURNAL OF PHARMACY AND PHARMACOLOGY. 17:59-60, 1965.

"Determination of amphetamine by ultraviolet spectrophotometry," by Wallace, Jack E., et al. ANALYTICAL CHEMISTRY. 40(14):2207-2210, Dec., 1968.

"Determination of amphetamines in urine by gas phase chromatography," by Lebbe, J. ARCHIVES DES MALADIES PROFESSIONNELLES DE MEDECINE DU TRAVAIL ET DE SECURITE SOCIALE. 26:221-224, 1965.

"Development of scales based on patterns of drug effects, using the Addiction Research Center Inventory (ARCI)," by Haertzen, Charles A. PSYCHOLOGICAL REPORTS. 18(1): 163-194, 1966.

"Differences in sedative susceptibility between types of depression," by Perez-Reyes, Mario. ARCHIVES OF GENERAL PSYCHIATRY. 19(1):64-71, 1968.

"Differential diagnosis in amphetamine psychosis," by Weiner, I.B. PSYCHIATRIC QUARTERLY. 38(4):707-714, 1964.

"Differential effects of amphetamine on food and water intake in rats with lateral hypothalamic lesions," by Carlisle, Harry J. JOURNAL OF COMPARATIVE AND PHYSIOLOGICAL PSYCHOLOGY. 58(1): 47-54, 1964.

"Differential effects of two amphetamine-barbiturate mixtures in man," by Dickens, D., et al. BRITISH JOURNAL OF PHARMACOLOGY. 24:14-23, 1965.

"Diffuse systems of the brain: physiological and pharmacological mechanisms," by Bradley, P.B. DEVELOPMENTAL MEDICINE AND CHILD NEUROLOGY. 4(1):49-54, 1962.

"Dilution of dose and acute oral toxicity," by Ferguson, H.C. TOXICOLOGY AND APPLIED PHARMACOLOGY. 4:759-762, 1962.

"The disadvantages of various drugs in prolonged use. Diseases due to laxatives, nose drops, chronic argyrism, amphetamines," by Labram, C. CONCOURS MEDICAL. 85:365-368, 1963.

"Discriminative control of dl-amphetamine and saline of lever choice and response patterning," by Harris, R.T. and Balster, R.L. PSYCHONOMIC SCIENCE. 10(3):105-106, 1967.

"Dose-response relations of amphetamine-barbiturate mixtures," by Rushton, R., and Steinberg, H. NATURE. 197: 1017-1018, 1963.

"Drug-behavior interaction affecting development of tolerance to d-amphetamine as observed in fixed tolerance ratio behavior of rats," by Brown, Hugh. PSYCHOLOGICAL REPORTS. 16(3,pt.1):917-921, 1965.

"Drug effects in fixed ratio matching to sample," by Mentz, Donald E., et al. PSYCHONOMIC SCIENCE. 12(5):171-172, 1968.

"Drug-induced hyperthermia and amphetamine toxicity," by Wolff, J., et al. JOURNAL OF PHARMACEUTICAL SCIENCES. 53:748-752, 1964.

"Drug withdrawal and fighting in rats," by Florea, J. and Thor, D.H. PSYCHONOMIC SCIENCE. 12(1):33, 1968.

"Drugs and judgement: Effects of amphetamine and secobarbital on self-evaluation," by Smith, Gene Marshall and Beecher, Henry K. JOURNAL OF PSYCHOLOGY. 58(2): 397-

13

405, 1964.
"Drugs and personality. The effects of stimulant and depressant drugs upon kinaesthetic figural after-effects," by Eysenck, H., and Easterbrook, J. JOURNAL OF MENTAL SCIENCE. 106:852-854, 1960.
"Drugs and personality. The effects of stimulant and depressant drugs on visual after-effects of a rotating spiral," by Eysenck, H., and Easterbrook. J. JOURNAL OF MENTAL SCIENCE. 106:842-844, 1960.
"Drugs and personality. The effects of stimulant and depressant drugs upon visual figural after-effects," by Eysenck, H., and Easterbrook, J. JOURNAL OF MENTAL SCIENCE. 106:845-851, 1960.
"Drugs and personality. The effects of stimulant and depressant drugs upon body sway (static ataxia)," by Eysenck, H., and Easterbrook, J. JOURNAL OF MENTAL SCIENCE. 106:831-834, 1960.
"Drugs and personality. The effects of stimulant and depressant drugs upon pupillary reactions," by Eysenck, H., and Easterbrook, J. JOURNAL OF MENTAL SCIENCE. 106: 835-841, 1960.
"Drugs and placebos: a model design," by Ross, Sherman, et al. PSYCHOLOGICAL REPORT. 10(2):383-392, 1962.
"Drugs and placebos: the effects of instructions upon performance and mood under amphetamine sulfate and chloral hydrate," by Lyerly, Samuel B., et al. JOURNAL OF ABNORMAL AND SOCIAL PSYCHOLOGY. 68(3):321-327, 1964.
"Drugs and placebos: Effects of instructions upon performance and mood under amphetamine sulfate and chloral hydrate with younger subjects," by Krugman, A.D., et al. PSYCHOLOGICAL REPORTS. 15(3):925-926, 1964.
"Drugs on cortical D.C. potentials and behavior of rats with septal area lesions," by Pirch, James H., and Norton, Stata. PHYSIOLOGY AND BEHAVIOR. 2(2):121-125, 1967.
"The EEG of the olfactory bulb of the rabbit and its reaction to psychopharmacological agents," by Khazan, N., et al. PSYCHOPHARMACOLOGIA. 10(3):226-236, 1967.
"The effect of amphetamine on established hoarding in the rat," by Zucker, Irving and Milner, Peter. PSYCHONOMIC SCIENCE. 1(12):367, 1964.
"Effect of amphetamine on the detectability of signals in a vigilance task," by Mackworth, Jane F. CANADIAN JOURNAL OF PSYCHOLOGY. 19(2):104-110, 1965.
"The effect of amphetamine on the sleep cycle," by Rechtschaffen, Allan and Maron, Louise. ELECTROENCEPHALOGRAPHY AND CLINICAL NEUROPHYSIOLOGY. 16(5):438-445, 1964.
"The effect of amphetamine upon cats with lesions in the ventromedial hypothalamus," by Sharp, Joseph et al. JOURNAL OF COMPARATIVE AND PHYSIOLOGICAL PSYCHOLOGY. 55(2):198-200, 1962.
"Effect of chlorpromazine and amphetamine on conditioned DC shifts in septal rats," by Pirch, J.H., and Norton, Stata. INTERNATIONAL JOURNAL OF NEUROPHARMACOLOGY. 6(2):125-132, 1967.
"Effect of dextroamphetamine on children: studies on sub-

14

jects with learning disabilities and school behavior problems," by Conners, C. Keith, et al. ARCHIVES OF GENERAL PSYCHIATRY. 17(4):478-485, 1967.

"The effect of dextroamphetamine sulfate on the behavior of REM sleep deprived rats," by Ferguson, James, and Dement, William. PSYCHOPHYSIOLOGY. 3: no. 4, p.380, 1968.

"Effect of drugs and illumination change on activity in the turtle," by Spigel, Irwin M. PSYCHOLOGICAL RECORD. 14(3):305-310, 1964.

"The effect of forced exercise on body temperature and amphetamine toxicity," by Hardinge, M.G., et al. JOURNAL OF PHARMACOLOGY AND EXPERIMENTAL THERAPEUTICS. 145:47-51, 1964.

"Effect of illumination and d-amphetamine on activity of the rhesus macaque," by Alexander, Margery and Isaac, Walter. PSYCHOLOGICAL REPORTS. 16(1):311-313, 1965.

"Effect of imipramine, physostigmine and amphetamine on the electrical activity of the brain in the cat," by Dasberg, H., and Feldman, S. PSYCHOPHARMACOLOGIA. 13 (2):129-139, 1968.

"The effect of LSD, mescaline, and d-amphetamine on the evoked 'secondary discharge'," by Roth, W.T. PSYCHOPHARMACOLOGIA. 9(3):253-258, 1966.

"Effect of leteral hypothalamic stimulation on amphetamine-induced anorexia," by Thode, Walter F., and Carlisle, Harry J. JOURNAL OF COMPARATIVE AND PHYSIOLOGICAL PSYCHOLOGY. 66(2):547-548, 1968.

"Effect of psilocybin, dextroamphetamine and placebo on performance of the Trail Making Test," by Duke, R.B., and Keeler, M.H. JOURNAL OF CLINICAL PSYCHOLOGY. 24 (3):316-317, 1968.

"The effect of REM sleep deprivation on the lethality of dextroamphetamine sulfate in grouped rats," by Ferguson, James and Dement, William. PSYCHOPHYSIOLOGY. 4: no. 3, p. 380, 1968.

"Effect of sensory stimuli on amphetamine toxicity in aggregated mice," by Cohen, M., et al. NATURE. 201:1037, 1964.

"The effect of some drugs on hippocampal arousal," by Bradley, P.B., and Nicholson, A.N. ELECTROENCEPHALOGRAPHY AND CLINICAL NEUROPHYSIOLOGY. 14:824-834, 1962.

"The effect of some drugs on the maximal capacity of athletic performance in man," by Margaria, R., et al. INTERNATIONALE ZEITSCHRIFT FUR ANGEWANDTE PHYSIOLOGIE EINSCHLIESSLICH ARBEITSPHYSIOLOGIE. 20:281-287, 1964.

"Effect of thioridazine, amphetamine and placebo on the hyperkinetic syndrome and cognitive area in mentally deficient children," by Alaxandris, Athina and Lundell, Frederick W. CANADIAN MEDICAL ASSOCIATION JOURNAL. 98 (2):92-96, 1968.

"Effects of a single experience on subsequent reactions to drugs," by Rushton, R., Steinberg, H., and Tinson, C. BRITISH JOURNAL OF PHARMACOLOGY. 20:99-105, 1963.

"Effects of aggression and early handling on amphetamine

toxicity in CBA/J inbred mice," by Thiessen, D.D., et al. JOURNAL OF COMPARATIVE AND PHYSIOLOGICAL PSYCHOLOGY. 64(3):532-534, 1967.
"Effects of amphetamine and pentobarbitone on exploratory behavior in rats," by Stretch, R.,NATURE. 199:787-789, 1963.
"Effects of amphetamine, Dexamyl and meprobamate on poor shuttle-box avoidance performers," by Kamano, Dennis K., et al. PSYCHONOMIC SCIENCE. 8(3):119-120, 1967.
"Effects of amphetamine on selective attention," by Day, H., and Thomas, E.L. PERCEPTUAL AND MOTOR SKILLS. 24(3, Pt. 2):1119-1125, 1967.
"Effects of amphetamine on the monkey's visual threshold," by Thurmond, John B. PSYCHONOMIC SCIENCE. 3(3):115-116, 1965.
"The effects of amphetamine on the sleep-wakefulness cycle of developing kittens," by Shimizu, A., and Himwich, H.E. PSYCHOPHARMACOLOGIA. 13(2):161-169, 1968.
"Effects of amphetamine therapy on hyperkinetic children," by Burks, Harold F. GENERAL PSYCHIATRY. 11(6):604-609, 1964.
"Effects of amphetamine sulfate on activity level of green sunfish," by Damkot, D.K. PSYCHOLOGICAL RECORD. 17(4): 509-513, 1967.
"Effects of amphetamine sulfate (Benzedrine) on the behavior of paired rats in a competitive situation," by Heimstra, N.W. PSYCHOLOGICAL RECORD. 12:25-34, 1962.
"Effects of brief psychotherapy, drugs, and type of disturbance on Holtzman Inkblot Scores in children," by Conners, C. Keith. PROCEEDING OF THE 73RD ANNUAL CONVENTION OF THE AMERICAN PSYCHOLOGICAL ASSOCIATION. 201-202, 1965.
"Effects of chlorpromazine and d-amphetamine on escape and avoidance behavior under a temporally defined schedule of negative reinforcement," by Sidley, N.A., and Schoenfeld, W.N. JOURNAL OF EXPERIMENTAL ANALYSIS OF BEHAVIOR. 6(2):293-295, 1963.
"The effects of chlorpromazine and methamphetamine on visual signal-from-noise detection," by Kopell, Bert S., and Wittner, William K. JOURNAL OF NERVOUS AND MENTAL DISEASES. 147(4):418-424, 1968.
"Effects of chronic administration of the amphetamines and other stimulants on behavior," by Kosman, M., et al. CLINICAL PHARMACOLOGY AND THERAPEUTICS. 9:240-254, Mar.-Apr., 1968.
"Effects of d-amphetamine on multiple schedule performance in the pigeon," by Gibson, David A. PSYCHONOMIC SCIENCE 7(1):3-4, 1967.
"Effects of d-amphetamine on performance under a multiple schedule in the rat," by Clark, Fogle C., and Steele, Bobby J. PSYCHOPHARMACOLOGIA. 9(2):157-169, 1966.
"The effects of d-amphetamine on risk taking," by Hurst, P.M. PSYCHOPHARMACOLOGIA. 3:283-290, 1962.
"Effects of d-amphetamine sulfate, caffeine, and high temperature on human performance," by Lovingood, B.W., et al. AMERICAN ASSOCIATION FOR HEALTH, PHYSICAL EDUCATION,

16

RECREATION. RESEARCH QUARTERLY. 38(1):64-71. Mar., 1967.
"The effects of DL-amphetamine and reserpine on runaway per-
formance," by Carlson, Nils J., et al. PSYCHOPHARMACOL-
OGIA. 8(3):157-173, 1965.
"Effects of dl-amphetamine under concurrent VI DRL rein-
forcement," by Segal, E.F. JOURNAL OF EXPERIMENTAL ANAL-
YSIS OF BEHAVIOR. 5(1):105-112, 1962.
"Effects of dl-amphetamine upon placing responses in neo-
decorticate cats," by Meyer, Patricia M., et al. JOUR-
NAL OF COMPARATIVE AND PHYSIOLOGICAL PSYCHOLOGY. 56(2):
402-404, 1963.
"The effects of depressant and stimulant drugs on the re-
lationship between reaction and stimulus light intensity,"
by Costello, C.G. BRITISH JOURNAL OF SOCIAL AND CLINICAL
PSYCHOLOGY. 3(1):1-5, 1964.
"The effects of dextroamphetamine and phenobarbital on a
simplified standardized CFF measure," by Misiak, H., and
Rizy, E.F. PSYCHOPHARMACOLOGIA. 13(4):346-353, 1968.
"The effects of drugs and their combinations on the rear-
ing response in two strains of rats," by Gupta, B.D.,
and Gregory, K. PSYCHOPHARMACOLOGIA. 11(4):365-371,
1967.
"Effects of drugs on conditioned 'anxiety'," by Blackman,
Derek. NATURE. 217(5130):769-770, 1968.
"Effects of early drug treatment on adult dominance behav-
ior in rats," by Heimstra, Norman W., and Sallee, Stella
J. PSYCHOPHARMACOLOGIA. 8(4):235-240, 1965.
"The effects of exercise and limitation of movement on amphetamine toxicity," by Harding, M.G. JOURNAL OF PHAR-
MACOLOGY AND EXPERIMENTAL THERAPEUTICS. 141:260-265,
1963.
"Effects of magnesium pemoline and dextroamphetamine on
human learning," by Burns, J.T., et al. SCIENCE. 155:
849-851, Feb. 17, 1967.
"The effects of meprobamate, d-amphetamine, and placebo on
disjunctive reaction time to taboo and nontaboo words,"
by Peterson, E.A., et al. PSYCHOPHARMACOLOGIA. 3(3):
173-187, 1962.
"The effects of messaline, amphetamine, and four-ring substituted amphetamine derivatives on spontaneous brain
electrical activity in the cat," by Fairchild, M.D., et
al. INTERNATIONAL JOURNAL OF NEUROPHARMACOLOGY. 6(3):
151-167, 1967.
"Effects of methamphetamine on hunger and thirst motivated
variable-interval performance," by Poschel, B.P.H.
JOURNAL OF COMPARATIVE AND PHYSIOLOGICAL PSYCHOLOGY.
56(6):968-973, 1963.
"Effects of placebo, dexamyl, and lucofen on moods, emotions, and motivations," by Cameron, Jean S., et al.
JOURNAL OF PSYCHOLOGY. 66(2):199-209, 1967.
"The effects of prenatal injections of adrenalin chloride
and d-amphetamine sulfate on subsequent emotionality
and ulcer-proneness of offspring," by Bell, R.W., et al.
PSYCHONOMIC SCIENCE. 2(9):269-270, 1965.
"Effects of previous radiation exposure on the activity re-

17

sponse to d-amphetamine hydrochloride," by McDowell, A.A., et al. JOURNAL OF GENETIC PSYCHOLOGY. 111(2): 241-243, 1967.

"Effects of secobarbital and d-amphetamine on psychomotor performance of normal subjects," by Goldstein, Avram, et al. JOURNAL OF PHARMACOLOGY AND EXPERIMENTAL THERAPEUTICS. 130:55-58, 1960.

"The effects of secobarbital and dextroamphetamine upon time judgment: intersensory factors," by Goldstone, S., and Kirkham, J.E. PSYCHOPHARMACOLOGIA. 13(1):65-73, 1968.

"The effects of shock intensity and d-amphetamine on avoidance learning," by Cicala, George A., and Kremer, Edwin. PSYCHONOMIC SCIENCE. 14(1):41-42, 1969.

"Effects of sodium pentobarbital and d-amphetamine on latency of the escape response in the rat," by Mize, Donna and Isaac, Walter. PSYCHOLOGICAL REPORTS. 10:643-645, 1962.

"Effects of some stimulant and depressant drugs on sleep cycles of cats," by Jewett, Robert E., and Norton, Stata. EXPERIMENTAL NEUROLOGY. 15(4):463-474, 1966.

"Effects of stimulants on rotarod performance of mice," by Plotnikoff, N., Reinke, D., and Firzloff, J. JOURNAL OF PHARMACEUTICAL SCIENCES. 51:1007-1008, 1962.

"Effects of two meprobamate-amphetamine combinations on moods, emotions, and motivations," by Cameron, Jean S., et al. JOURNAL OF PSYCHOLOGY. 67(1):169-181, 1967.

"Effects of two slimming drugs on sleep." by Oswald, Ian, et al. BRITISH MEDICAL JOURNAL. 1(5595):796-799, 1968.

"Effects of unwanted signals and d-amphetamine sulfate on observer responses," by Weiner, H., and Ross, S. JOURNAL OF APPLIED PSYCHOLOGY. 46:135-141, Apr., 1962.

"Enhancement of amphetamine sulphate effects by atropine in a social situation," by Rumelhart, David E., and Mueller, Marvin R. PSYCHOLOGICAL REPORTS. 12(1):251-254, 1963.

"Enhancement of human performance by caffeine and the amphetamines," by Weiss, Bernard and Laties, Victor G. PHARMACOLOGICAL REVIEWS. 14:1-36, 1962.

"Evidence that the central action of (+)-amphetamine is mediated via catecholamines," by Hanson, L.C. PSYCHOPHARMACOLOGIA. 10(4):289-297, 1967.

"Facilitating effects of d-amphetamine on discriminated-avoidance performance," by Hearst, E., and Whalen, R.E. JOURNAL OF COMPARATIVE PHYSIOLOGY AND PSYCHOLOGY. 56 (1):124-128, 1963.

"Facilitation of avoidance learning by d-amphetamine," by Kulkarni, A.L., and Job, William M. LIFE SCIENCES. 6(15):1579-1587, 1967.

"Facilitative effects of amphetamine on avoidance conditioning in relation to age and problem difficulty," by Doty, Barbara A., and Doty, L.A. PSYCHOPHARMACOLOGIA. 9(3):234-241, 1966.

"Further support for a placebo effect," by Ross, Sherman. PSYCHOLOGICAL REPORTS. 13(2):461-462, 1963.

18

"The hyperkinetic child: A forgotten entity. Its diagnosis and treatment," by Levy, Sol. INTERNATIONAL JOURNAL OF NEUROPSYCHIATRY. 2(4):330-336, 1966.

"Hyperpyrexia as a contributory factor in the toxicity of amphetamine to aggregated mice," by Askew, B.M. BRITISH JOURNAL OF PHARMACOLOGY. 19:245-247, 1962.

"Increased sensitivity of measurement of drug effects in expert swimmer," by Smith, G.M., Weitzner, M., and Beecher, H.K. JOURNAL OF PHARMACOLOGY AND EXPERIMENTAL THERAPEUTICS. 139:114-119, 1963.

"Increased suppression of food intake by amphetamine in rats with anterior hypothalamic lesions," by Cole, Sherwood O. JOURNAL OF COMPARATIVE AND PHYSIOLOGICAL PSYCHOLOGY. 61(2):302-305, 1966.

"Influence of amphetamine and scopolamine on the catalepsy induced by diencephalic lesions in rats," by Delini-Stula, A., and Morpurg0, C. INTERNATIONAL JOURNAL OF NEUROPHARMACOLOGY. 7(4):391-394, 1968.

"The influence of dl-, d-, and l-amphetamine and d-methamphetamine on a fixed ratio schedule," by Owen, John E., Jr. JOURNAL OF EXPERIMENTAL ANALYSIS OF BEHAVIOR. 3:293-309, 1960.

"The influence of serotonine and amphetamine on analgesic effect of morphine after reserpine premedication in rats and mice," by Nicak, A. MEDICINA ET PHARMACOLOGIA EXPERIMENTALS. 13:43-48, 1965.

"Influence of some psychotropic and andrenergic blocking agents upon amphetamine stereotyped behavior in white rats," by Zbigniew, H.L. PSYCHOPHARMACOLOGIA. 11(2):136-142, 1967.

"The interaction of amphetamine and eserine on the EEG," by Barnes, Charles D. LIFE SCIENCES. 5(20):1897-1902, 1966.

"Interaction of amphetamine with conditions of food deprivation," by Cole Sherwood O. PSYCHOLOGICAL REPORTS. 13(2):387-390, 1963.

"Interaction of asarone with mescaline, amphetamine and tremorine," by Danduja, D.C., and Menon, M.K. LIFE SCIENCES. 4(17):1635-1641, 1965.

"Interaction of d-amphetamine and food deprivation on fixed ratio behavior of pigeons," by Meginniss, Richard F. PSYCHOLOGICAL REPORTS. 20(2):355-358, 1967.

"Interaction of the effects of tyramine, amphetamine, and reserpine in man," by Gelder, M., and Vane, J. PSYCHOPHARMACOLOGIA. 3:321-241, 1962.

"The interactive effect of amphetamine on the activity level of rats with lesions in the septum," by Pike, R.O., and Greenberg, Issac. PSYCHONOMIC SCIENCE. 14(5):216-217, 1969.

"Magnesium pemoline: effect on acquisition and retention of discriminated avoidance behavior," by Filby, Yasuko, et al. PSYCHONOMIC SCIENCE. 9(3):131-132, 1967.

"Mechanism of action of cocaine and amphetamine in the brain," by Van Rossum, J.M., et al. EXPERIENTIA. 18(5):229-231, 1962.

"Methamphetamine and pentobarbital effects on human motor performance," by Talland, George A., and Quarton, Gardner C. PSYCHOPHARMACOLOGIA. 8(4):241-250, 1965.

"Methamphetamine reinforcement in rats," by Pickens, Roy, et al. PSYCHONOMIC SCIENCE. 8(9):371-372, 1967.

"Methods and problems of measuring drug-induced changes in emotions and personality," by Steinberg, H. REVUE DE PSYCHOLOGIE APPLIQUEE. 11:361-372, 1961.

"Mode of action of apomorphine and dexa-amphetamine on gnawing compulsion in rats," by Ernst, A.M. PSYCHOPHARMACOLOGIA. 10(4):316-323, 1967.

"Modification of affect, social behavior and performance by sleep deprivation and drugs," by Laties, Victor G. JOURNAL OF PSYCHIATRIC RESEARCH. 1(1):12-24, 1961.

"Modification of the effect of some central stimulants in mice pretreated with a-methyl-1-tyrosine," by Menon, M.K., et al. PSYCHOPHARMACOLOGIA. 10(5):437-444, 1967.

"Modification of the effects of amphetamine sulphate by past experience in the hooded rat," by Kiernan, C.C. PSYCHOPHARMACOLOGIA. 8(1):23-31, 1965.

"Narcotic and methamphetamine use during pregnancy. Effect on newborn infants," by Sussman, S. AMERICAN JOURNAL OF DISEASES OF CHILDREN. 106:325-330, 1963.

"Non-random oscillation in the response duration curve of electrographic activation," by Morrell, Leonore and Morrell, Frank. ELECTROENCEPHALOGRAPHY AND CLINICAL NEUROPHYSIOLOGY. 14:724-730, 1962.

"On a new method of recording movement in the environment--its application to the study of some behavior-modifying agents," by Dumont, C., et al. ARCHIVES INTERNATIONALES DEPHARMACODYNAMIE ET DE THERAPIE. 151:60-75, 1964.

"On the effect of addiction and tolerance observed from brain waves in animals, with special reference to continuous administration of morphine and methamphetamine," by Ishikawa, T. FOLIA PHARMACOLOGICA JAPONICA / NIHON YAKURIGAKU ZASSHI. 59:187-205, 1963.

"Pathologic dental manifestations poisoning with amphetaminic substances. Clinical and experimental studies," by Rossi, A. MONDO ODONTOSTOMATOLOGICO. 8:183-188, 1966.

"Pentobarbital and dextroamphetamine sulfate: effects of the sleep cycle in man," by Baekeland, F. PSYCHOPHARMACOLOGIA. 11(5):388-396, 1967.

"Performances as a function of drug, dose, and level of training," by Ray, O.S., and Bivens, L.W. PSYCHOPHARMACOLOGIA. 10(2):103-109, 1966.

"Pharmacodynamic reactivity in mental patients measured by fractioned 'Weckanalyse'," by Frazio, C., et al. COMPREHENSIVE PSYCHIATRY. 4(4):246-255, 1963.

"Pharmacologic influences on mating behavior in the male rat," by Bignami, G. PSYCHOPHARMACOLOGIA. 10(1):44-58, 1966.

"Pharmacological modification of the effects of spaced occipital ablations," by Cole, D.D. et al. PSYCHOPHARMACOLOGIA. 11(4):311-316, 1967.

"Physical and psychologic factors in glue sniffing," by Massengale, O.N., et al. NEW ENGLAND JOURNAL OF MEDICINE. 269(25):1340-1344, 1963.

"Potentiation of amphetamine and pethidine by monoamine-oxidase inhibitors," by Brownlee, G., and Williams, G.W. LANCET. 1:669, 1963.

"Potentiation of evoked cortical responses in the rabbit by methamphetamine and antidepressants," by Plotnikoff, N., and Everett, G.M. LIFE SCIENCES. 4(11):1135-1147, 1965.

"Preferences for punished and unpunished schedules of reinforcement under oxazepam, chlordiazepoxide, and amphetamine," by Margules, D.L., and Stein, Larry. PROCEEDINGS OF THE 74TH ANNUAL CONVENTION OF THE AMERICAN PSYCHOLOGICAL ASSOCIATION. 113-114, 1966.

"Prior social experience and amphetamine toxicity in mice," by Mast, Truman M., and Heimstra, Norman. PSYCHOLOGICAL REPORTS. 11(3):809-812, 1962.

"Psychiatric complications of amphetamine substances," by Johnson, J., et al. ACTA PSYCHIATRICA SCANDINAVICA. 42:252-263, 1966.

"A psychopharmacologic experiment in a training school for delinquent boys: methods, problems, findings," by Eisenberg, L., Lachman, R., Molling, P.A., Mizelle, J.D., and Conners, C.K. AMERICAN JOURNAL OF ORTHOPSYCHIATRY. 33:431-447, 1963.

"A psychpharmacological comparison or operant and classical conditioning," by Bridger, Wagner H. CONDITIONAL REFLEX. 2(2):169, 1967.

"The psychopharmacological profile: a systematic approach to the interaction of drug effects and personality traits," by Lehmann, H.E., and Knight, D.A. REVUE CANADIENNE DE BIOLOGIE. 20:631-641, 1961.

"Quantitative comparisons of the electroencephalographic stimulant effects of deanol, choline, and amphetamine," by Pfeiffer, C., et al. CLINICAL PHARMACOLOGY AND THERAPEUTICS. 4:461-466, 1963.

"Reduction of freezing behavior and improvement of shock avoidance by d-amphetamine," by Krieckhaus, E.E., et al. JOURNAL OF COMPARATIVE AND PHYSIOLOGICAL PSYCHOLOGY. 60(1):36-40, 1965.

"The relation role of storage and synthesis of brain norepinephrine in the psychomotor stimulation evoked by amphetamine or by desipramine and tetrabenazine," by Sulser, F., et al. PSYCHOPHARMACOLOGIA. 12(4):322-332, 1968.

"Release of norepinephrine from hypothalamus and amygdala by rewarding medial forebrain bundle stimulation and amphetamine," by Stein, Larry and Wise, C. David. JOURNAL OF COMPARATIVE AND PHYSIOLOGICAL PSYCHOLOGY. 67 (2, Pt.1):189-198, 1969.

"A research note: Effects of dextro-amphetamine and meprobamate on problem-solving and mood of aged subjects," by Krugman, A., et al. JOURNAL OF GERONTOLOGY. 15:

419-420, 1960.

"Responses of the habituated vestibulo-ocular reflex arc to drug stress," by Dowd, Patrick J. UNITED STATES AIR FORCE SCHOOL OF AVIATION MEDICINE TECHNICAL DOCUMENTARY REPORT. No. 64-72.

"Rhythmic urinary excretion of amphetamine in man," by Beckett, A.H. NATURE. 204:1203, 1224, 1964.

"Scopolamine, amphetamine and light-reinforced responding," by Carlton, Peter L. PSYCHONOMIC SCIENCE. 5(9):347-348, 1966.

"Self-stimulation of the brain by cats: effects of imipramine, amphetamine and chlorpromazine," by Horovitz, Z., et al. PSYCHOPHARMACOLOGIA. 3:455-462, 1962.

"Self-stimulation of the brain by cats: technique and preliminary drug-effects," by Horovitz, Z.P., Chow, M.E., and Carlton, P.L. PSYCHOPHARMACOLOGIA. 3:449-454, 1962.

"Social influence on the response to drugs: IV. Stimulus factors," by Heimstra, N.W., and McDonald, A.L. PSYCHOLOGICAL RECORD. 12(4):383-386, 1962.

"Some effects of amphetamine and chlorpromazine upon the acquisition of an avoidance escape response in the albino rat," by Loiselle, R., et al. PSYCHIATRIC COMMUNICATIONS. 7:23-26, 1964.

"Some effects of morphine and amphetamine on intellectual functions and mood," by Evans, W.O. PSYCHOPHARMACOLOGIA. 6:49-56, 1964.

"Some new behavior-disrupting amphetamines and their significance," by Smythies, J.R., et al. NATURE. 216 (5111):128-129, 1967.

"Spaced responding in multiple DRL schedules," by Zimmerman, J., and Schuster, C.R. JOURNAL OF EXPERIMENTAL ANALYSIS OF BEHAVIOR. 5(4):497-504, 1962.

"A specific method for the determination of amphetamine in urine," by Beckett, A.H., et al. JOURNAL OF PHARMACY AND PHARMACOLOGY. 16(Suppl.):2703 1T, 1964.

"Standardization of scales which evaluate subjective effects of morphine, amphetamine, pentobarbital, alcohol, LSD-25, pyrahexl and chlorpromazine." PSYCHOPHARMACOLOGIA. 4(3):184-205, 1963.

"Stereotyped activities produced by amphetamine in several animal species and man," by Randrup, A., and Munkvad, I. PSYCHOPHARMACOLOGIA. 11(4):300-310, 1967.

"Stereotyped movements of mental defectives: VI. No effect of amphetamine or a barbiturate," by Berkson, Gershon. PERCEPTUAL AND MOTOR SKILLS. 21(3):698, 1965.

"Studies in activity level: VII. Effects of amphetamine drug administration on the activity of retarded children," by McConnell, Thomas R., Jr., et al. AMERICAN JOURNAL OF MENTAL DEFICIENCY. 68(5):647-651, 1964.

"Studies in hyperkinetic behavior: II. Laboratory and clinical evaluation of drug treatments," by Millichap, J. Gordon, and Boldrey, Edwin E. NEUROLOGY. 17(5):467-471, 1967.

"Studies on mescaline XIX: a new theory concerning the nature of schizophrenia," by Denber, H.C., and Teller, D.N. PSYCHOSOMATICS. 9(3):145-151, 1968.
"Study on the excitation induced by amphetamine, cocaine and a-methyltryptamine," by Glambos, Eva, et al. PSYCHOPHARMACOLOGIA. 11(2):122-129, 1967.
"Successful treatment of amphetamine addiction in a schizophrenic woman," by Seelye, Edward E.. AMERICAN JOURNAL OF PSYCHOTHERAPY. 21(2):295-301, 1967.
"Time estimation, knowledge of results and drug effects," by Rutschmann, J., and Rubinstein, L. JOURNAL OF PSYCHIATRIC RESEARCH. 4(2):107-114, 1966.
"Time relations of objective and subjective reactions to d-amphetamine and pentobarbitone," by Frankenhaeuser,M., and Post, B. SCANDINAVIAN JOURNAL OF PSYCHOLOGY. 5(2):99-107, 1964.
"Timing behavior during prolonged treatment with dl-amphetamine," by Schuster, C.R., and Zimmerman, J. JOURNAL OF THE EXPERIMENTAL ANALYSIS OF BEHAVIOR. 4:327-330, 1961.
"Tolerance and cross-tolerance among psychotomimetic drugs," by Appel, J.B., and Freedman, D.X. PSYCHOPHARMACOLOGIA. 13(3):267-274, 1968.
"Toxicity and catecholamine releasing actions of d- and l-amphetamine in isolated and aggregated mice," by Moore, K.E. JOURNAL OF PHARMACOLOGY AND EXPERIMENTAL THERAPEUTICS. 142:6-12, 1963.
"2, 5-dimethoxy-4-methyl-amphetamine, STP: a new hallucinogenic drug," by Snyder, S.H., et al.; reply with rejoinder," by Cabe, P.A. SCIENCE. 159:1491-1492, Mar. 29, 1968.
"Urinary excretion kinetics of amphetamine in man," by Beckett, A.H., and Rowland, M. JOURNAL OF PHARMACY AND PHARMACOLOGY. 17:628-639, 1965.
"Urinary excretion of methylamphetamine in man," by Beckett, A.H. NATURE. 206:1260-1261, 1965.
"Use of peritoneal dialysis in experimental amphetamine poisoning," by Zalis, E.G., Cohen, R.J., and Lundberg, G.D. PROCEEDINGS OF THE SOCIETY FOR EXPERIMENTAL BIOLOGY AND MEDICINE. 120:278-281, 1965.
"Workshop on the detection and control of abuse of narcotics, barbiturates, and amphetamines: San Juan, Puerto Rico, December 13-15, 1965," by Leonard, Frederick. PSYCHOPHARMACOLOGY BULLETIN. 3(4):21-26, 1966.

BARBITURATES AND TRANQUILIZING DRUGS: BOOKS

Eichlenlaub, John E. ALCOHOL, TRANQUILIZERS, SEDATIVES, AND NARCOTICS. New York: Macmillan, 1962.
Fraser, H.F., et al. ADDICTIVENESS OF NEW SYNTHETIC ANALGESICS, Mintues of the 21st Meeting of the Committee

on Drug Addiction and Narcotics, National Research
Council, Washington, D.C., National Academy of Sci-
ences, January 11-12, 1960.
Fraser, H.F., et al. PRELIMINARY REPORT ON THE HUMAN
PHARMACOLOGY AND ADDICTION LIABILITY OF 2-CYCLOPRO-
PYLMETHYL-2-HYDROXY-5, 9-DIMETHYL-6, 7-BENZOMORPHAN
(ARC-II-C-3; Win 20, 740), Appendix 8 to the Minutes
of the 25th Meeting of the Committee on Drug Addiction
and Narcotics, National Academy of Science and National
Research Council, 1963, pp. 3237-3249.
United Nations. Secretary-General, 1961- (Thant). BAR-
BITURATES. New York: United Nations Economic and So-
cial Council, Commission on Narcotic Drugs, 1962. (Doc-
ument. E/CN. V417).
U.S. Department of Health, Education, and Welfare. BARBIT-
URATES AS ADDICTING DRUGS. Washington, D.C.: United
States Public Health Service Publication No. 545; Super-
intendent of Documents, Rev. 1965.
U.S. Department of Health, Education, and Welfare. THE UP
AND DOWN DRUGS: AMPHETAMINES AND BARBITURATES. United
States Public Health Service Publication No. 1830. Wash-
ington, D.C.: Government Printing Office, 1969.

BARBITURATES AND TRANQUILIZING DRUGS: Doctoral Dissertations

Thompson, Tracis Irving. "The effect of two phenothiazines
and a barbiturate on extinction-induced rate increase of
a free operant." (Thesis, unpublished, University of
Minnesota). DISSERTATION ABSTRACTS. 22(8):2889, 1962.

BARBITURATES AND TRANQUILIZING DRUGS: Periodical Literature

General Publications

"Abuse of barbiturates and amphetamines," by Seevers, M.H.
POSTGRADUATE MEDICINE. 37:45-51, Jan., 1965.
"The abuse of barbiturates by heroin addicts," by Cumber-
lidge, M.C. CANADIAN MEDICAL ASSOCIATION JOURNAL. 98
(22):1045-1049, June 1, 1968.
"Abuse of barbiturates, stimulants, LSD, as great a danger
as illegal narcotics," by Braude, A. AMERICAN ASSOCIA-
TION OF INDUSTRIAL NURSES JOURNAL. 15:40-41, Jan., 1967.
"Acute barbiturate poisoning and its treatment," by Oner, C.
TURK TIB CEMIYETI. 31:219-227, 1965.
"Acute psychotic reaction following ingestion of phenter-
mine," by Rubin, R.T. AMERICAN JOURNAL OF PSYCHIATRY.

24

120:1124-1125, 1964.
"The addiction potential of oxycodone (percodan)," by
Bloomquist, E.R. CALIFORNIA MEDICINE. 99:127-130, 1963.
"Addiction to long-acting barbiturates," by Remmer, H.,
Siegert, M., Nitze, H.R., and Kerstein, I. NAUNYN-
SCHMIEDEBERGS ARCHIV FUER PHARMAKOLOGIE UND EXPERIMENT-
ELLE PATHOLOGIE. 243:468-478, 1962.
"Amphetamine and barbiturate abuse," by Mansfield, N.J.H.
CANADA'S MENTAL HEALTH. 17:2-5, Sept.-Oct., 1969.
"Amphetamines and barbiturates; the up and down drugs."
TODAY'S EDUCATION. 58:42-44, Mar., 1969.
"Analgesia and addiction," by Mellet, L.B. ARZNEIMITTEL-
FORSCHUNG. 5:155-267, 1963.
"Analytical investigations of barbiturate poisoning - De-
scription of methods and a survey of results," by Bogan,
James, et al. JOURNAL OF THE FORENSIC SCIENCE SOCIETY.
7(1):37-45, Jan., 1967.
"Aortic disease: barbiturate poisoning." BRISTOL MEDICO-
CHIRURGICAL JOURNAL. 80:29-33, 1965.
"Appetite suppressing drugs as an etiologic factor in men-
tal illness," by Breitner, C. PSYCHOSOMATICS. 4:327-
333, 1963.
"Apropos of a widespread warning against the abuse of anal-
gesics in Switzerland," by Cheymol, J. THERAPIE. 19:
1323-1330, 1964.
"Barbiturate abstinence syndrome," by Westgate, H.D. ANES-
THESIOLOGY. 25:403-406, 1964.
"Barbiturate abuse: an iatrogenic disorder," by Halliday,
Robert. BRITISH COLUMBIA MEDICAL JOURNAL. 9:374-378,
Oct., 1967.
"Barbiturate addiction and sensitivity," by Armitage, G.H.,
and Sim, M. BRITISH JOURNAL OF MEDICAL PSYCHOLOGY. 33:
149-155, 1960.
"Barbiturate curbs to go into effect; producers and distrib-
utors of barbiturates, amphetamines and drugs must keep
records." OIL, PAINT AND DRUG REPORT. 188:7 passim,
Dec. 27, 1965.
"Barbiturate intoxication," by Mullan, D., et al. LANCET.
1:705, 1965.
"Barbiturate poisoning," by Clifton, B.S., et al. MEDICAL
JOURNAL OF AUSTRALIA. 1:63-67, 1965.
"Barbiturate poisoning," by Leclercq, A. GAZETTE MEDICALE
DE FRANCE. 71:2891-2906, 1964.
"Barbiturate poisoning," by McBay, A.J. NEW ENGLAND JOUR-
NAL OF MEDICINE. 273:38-39, 1965.
"Barbiturate poisonings," by Jacobziner, H., and Raybin,
H.W. NEW YORK JOURNAL OF MEDICINE. 62:3612-3614, 1962.
"Barbiturate poisonings," by Jacobziner, H., and Raybin,
H.W. NEW YORK JOURNAL OF MEDICINE. 63:713-714, 1963.
"Barbiturate toxicity," by Tattersall, R. PRACTITIONER.
194:68-71, 1965.
"Barbiturate use in narcotic addicts," by Hamburger, E.
JOURNAL OF THE AMERICAN MEDICAL ASSOCIATION. 189(5):
366-368, 1964.

"Barbiturates and amphetamines bill; do not overlook the competitors." OIL, PAINT AND DRUG REPORT. 187:4 passim, Feb. 8, 1965.

"Barbiturates and amphetamines bill; House leadership clears decks." OIL, PAINT AND DRUG REPORT. 187:5, Mar. 8, 1965.

"Barbiturates and synergistic drugs," by Whitley, E.K. MEDICO-LEGAL BULLETIN. 126: 1-4, 1963.

"Barbiturates as addicting drugs. INDUSTRIAL MEDICINE AND SURGERY. 35:111-112, 1966.

"Barbiturates, automatism and suicide," by Long, R.H. POST-GRADUATE MEDICINE. 28:A56-72, 1960.

"Barbiturates suppress cell division." THE AMERICAN BIOLOGY TEACHER. 30:848, Dec., 1968.

"Chlorphentermine," by Craig, D.D. BRITISH MEDICAL JOURNAL. 5367:1269, 1963.

"Chronic intoxication with sedatives." LANCET. 2:1368, 1962.

"Chronic use of barbiturates and chloral hydrate," by Domino, E.F. JOURNAL OF THE AMERICAN MEDICAL ASSOCIATION. 183:816-817, 1963.

"Clinical aspects of barbiturate and sedative drug abuse," by Essig, C.F. AMERICAN JOURNAL OF HOSPITAL PHARMACY. 22:140-143, 1965.

"Dependence on barbiturates and other sedative drugs. JOURNAL OF THE AMERICAN MEDICAL ASSOCIATION. 193:673-677, 1965.

"Dependency on methaqualone hydrochloride (Melsedin)," by Martin, G.J. BRITISH MEDICAL JOURNAL. 5505:114, 1966.

"Dependency upon tranquilizers," by Siegel, I. JOURNAL OF THE AMERICAN MEDICAL ASSOCIATION. 191:352, Jan. 25, 1965.

"Diagnosis and treatment of drug dependence of the barbiturate type," by Wikler, A. AMERICAN JOURNAL OF PSYCHIATRY. 125:758-765, Dec., 1968.

"Don't dodge the drug questions; depressants," by Hawkins, M.E. SCIENCE TEACHER. 33:34, Nov., 1966.

"Drug abuse law; over-the-counter barbiturates given more time." OIL, PAINT AND DRUG REPORT. 189:4, Jan. 17, 1966.

"Drug intoxication: barbiturates and tranquilizers," by Smith, D.R. APPLIED THERAPY. 6:219-222, Mar., 1964.

"Drug makers, druggist rebuffed on pills stand." OIL, PAINT AND DRUG REPORT. 187:3 passim, Mar. 1, 1965.

"Drug profiles. The barbiturates," by Prichard, E.N. MEDICAL WORLD. 99:41-50, 1963.

"FDA sets date for speaking up by drug people (Barbiturates and amphetamines involved)." OIL, PAINT AND DRUG REPORT. 189:4, Feb. 28, 1966.

"First aid: depressant drug overdose," by Potthoff, C.J. TODAY'S HEALTH. 47(11):74, Nov., 1969.

"Five weeks to escape the sleeping pill habit," by Oswald, I., and Priest, R.G. BRITISH MEDICAL JOURNAL. 5470: 1093-1095, 1965.

"Hypnotics. I. Barbiturates." BRITISH MEDICAL JOURNAL. 5322:39-40, 1963.

"Infringement of traffic safety by barbiturate medication and the barbiturate/alcohol combination," by Doenicke, A. ARZNEIMITTEL-FORSCHUNG. 12:1050-1054, 1962.

"Learning and drugs," by Bustamane, J.A., et al. PHYSIOLOGY AND BEHAVIOR. 3(4):553-555, 1968.

"Learning and phenobarbital," by Lampe, J.M. JOURNAL OF SCHOOL HEALTH. 34:392, Oct., 1964.

"Misuse of dristan inhaler," by Greenberg, H.R. NEW YORK JOURNAL OF MEDICINE. 66:613-617, 1966.

"Misuse of thiobarbiturates and of the recovery room," NEW YORK JOURNAL OF MEDICINE. 62:3458-3459, 1962.

"Misuse of valuable therapeutic agents: barbiturates, tranquilizers and amphetamines." BULLETIN OF THE NEW YORK ACADEMY OF MEDICINE. 40:972-979, 1964.

"More and more barbiturates," by Brooke, E.M., et al. MEDICINE, SCIENCE AND THE LAW. 4:277-282, 1964.

"Motivation enhancement produced by injections of phenobarbital," by Stewart, Alan L., and Schmidt, Hans. PROCEEDINGS OF THE 73RD ANNUAL CONVENTION OF THE AMERICAN PSYCHOLOGICAL ASSOCIATION. 117-118, 1965.

"Newer sedative drugs that can cause intoxication and dependence of barbiturate type," by Essig, C.F. JOURNAL OF THE AMERICAN MEDICAL ASSOCIATION. 196:714, May, 1966.

"'Nil nocere,' Barbital poisoning caused by cough syrup," by Oster, H. MUENCHENER MEDIZINISCHE WOCHENSCHRIFT. 104:1941, 1962.

"On gracidinomania," by Nemirovskii, D.E. VRACHEBNOC DELO. 7:145-147, 1965.

"On psychoses after over-doses of anorexic substances," by Takacs, L. PSYCHIATRIE, NEUROLOGIE UND MEDIZINISCHE PSYCHOLOGIE. 17:183-185, 1965.

"On the problem of development of addiction by appetite depressants," by Klinger, W. ZEITSCHRIFT ARZNEIMITTEL FUER AERTZLICHE FORTBILDUNG. 59:49-50, 1965.

"On the use of so-called anorexigenic drugs," by Lachnit, V. WIENER ZEITSCHRIFT FUER INNERE MEDIZIN UND IHRE GRENZGEBIETE. 46:248-254, 1965.

"Patients receiving barbiturates in an urban general practice," by Adams, B.G., et al. JOURNAL OF THE COLLEGE OF GENERAL PRACTITIONERS. 12:24-31, Jul., 1966.

"Pep pills and barbiturates. Instant happiness-mood medicine," by Brierley, C. AMERICAN ASSOCIATION OF INDUSTRIAL NURSES JOURNAL. 14:23, 1966.

"Pep pills and barbiturates. Use and abuse," by Jackson, A.T. AMERICAN ASSOCIATION OF INDUSTRIAL NURSES JOURNAL. 14:22, 1966.

"Phenacetin cyanosis, barbiturate habituation and cardiac arrest," by Dwyer, B., and Gunner, B. MEDICAL JOURNAL OF AUSTRALIA. 1:13-14, 1963.

"Pills bill passes Senate, some ironing-out needed. (Controls over production and marketing of barbiturates, amphetamines, etc.)." OIL, PAINT AND DRUG REPORT. 187:3 passim, June 28, 1965.

"Pills measure moves to the half-way point. (Barbiturates

and amphetamines)." OIL, PAINT AND DRUG REPORT. 187:5
passim, Mar. 15, 1965.
"Pills traffic results in pelting for FDA." OIL, PAINT AND
DRUG REPORT. 187:3 passim, Feb. 15, 1965.
"The problem of barbiturate poisoning," by Murchison, G.C.,
Jr, JOURNAL OF THE MEDICAL ASSOCIATION OF ALABAMA. 32:
345-352, 1963.
"The problem of barbiturates in the United States of Amer-
ica," by Fort, J. BULLETIN ON NARCOTICS. 16:17-35, Jan.,
1964.
"The problem of phenmetrazine addiction," by Vencovsky, E.
CESKOSLOVENSKA PSYCHIATRIE. 61:411-414, 1965.
"Procedure for withdrawal of barbiturates," by Blachly, P.H.
AMERICAN JOURNAL OF PSYCHIATRY. 120:894-895, 1964.
"Propoxyphene hydrochloride, a drug of abuse," by Claghorn,
J., and Schoolar, J. JOURNAL OF THE AMERICAN MEDICAL
ASSOCIATION. 196:137-139, 1966.
"Psychological effects of amphetamines and barbiturates,"
by Nash, Harvey. JOURNAL OF MENTAL AND NERVOUS DISEASES.
134(3): 203-217, 1962.
"Psychological effects of drugs," by Steinberg, Hannah.
GAWEIN. 11(5-6):384-413, 1963.
"The rapid development of physical dependence on barbitur-
ates," by Jaffe, J.H., et al. JOURNAL OF PHARMACOLOGY
AND EXPERIMENTAL THERAPEUTICS. 150:140-145, Oct., 1965.
"Some clinical aspects of addiction to narcotic analgesics,"
by Martin, W.R. AMERICAN JOURNAL OF HOSPITAL PHARMACY.
22:133-139, 1965.
"Some problems of barbiturate and alcoholic intoxication,"
by Teare, R.D. MEDICO-LEGAL JOURNAL. 34:4-10, 1966.
"The story of tranquilizers." TODAY'S HEALTH. pp. 32-33,
56-59, Nov., 1960.
"Tranquilizer affects eyes," by McBroom, P. SCIENCE NEWS.
89:235, Apr. 9, 1966.
"Tranquilizer poisoning; an example of child abuse," by
Dine, M.S. PEDIATRICS. 36:782-785, 1965.
"The use and abuse of hypnotics," by Exton-Smith, A.N.
GERONTOLOGIA CLINICA. 9:264-269, 1967.
"Use and abuse of pervitin," by Wolffenbuttel, E. REVISTA
BRASILEIRA DE MEDICINA. 20:166, 1963.
"Use of barbiturates by heroin addicts," by Cumberlidge,
M.C. CANADIAN MEDICAL ASSOCIATION JOURNAL. 98:1045-1049,
June 1, 1968.
"The uses and abuses of appetite suppressants," by Seaton,
D.A., et al. BRITISH JOURNAL OF CLINICAL PRACTICE. 19:
89-93, 1965.
"What you should know about tranquilizers," by Hartley,W.,
and Hartley, E. READER'S DIGEST. July, 1962.
"Why millions of Americans use sleeping pills." Good House-
KEEPING. 168:135-137, Jan., 1969.
"Withdrawal fits in barbiturate addicts," by Gardner, A.J.
LANCET. 2:337-338, Aug. 12, 1967; also in: BULLETIN ON
NARCOTICS. 21(1):40, Jan./Mar., 1969.

"Action of enionic and cationic nerve-blocking agents: experiment and interpretation," by Blaustein, M.P., and Goldman, D.E.   SCIENCE.   153:429-432, July 22, 1966.
"Acute barbiturate and glutethimide intoxication.   Management by hemodialysis and peritoneal dialysis," by Del Greco, F., Arieff, A.J., and Simon, N.M.   QUARTERLY BULLETIN OF THE NORTHWESTERN UNIVERSITY MEDICAL SCHOOL. 36:306-315, 1962.
"Acute effects of phenobarbital upon a locomotor response," by Schmidt, H., and Stewart, A.L.   PHYSIOLOGY AND BEHAVIOR.   2(4):403-407, 1967.
"Acute myopathy associated with barbiturate withdrawal," by Hess, Joseph W., and Stoffer, Sheldon.   THE INTERNATIONAL JOURNAL OF THE ADDICTIONS.   3:319-327, Spring, 1968.
"Acute pulmonary edema caused by barbiturate poisoning: a consideration of its genesis and therapy," by Schoenfeld, M.R.   ANGIOLOGY.   15:445-453, 1964.
"Amobarbital effects on extinction and spontaneous recovery of active avoidance," by Kamano, Dennis K., et al.   PSYCHOLOGICAL RECORD.   17(1):97-102, 1967.
"Amobarbital sodium and instrumental performance changes following an increase in reward magnitude," by Ison, James R., and Northman, Joan.   PSYCHONOMIC SCIENCE.   12 (5):185-186, 1968.
"Analgesics and their antagonists: biochemical aspects and structure-activity relationships," by Beckett, A.H., and Casy, A.F.   PROGRESS IN MEDICINAL CHEMISTRY.   4:171-228, 1965.
"Analysis for narcotic analgesics and barbiturates in urine by thin-layer chromatographic techniques without previous extraction and concentration," by Cochin, J.   PSYCHOPHARMACOLOGY BULLETIN; National Clearinghouse for Mental Health Information.   3:53-60, 1966.
"Artificial dialysis of a case of severe barbiturate poisoning," by Eliahou, H.E., and Frensdorf, A.   HAREFUAH.   64: 255-256, 1963.
"Barbiturate-induced dissociation of acquisition and extinction: role of movement-initiating processes," by Bindra, Dalbir, et al.   JOURNAL OF COMPARATIVE AND PHYSIOLOGICAL PSYCHOLOGY.   60(2):223-228, 1965.
"Barbiturate sensitization or shift of adoption level?" by Douthitt, Thomas C., et al.   PROCEEDINGS OF THE 73RD ANNUAL CONVENTION OF THE AMERICAN PSYCHOLOGICAL ASSOCIATION.   119-120, 1965.
"Barbiturate withdrawal convulsions in decerebellate dogs," by Essig, C.F.   INTERNATIONAL JOURNAL OF NEUROPHARMACOLOGY.   3:453-456, 1964.
"Barbiturates, lysergic acid diethylamide, and the social

behavior of laboratory rats," by Silverman, A.P. PSY-
CHOPHARMACOLOGIA. 10(2):155-171, 1966.
"Bullous lesions in acute barbiturate intoxication," by
Beveridge, G.W., et al. BRITISH MEDICAL JOURNAL. 5452:
48, 1965.
"Bullous lesions in acute barbiturate intoxication," by
Bywaters, E.G. BRITISH MEDICAL JOURNAL. 5453:106-107,
1965.
"Bullous lesions in acute barbiturate intoxication," by
Freeman, D.M., et al. BRITISH MEDICAL JOURNAL. 5448:
1495-1496, 1965.
"Bullous lesions in acute barbiturate intoxication," by
Spillane, J.D. BRITISH MEDICAL JOURNAL. 5445:1308,
1965.
"Bullous lesions in acute barbiturate intoxication," by
Warnock, G. BRITISH MEDICAL JOURNAL. 5443:1188, 1965.
"Cardiovascular actions of narcotic analgesics," by Elliott,
H.W., and Adawi, Abdel. AMERICAN HEART JOURNAL. 69(4):
567-568, 1965.
"A case of primary addiction to meprobamate," by Little,
J.C. BRITISH MEDICAL JOURNAL. 5360:794, 1963.
"The cause of tolerance to oxidizable barbiturates," by
Remmer, H. NAUNYN-SCHMIEDEBERGS ARCHIV FUER EXPERIMENT-
ELLE PATHOLOGIE UND PHARMAKOLOGIE. 244:311-333, 1963.
"Chromatographic separation and microdetermination of pheno-
barbital, methylphenobarbital, butobarbital and pheny-
toin," by Westernik, D. PHARMACEUTISCH WEEKBLAD. 97:
849-856, 1962.
"Clinical pharmacology of hypnotics and sedatives," by
Shideman, F.E. CLINICAL PHARMACOLOGY AND THERAPEUTICS.
2:313-344, 1961.
"Comparison of phenobarbital and pentobarbital actions upon
water ingestion," by Schmidt, H., Jr., and Dry, L.
JOURNAL OF COMPARATIVE AND PHYSIOLOGICAL PSYCHOLOGY.
56(1):179-182, 1963.
"A comparison of the effects of meprobamate, phenobarbital
and d-amphetamine on two psychological tests," by Townsend, Arthur M., and Mirsky, Allan F. JOURNAL OF NER-
VOUS AND MENTAL DISEASE. 130:212-216, 1960.
"Compendium of neuropsychopharmacology. Analgesics," by
LaVerne, A.A. JOURNAL OF NEUROPSYCHIATRY. 5:201-211,
1964.
"Competing voice messages: Effects of message load and drugs
on the ability of acute schizophrenics to attend," by
Rappaport, Maurice. ARCHIVES OF GENERAL PSYCHIATRY.
17(1):97-103, 1967.
"Complex response patterns during temporally spaced respond-
ing," by Hodos, William, et al. JOURNAL OF EXPERIMENTAL
ANALYSIS OF BEHAVIOR. 5(4):473-479, 1962.
"The concept of the past, present and future of the self
under the effect of intravenous injection of pentobar-
bital calcium," by Harui, Tohru. TOHOKU PSYCHOLOGICA
FOLIA. 22(1-2):49-55, 1963.
"Considerations on intoxication due to barbiturates and

neuroplegics: therapy and resuscitation," by Savioli, A. ACTA ANAESTHESIOLOGICA (Padua). 15:787-798, 1964.
"Control for stimulus change while testing effects of amobarbital on conflict," by Barry, Herbert, III, et al. JOURNAL OF COMPARATIVE AND PHYSIOLOGICAL PSYCHOLOGY. 55(6):1071-1074, 1962.
"A controlled study of induced diuresis in barbiturate intoxication," by Bunn, H.F., et al. ANNALS OF INTERNAL MEDICINE. 62:246-251, 1965.
"Convulsive and sham rage behaviors in decorticate dogs during barbiturate withdrawal," by Essig, C.F. ARCHIVES OF NEUROLOGY. 7:471-475, 1962.
"Cough syrup containing diphenhydramine causing toxicomania and acute psychosis," by Harenko, A. SUOMEN LAAKARILEHTI (Finlands Lakartidning). 20:1100-1103, 1965.
"Current view on the physiopathology, clinical aspects and therapy of acute barbiturate poisoning," by Valenti, F. RASSEGNA DI CLINICA TERAPIA E SCIENZE AFFINI. 62:13-24, 1963.
"Data on the psychopathological symptoms caused by anorexigenics," by Takacs, L. ORVOSI HETILAP. 106:1611-1613, 1965.
"Death after withdrawal of meprobamate," by Swanson, L.A. and Okada, T. JOURNAL OF THE AMERICAN MEDICAL ASSOCIATION. 184:780-781, 1963.
"Deprivation and drug effects on prepyriform cortex electrical activity in rats," by Sutton, Dwight. PHYSIOLOGY AND BEHAVIOR. 2(2):139-144, 1967.
"Determinants of polydipsia: Effects of amphetamine and pentobarbital," by Segal, Evalyn F., et al. PSYCHONOMIC SCIENCE. 3(1):33-34, 1965.
"Dextromethorphan [Romilar] as an intoxicating agent," by Degkwitz, R. NERVENARZT. 35:412-414, 1964.
"Dextropropoxyphene addiction. Observations of a case," by Elson, A., and Domino, E.F. JOURNAL OF THE AMERICAN MEDICAL ASSOCIATION. 183:482-485, 1963.
"Drug administration to cerebral cortex of freely moving dogs," by Kobayasshi, Tsukasa. SCIENCE. 135(3509): 1126-1127, 1962.
"Drug interaction in the field of analgesic drugs," by Lasagna, L. PROCEEDINGS OF THE ROYAL SOCIETY OF MEDICINE. 58(11, Pt. 2):978-983, 1965.
"Drugs and dreams," by Whitman, R.M., et al. COMPREHENSIVE PSYCHIATRY. 2(4):219-226, 1961.
"The EEG of the olfactory bulb of the rabbit and its reaction to psychopharmacological agents," by Khazan, N., et al. PSYCHOPHARMACOLOGIA. 10(3):226-236, 1967.
"The effect of chronic administration of barbitone sodium on the behaviour of the rat," by Leonard, B.E. INTERNATIONAL JOURNAL OF NEUTOPHARMACOLOGY. 6(1):63-70, 1967.
"Effect of chronic administration and withdrawal of barbiturates upon drinking in the rat," by Schmidt, H., Jr., et al. ARCHIVES INTERNATIONALES DE PHARMACODYNAMIE ET DE THERAPIE. 151:142-149, 1964.

31

"The effect of four drugs on sleep patterns in man," by
Hartmann, E. PSYCHOPHAMRMACOLOGIA. 12(4):346-353, 1968.
"Effect of prior injection upon subsequent drinking of
phenobarbital in the rat," by Kleinman, K.M. JOURNAL OF
COMPARATIVE AND PHYSIOLOGICAL PSYCHOLOGY. 61:402-405,
1966.
"The effect of two phenothiazines and a barbiturate on ex-
tinction-induced rate increase of a free operant," by
Thompson, Travis. JOURNAL OF COMPARATIVE AND PHYSIOLOG-
ICAL PSYCHOLOGY. 55(5):714-718, 1962.
"Effects of amobarbital on discrimination acquisition and
reversal,by Caul, W. PSYCHOPHARMACOLOGIA. 11(5):414-
421, 1967.
"Effects of amobarbital sodium on avoidance performances
of rats differing in emotionality," by Martin, Louis K.,
et al. PROCEEDINGS OF THE 74TH ANNUAL CONVENTION OF THE
AMERICAN PSYCHOLOGICAL ASSOCIATION. 125-126, 1966.
"The effects of amobarbital sodium on differential instru-
mental conditioning and subsequent extinction," by Ison,
J.R., and Rosen, A.J. PSYCHOPHARMACOLOGIA. 10(5):417-
425, 1967.
"Effects of barbiturates and a tetrahydrocannabinol derivative on recovery cycles of medial lemniscus, thalamus,
and reticular formation in the cat," by Boyd, E., and
Meritt, D. JOURNAL OF PHARMACOLOGY AND EXPERIMENTAL
THERAPEUTICS. 151:376-384, 1966.
"Effects of carotid infusion of thiopental on learned be-
havior and EEG in goats," by Baldwin, Basil A., et al.
PHYSIOLOGY AND BEHAVIOR. 2(1):23-31, 1967.
"Effects of depressant drug as modified by experimentally-
included expectation," by Frankenhaeuser, Marianne, et
al. PERCEPTUAL AND MOTOR SKILLS. 18(2):513-522, 1964.
"Effects of dexedrine, ephedrine, phenobarbitone and chlor-
promazine on the latency of auto-kinetic movement," by
Lingh, S.D. PSYCHOLOGICAL STUDIES (Mysore). 8(1):7-14,
1963.
"The effects of dextroamphetamine and phenobarbital on a sim-
plified standardized CFF measure," by Misiak, H., and
Rizy, E.F. PSYCHOPHARMACOLOGIA. 13(4):346-353, 1968.
"Effects of drugs on approach-avoidance conflict tested re-
peatedly by means of a 'telescope alley'," by Barry, H.,
and Miller, N.E. JOURNAL OF COMPARATIVE AND PHYSIOLOG-
ICAL PSYCHOLOGY. 55(2):201-210, 1962.
"Effects of meprobamate and prochlorperasine on positive
and negative conditioning," by Uhr, L., et al. JOURNAL
OF ABNORMAL AND SOCIAL PSYCHOLOGY. 63(3):546-551, 1961.
"Effects of meprobamate, chlordiazepoxide, diazepan, and
sodium pentobarbital on visually evoked responses in the
tectotegmental area of the rat," by Olds, M.E., and Baldrighi, G. INTERNATIONAL JOURNAL OF NEUROPHARMACOLOGY.
7(3):231-239, 1968.
"Effects of methylphenidate, pentobarbital, and reserpine
on behavior controlled by a schedule of interresponse
time reinforcement," by Stretch, R., and Dalrymple, D.
PSYCHOPHARMACOLOGIA. 13(1):49-64, 1968.

"The effects of mono-urethans, di-urethans and barbiturates on a punishment discrimination," by Geller, I., and Seifter, J. JOURNAL OF PHARMACOLOGY AND EXPERIMENTAL THERAPEUTICS. 136(3):284-288, 1962.
"Effects of morphine and pentobarbital on conditioned electroderman responses and basal conductance in man," by Jones, B.E., et al. PSYCHOPHARMACOLOGIA. 7(3):159-174, 1965.
"Effects of pentobarbital on fixed ratio reinforcement," by Waller, Marcus B. and Morse, W.H. JOURNAL OF THE EXPERIMENTAL ANALYSIS OF BEHAVIOR. 6(1):125-130, 1963.
"Effects of placebo, dexamyl, and lucofen on moods, emotions, and motivations," by Cameron, Jean S., et al. JOURNAL OF PSYCHOLOGY. 66(2):199-209, 1967.
"The effects of secobarbital and d-amphetamine on performance during a simulated tactical air mission," by McKenzie, Richard E., and Elliott, Lois L. UNITED STATES AIR FORCE SCHOOL OF AVIATION MEDICINE TECHNICAL DOCUMENTARY REPORT. No. 64-79.
"The effects of secobarbital and dextroamphetamine upon time judgment: intersensory factors," by Goldstone, S., and Kirkham, J.E. PSYCHOPHARMACOLOGIA. 13(1):65-73, 1968.
"Effects of several drugs on relevant and irrelevant behavior components in a lever-pressing situation," by Bindra, D. PSYCHOLOGICAL REPORTS. 11(2):307-310, 1962.
"Effects of sodium pentobarbital and d-amphetamine on latency of the escape response in the rat," by Mize, Donna, and Isaac, Walter. PSYCHOLOGICAL REPORTS. 10:643-645, 1962.
"Effects of sodium pentobarbital on brain self-stimulation," by Mogenson, G.J. JOURNAL OF COMPARATIVE AND PHYSIOLOGICAL PSYCHOLOGY. 58(3):461-462, 1964.
"Effects of unilateral hypothalamic destruction upon some facets of water ingestion," by Wolff, Susan M., and Schmidt, Hans, Jr. PROCEEDINGS OF THE 74TH ANNUAL CONVENTION OF THE AMERICAN PSYCHOLOGICAL ASSOCIATION. 119-120, 1966.
"Efficiency in traffic under the influence of anesthetics, hypnotics, analgesics, and ataractics," by Kreuscher, H., and Frey, R. ARZNEIMITTEL-FORSCHUNG. 12:1056-1059, 1962.
"Electroencephalographic correlates of temporally spaced responding and avoidance behavior," by Ross, Gilbert S., et al. JOURNAL OF THE EXPERIMENTAL ANALYSIS OF BEHAVIOR. 5(4):467-472, 1962.
"Enhancement of the drinking response to phenobarbital after a previous course of barbiturates," by Schmidt, H., Jr., et al. PHYSIOLOGY AND BEHAVIOR. 2(3):265-271, 1967.
"Enzyme changes in neurons and glia during barbiturate sleep," by Hamberger, A., et al. SCIENCE. 151:1394-1395, Mar. 18, 1966.
"Evidence that the cat's electroretinogram is not influenced by impulses passing to the eye along the optic nerve,"

by Brindley, G.S., and Hamasaki, D.I. JOURNAL OF PHY-
SIOLOGY (London). 163(3):558-565, 1962.
"Experimental evaluation of some common analgesics on medical students," by Vad, B.G., et al. JOURNAL OF EXPER-
IMENTAL MEDICAL SCIENCES. 6(4):109-111, 1963.
"Experimental study of the habituation to psychosomatic
disorders and the physical dependence induced by dextro-
morphane in monkeys," by Mercier, J. THERAPIE. 21:183-
186, 1966.
"Experimental study of habituation to psychosomatic disturbances and of the physical dependency induced by d-propoxyphene (d-4-dimethylamino-1, 2-diphenyl-2-methyl-2-
propionoxybutane HCL) in the monkey," by Etzensperger,
P., and Mercier, J. THERAPIE. 18:475-493, 1963.
"Extraction of narcotic drugs, tranquilizers, and barbiturates by cation-exchange paper, and detection on a thin-
layer chromatogram by a series of reagents," by Dole,
V.P., et al. PSYCHOPHARMACOLOGY BULLETIN; National Clearinghouse for Mental Health Information. 3:45-48, 1966.
"Failure of chlorpromazine to prevent barbiturate-withdraw-
al convulsions," by Essig, C.F. CLINICAL PHARMACOLOGY
AND THERAPEUTICS. 7:466-469, 1966.
"Failure of diphenylhydantoin in preventing barbiturate withdrawal convulsions in the dog," by Essig, C.F., and Car-
ter, W.W. NEUROLOGY. 12:481-484, 1962.
"Failure rate of tranquilizers as an index of drug effect,"
by Boswell, J.I. JOURNAL OF NEW DRUGS. 3(2):96-105,
1963.
"Fear and pain: their effect on self-injection of amobarbi-
tal sodium by rats," by Davis, John D., and Miller Neal E.
SCIENCE. 141(Whole No. 3587):1286-1287, 1963.
"Focal convulsions during barbiturate abstinence in dogs
with cerebro-cortical lesions," by Essig, C.F. PSYCHO-
PHARMACOLOGIA. 3:432-437, 1962.
"Habituation to diethylpropion (tenulate)," by Caplan, J.
CANADIAN MEDICAL ASSOCIATION JOURNAL. 88:943-944, 1963.
"Human pharmacology and addiction liabilities of phenzocine
and levophenacylmorphan," by Fraser, H.F., and Isbell, H.
BULLETIN OF NARCOTICS. 12:15-23, 1960.
"The identification of barbiturates in forensic toxicology:
Considerations on the results of chemico-toxological in-
vestigations in 19 cases of fatal poisoning by 5,5 sub-
stituted barbiturates," by Marozzi, E. ZACCHIA. 26:
146-162, 1963.
"Incorporation of barbital C-14 in rats in conditions of
habituation to certain barbiturates," by Timar, M. MED-
ICINA ET PHARMACOLOGIA EXPERIMENTALS. 14:24-30, 1966.
"Induced hypersensitivity to barbital in the female rat,"
by Aston, Roy, and Hibbeln, Phyllis. SCIENCE. 157(3795):
1463-1464, 1967.
"The influence of sodium pentobarbital on vocal behavior,"
by Starkweather, John A., and Hargreaves, William A.
JOURNAL OF ABNORMAL AND SOCIAL PSYCHOLOGY. 69(1):123-
126, 1964.

"The influence of subchronic alcohol doses on barbiturate narcosis in the guinea pig," by Frahm, M., Loebkens, K., and Soehring, K. ARZNEIMITTEL-FORSCHUNG. 12:1055-1056, 1962.

"Inhibition of pentobarbital and meprobamate metabolism by some 'inducers' of drug-metabolizing enzymes," by Kato, R., et al. EXPERIENTIA. 18(10):453-454, 1962.

"Low addictiveness of two analgesics in the benzomorphan series," by Fraser, H.F., and Rosenberg, D.E. BIOCHEMICAL PHARMACOLOGY (Conference issue). 12:6, 1963 (abstract).

"The mechanism of shock following suicidal doses of barbiturates, narcotics and tranquillizer drugs, with observations on the effects of treatment," by Shubin, H., and Weil, M.H. AMERICAN JOURNAL OF MEDICINE. 38(6):853-863, 1965.

"Mediation of shock and drug-produced effects on avoidance responding," by Martin, L.K., et al. PSYCHONOMIC SCIENCE. 9(1):3-4, 1967.

"Melancholia and barbiturates: a controlled EEG, body and eye movement study of sleep," by Oswald, Ian, et al. BRITISH JOURNAL OF PSYCHIATRY. 109(Whole No. 458), 1963.

"Meprobamate and absolute auditory thresholds," by Van Houten, P., and Zenhausern, R. JOURNAL OF AUDITORY RESEARCH. 7(3):253-257, 1967.

"Meprobamate and chlorpromazine in psychotherapy: some effects on anxiety and hostility of outpatients," by Lorr, Maurice, et al. ARCHIVES OF GENERAL PSYCHIATRY. 4:381-389, 1961.

"Metabolism of barbiturates in man," by Mark, L.C. CLINICAL PHARMACOLOGY AND THERAPEUTICS. 4:504-530, 1963.

"Mild analgesics. A review of their clinical pharmacology. II. (Continued from Nov., 1965 issue)," by Beaver, W.T. AMERICAN JOURNAL OF THE MEDICAL SCIENCES. 251(5):576-599, 1966.

"Modified method for studying anorexigenic agents in dogs," by Adams, H.J., et al. JOURNAL OF PHARMACEUTICAL SCIENCES. 53:1405-1406, 1964.

"Narcotic analgesics: Possibility of broadening the structural basis of analgesics," by Wilson, A., and Pircio, A.W. NATURE. 206(4989):1151-1152, 1965.

"The nature of dissociation: Effects of transitions between normal and barbiturate-induced states on reversal learning and habituation," by Bindra, D., and Reichert, H. PSYCHOPHARMACOLOGIA. 10(4):330-344, 1967.

"Nonnarcotic addiction. Newer sedative drugs that can cause states of intoxication and dependence of barbiturate type," by Essig, C.F. JOURNAL OF THE AMERICAN MEDICAL ASSOCIATION. 196:714-717, May 23, 1966.

"On a case of confusional excitation of an amentia type with residual hallucinatory delusion [induced by a sympathomimetic appetite depressant]," by Monteverdi, T. RASSEGNA DI STUDI PSICHIATRICI. 51:527-542, 1962.

"Papillary necrosis and abuse of analgesics," by Sokeland, J.

UROLOGE. 4:23-27, 1965.
"Paranoid psychosis associated with phenmetrazine addiction," by Mendels, J. BRITISH JOURNAL OF PSYCHIATRY. 110:865, 1964.
"Pentobarbital and dextroamphetamine sulfate: effects of the sleep cycle in man," by Baekeland, F. PSYCHOPHARMACOLOGIA. 11(5):388-396, 1967.
"Perceptual-motor behavior in relation to blood phenobarbitone level: A preliminary report," by Hutt, S.J., et al. DEVELOPMENTAL MEDICINE AND CHILD NEUROLOGY. 10(5):626-632, 1968.
"Performance decrement after intake of meprobamate as a function of task difficulty and learning level," by Frankenhaeuser, Marianne, and Myrsten, Anna L. PERCEPTUAL AND MOTOR SKILLS. 27(3, Pt. 1):839-843, 1968.
"The performance of x-ray irradiated rhesus monkeys before, during and following chronic barbiturate sedation," by Davis, R.T., et al. JOURNAL OF GENETIC PSYCHOLOGY. 93: 37-51, 1958.
"Phenmetrazine [preludin and gracidin] addiction and psychosis," by Varga, G., Floro, K., and Battay, I. ORVOSI HETILAP. 104:1378-1379, 1963.
"Phenobarbital improves retention and impairs learning of shock escape in the rat," by Coppock, H.W. PSYCHOLOGICAL RECORD. 12(4):367-372, 1962.
"Physiological and clinical effects of amylobarbitone sodium therapy in patients with anxiety states," by Wing, Lorna, and Lader, M.H. JOURNAL OF NEUROLOGY, NEUROSURGERY, AND PSYCHIATRY. 28(1):78-87, 1965.
"Physio-pathological treatment of barbiturate coma," by Mollaret, P. JORNAL DO MEDICO (Porto). 50:689-703, 1963.
"Polyneurtis secondary to massive meprobamate poisoning [unpublished case] with review of the literature of the complications caused by tranquilizers," by Bui-Quoc-Huong. SEMAINE DES HOPITAUX DE PARIS. 38:3730-3734, 1962.
"Possible idiosyncrasy to belladonna, phenobarbital, or paregoric," by Cohen, G.J. PEDIATRICS. 35:148-149, 1965.
"Postnatal behavioral effects of tranquillizers administered to the gravid rat," by Werboff, J., and Havlena, J. EXPERIMENTAL NEUROLOGY. 6(3):263-269, 1962.
"Predicting the relief of anxiety with meprobamate: nondrug factors in the response of psychoneurotic patients," by Uhlenluth, E.H., et al. ARCHIVES OF GENERAL PSYCHIATRY. 19(5):619-630, 1968.
"Quantitative estimation and identification of barbiturates in blood in emergency cases," by Street, H.V. NATURE. 199:456-459, 1963.
"Rapid differentiation of barbiturates in blood serum by thin-layer chromatography," by Lehmann, J., and Karamustafaoglu, V. SCANDINAVIAN JOURNAL OF CLINICAL AND LABORATORY INVESTIGATION. 14:554-558, 1962.
"Rapid identification of analgesic drugs in urine with thin-layer chromatography," by Cochin, J., and Daly, I.W. EXPERIENTIA. 18:294, 1962.

"A rapid method for determination of barbiturate in serum or urine," by Wallenius, G., Zaar, B., and Lausing, E. SCANDINAVIAN JOURNAL OF CLINICAL AND LABORATORY INVESTIGATION. 15(Suppl. 69):252-256, 1963.

"Rapid method of screening for barbiturates," by Curry, A.S. BRITISH MEDICAL JOURNAL. 5364:1040-1041, 1963.

"Reaction thresholds to pressure in edematous hindpaws of rats and responses to analgesic drugs," by Winter, C.A., and Flataker, L. JOURNAL OF PHARMACOLOGY AND EXPERIMENTAL THERAPEUTICS. 150(1):165-171, 1965.

"Recent research on the identification of barbiturates with the eyeball-touch method," by La Torraca, F. FOLIA MEDICA (Naples). 45:1123-1126, 1962.

"Recovery from acute phenobarbital intoxication after prolonged coma," by Vandam, L.D., and Collins, W.L. JOURNAL OF THE AMERICAN MEDICAL ASSOCIATION. 184:239-241, 1963.

"Relation of EEG and seizures to phenobarbital in serum," by Buchthal, F., et al. ARCHIVES OF NEUROLOGY. 19(6): 567-572, 1968.

"Renal papillary necrosis associated with analgesic abuse," by Plass, H.F. ANNALS OF INTERNAL MEDICINE. 60:111-114, 1964.

"Report on psychoses due to chronic abuse of antiasthma agents," by May, V. WIENER KLINISCHE WOCHENSCHRIFT. 75:929-932, 1963.

"Responses of the habituated vestibulo-ocular reflex arc to drug stress," by Dowd, Patrick J. UNITED STATES AIR FORCE SCHOOL OF AVIATION MEDICINE TECHNICAL DOCUMENTARY REPORT. No. 64-72.

"Rorschach performance under Ravona dosage," by Sato, Isao, et al. TOHOKU PSYCHOLOGICA FOLIA. 21(1-2-3):1-17, 1962/ 1963.

"Selective action of pentobarbital on a multiple schedule of reinforcement," by Stretch, R., et al. NATURE. 216 (5110):92-93, 1967.

"Separation of tabletted mixtures of barbiturates, aspirin, phenacetin, caffeine, codeine, and quinine by ion-exchange paper chromatography," by Street, H.V., and Niyogi, S.K. JOURNAL OF PHARMACEUTICAL SCIENCES. 51:666-668, 1962.

"Some human pharmacological studies of three psychotropic drugs: Thiothixine, Molindone, and W-1867," by Hollister, Leo E. JOURNAL OF CLINICAL PHARMACOLOGY AND THE JOURNAL OF NEW DRUGS. 8(2):95-101, 1968.

"The spectrophotometric determination of low levels of barbiturates in blood," by Stone, H.M., et al. JOURNAL OF THE FORENSIC SCIENCE SOCIETY. 7(1):51-54, Jan., 1967.

"Standardization of scales which evaluate subjective effects of morphine, amphetamine, pentobarbital, alcohol, LSD-25, pyrahexl and chlorpromazine." PSYCHOPHARMACOLOGIA. 4(3):184-205, 1963.

"State-dependent or 'dissociated' learning produced with pentobarbital," by Overton, Donald A. JOURNAL OF COMPARATIVE AND PHYSIOLOGICAL PSYCHOLOGY. 57(1):3-12, 1964.

"The structure-activity relationship in barbiturates and its similarities to that in other narcotics," by Hansch, C., and Anderson, S.M. JOURNAL OF MEDICINAL CHEMISTRY. 10(5):745-753, 1967.

"Studies in hyperkinetic behavior: II. Laboratory and clinical evaluations of drug treatments," by Millichamp, J. Gordon, and Baldrey, Edwin C. NEUROLOGY. 17(5):467-471, 1967.

"Studies of analgesic drugs: IX. Antagonism of narcotic antagonist-induced respiratory depression," by Telford, J., and Keats, A.S. CLINICAL PHARMACOLOGY AND THERAPEUTICS. 6(1):12-16, 1965.

"Studies on an almost specific test for regenon, regenon A and preludin in the urine," by Kamm, G. BEITRAEGE ZUR GERICHTLICHEN MEDIZIN. 23:119-124, 1965.

"Studies on glucuronic acid metabolism: Effects of carbohydrates with lactone rings on the action of lethal doses of barbital sodium," by Ito, H. FOLIA PHARMACOLOGICA JAPONICA. 58:467-471, 1962.

"Studies on the human addiction liability of 2'-hydroxy-5, 9-dimethyl-2, (3,3-dimethylallyl)-6, 7-benzomorphan (Win 20, 228): A weak morphine antagonist," by Fraser, H.F., and Rosenberg, D.E. JOURNAL OF PHARMACOLOGY AND EXPERIMENTAL THERAPEUTICS. 143:149-156, 1963.

"A study of the anti-barbiturate effects of bemegride," by Orwin, A., et al. BRITISH JOURNAL OF PSYCHIATRY. 11:531-533, 1965.

"Subjective estimation of drug-induced changes in activation level," by Dureman, I., and Scholander, T. SCANDINAVIAN JOURNAL OF PSYCHOLOGY. 1:36-40, 1960.

"Synergism of alcohol and sedatives," by Eerola, R., and Alha, A. DEUTSCHE ZEITSCHRIFT FUER DIE GESAMTE GERICHTLICHE MEDIZIN. 53:201-210, 1963.

"Therapy of barbiturate poisoning with massive doses of B-B-methyl-ethyl-glutarimide [Eukraton]," by Stanler, O., and Gletz, E. MUENCHENER MEDIZINISCHE WOCHENSCHRIFT. 105:1309-1311, 1963

"Time and dosage effects of meprobamate on simple behavioral tasks," by Uhr, Leonard. JOURNAL OF GENERAL PSYCHOLOGY. 68(2):317-323, 1963.

"Time estimation, knowledge of results and drug effects," by Rutschmann, J., and Rubinstein, L. JOURNAL OF PSYCHIATRIC RESEARCH. 4(2):107-114, 1966.

"The toxicity of some of the newer narcotic analgesics," by Lister, R.E. JOURNAL OF PHARMACY AND PHARMACOLOGY. 18(6):374-383, 1966.

"Tranquillizers, barbiturates, and the brain," by Himwich, H.E. JOURNAL OF NEUROPSYCHIATRY. 3:279-294, 1962.

"Treatment of barbiturate poisoning based on 271 cases," by Montani, S., and Perret, C. SCHWEIZERISCHE MEDIZINISCHE WOCHENSCHRIFT. 93:692-695, 1963.

"Treatment of barbiturate poisoning. The use of peritoneal dialysis," by Whiting, E.G., Jr., et al. CALIFORNIA MEDICINE. 102:367-369, 1965.

"Treatment of severe barbiturate poisoning," by Yatzidis,H., et al. LANCET. 2:216-217, 1965.
"Urea-induced, osmotic diuresis and alkalization of urine in acute barbiturate intoxication," by Myschetsky, A., and Lassen, N.A. JOURNAL OF THE AMERICAN MEDICAL ASSOC-IATION. 185:936-942, 1963.
"Use of a demographic index score as a control measure in psychiatric drug research," by Hanlon, T.E. PSYCHOLOGI-CAL REPORTS. 10(2):465-466, 1962.
"The use of a discriminant function in the assessment of analgesic drugs,: by Hill, G.B., et al. CLINICAL PHARM-ACOLOGY AND THERAPEUTICS. 8(4):532-547, 1967.
"Use of a reagent containing thiobarbituric acid for the de-tection of ketoses on chromatograms," by Percheron, F. BULLETIN DE LA SOCIETE DE CHIMIE BIOLOGIQUE. 44:1161-1165, 1962.
"The use of chlordiazepoxide (librium) in the barbiturate abstinence syndrome," by Remington, F.B. AMERICAN JOUR-NAL OF PSYCHIATRY. 120:402-403, 1963.
"The use of ethamivan in the treatment of barbiturate poi-soning," by Wheeldon, P.J., and Perry, A.W. CANADIAN MEDICAL ASSOCIATION JOURNAL. 89:20-22, 1963.
"Use of the Soviet preparation bemegride in barbiturate poi-soning," by Raevskaia, V.V. TERAPENTICHESKII ARKHIV. 36:105-108, 1964.
"The use of thin-layer chromatography for the analysis of drugs. Isolation and identification of barbiturates and non-barbiturate hypnotics from urine, blood and tissues," by Cochin, J., and Daly, J.W. JOURNAL OF PHARMACOLOGY AND EXPERIMENTAL THERAPEUTICS. 139:154-159, 1963.
"Use of tranquilizers in the treatment of stuttering; reser-pine, chlorpromazine, meprobamate, atarax," by Kent, L.R. JOURNAL OF SPEECH AND HEARING DISORDERS. 28:288-294, Aug., 1963.
"Value of forced diuresis in acute barbiturate poisoning," by Mawer, G.E., and Lee, H.A. BRITISH MEDICAL JOURNAL. 2(5608):790-793, 1968.
"Variations in survival time after whole-body radiation at 2 times of day," by Pizzarello, Donald J., et al. SCIENCE. 139(Whole no. 3552), 1963.
"Workshop on the detection and control of abuse of narcotics, barbiturates, and amphetamines: San Juan, Puerto Rico, December 13-15, 1965," by Leonard, Frederick. PSYCHO-PHARMACOLOGY BULLETIN. 3(4):21-26, 1966.

LYSERGIC ACID DIETHYLAMIDE: Books and Essays

Abood, L. "The biochemistry of psychoactive drugs," BACK-GROUND PAPERS ON STUDENT DRUG INVOLVEMENT, ed. Hollander, C. Washington: United States National Student Associa-tion, 1967, p. 151-158.

Abrams S. INFINITY ON TRIAL: a psychological study of LSD, cannabis, and other psychedelic agents. London, 1967.

Alexander, Marsha. SEXUAL PARADISE OF LSD. North Hollywood, California: Brandon House, 1969.

Alpert, R., and Cohen, S. LSD. New York: New American Library, 1966.

Andrews, George, and Vinkenoog, S. THE BOOK OF GRASS; an anthology on Indian hemp. New York: Grove Press, 1967.

Barron, F. "The effects of consciousness-altering drugs on creativity" [Paper read at 1962 Utah Conference on Creativity], WIDENING HORIZONS IN CREATIVITY, ed. Calvin W. Taylor. New York: Wiley, 1964.

Bestic, Alan. TURN ME ON, MAN. New York: Award Books, 1968.

Bischoff, William H. THE ECSTASY DRUGS. Delray Beach, Florida: University Circle Press, 1966.

Bishop, Malden G. THE DISCOVERY OF LOVE; a psychedelic experience with LSD-25. New York: Dodd, Mead and Company, 1963.

Blum, Richard. UTOPIATES; the use and users of LSD-25. New York: Atherton Press, 1965.

Blum, Richard H. "A history of hallucinogens," SOCIETY AND DRUGS. San Francisco: Jossey-Bass, 1969, pp. 117-133.

Blum, Richard, and Funkhouser-Balbaky, M. "Mind-altering drugs and dangerous behavior: dangerous drugs," NARCOTICS AND DRUG ABUSE. U.S. President's Commission on Law Enforcement and Administration of Justice: Task Force Report. Washington: Government Printing Office, 1967.

Blum, Richard, et al. "The natural history of LSD use," UTOPIATES, by R. Blum et al. New York: Atherton Press, 1964, pp. 90-117.

Braden, William. THE PRIVATE SEA: LSD and the search for God. Chicago: Quadrangle Books, 1967.

Burn, H. "Drugs producing hallucinations," DRUGS, MEDICINES AND MAN, by H. Burn. New York: Scribner's Sons, 1962, pp. 219-224.

Burroughs, William. "Points of distinction between sedative and consciousness-expanding drugs," LSD: THE CONSCIOUSNESS-EXPANDING DRUG, ed. D. Solomon. New York: Berkely Medallion, 1966, pp. 170-174.

Burroughs, William, and Ginsberg, A. THE YAGE LETTERS. San Francisco: City Lights Books, 1963.

Caldwell, William Vernon. LSD PSYCHOTHERAPY; an exploration of psychedelic and psycholytic therapy. New York: Grove Press, 1968.

Cashman, John. THE LSD STORY. Greenwich, Connecticut: Fawcett Publications, 1966

Castaneda, Carlos. THE TEACHING OF DON JUAN: a Yaqui way of knowledge. New York: Ballantine Books, 1969.

Charbonneau, Louis. PSYCHEDELIC-40. New York: Bantam Books, 1965.

Clark, W.H. "Psychotomimetic (hallucinogenic) drugs," LECTURES IN PSYCHOPHARMACOLOGY, ed. W. Clark, and K. Ditman. Sepulveda: Veterans Administration Hospital, 1964, 19p. [Each article begins with page 1].

40

Clark, W.H. "Theoretical issues raised by the psychological effects of the psychedelic drugs," [chapter in] RELIGION PONDERS SCIENCE, ed. Edwin P. Booth. New York: Appleton, 1964.

Cohen, A.S., and Schiller, L. LSD. New York: New American Library, 1966.

Cohen, Sidney. THE BEYOND WITHIN; the LSD story. New York; Atheneum, 1964.

Cohen, Sidney. DRUGS OF HALLUCINATION; the uses and misuses of lysergic acid diethylamide. London: Seker and Warburg, 1965.

Cohen, Sidney. "A quarter century of research with LSD," THE PROBLEMS AND PROSPECTS OF LSD, ed. J. Ungerleider. Springfield, Illinois: C.C. Thomas, 1968, pp. 22-44.

Conference on d-Lysergic Acid Diethylamide (LSD-25), Princeton, New Jersey, 1959. THE USE OF LSD IN PSYCHOTHERAPY; TRANSACTIONS, ed. Harold A. Abramson. New York: Josiah Macy, Jr. Foundation, 1960.

Conference on Parapsychology and psychedelics, New York, 1958. PROCEEDINGS OF TWO CONFERENCES ON PARAPSYCHOLOGY AND PHARMACOLOGY. New York: Parapsychology Foundation, 1961.

Crocket, Richard, et al. HALLUCINOGENIC DRUGS AND THEIR PSYCHOTHERAPEUTIC USE: Proceedings of the Quarterly Meeting of the Royal Medico-Psychological Association of London, Feb., 1961. Springfield, Illinois: C.C.Thomas, 1963.

Downing, D. "Psychotomimetic compounds," [chapter 13 in] PSYCHOPHARMACOLOGICAL AGENTS, V.1, ed. M. Gordon. New York: Academic Press, 1964, pp. 555-618.

Downing, Joseph J. ON THE MIND-ALTERING FUNCTION OF LSD-25. San Mateo County Mental Health Service, 1964.

Du Maurier, Daphne. THE HOUSE ON THE STRAND. Garden City, New York: Doubleday, 1969. [Fiction].

Dunlap, Jane. EXPLORING INNER SPACE: personal experiences under LSD-25. New York: Harcourt, Brace and World, 1961.

Ebin, David, ed. THE DRUG EXPERIENCE; first-person accounts of addicts, writers, scientists and others. New York: Orion Press, 1961.

Fort, J. "LSD and the mind-altering drug (m.a.d.) world," THE PROBLEMS AND PROSPECTS OF LSD, ed. J. Ungerleider. Springfield, Illinois: C.C.Thomas, 1968, pp. 3-21.

Geller, Allen, and Boas, Maxwell. DRUG BEAT; a complete survey of the history, distribution, uses and abuses of marijuana, LSD, and amphetamines. New York: Cowles Book Company, 1969.

Goldstein, Richard. ONE IN SEVEN: Drugs on campus. New York: Walker and Company, 1966.

Gustaitis, Rasa. TURNING ON. New York: Macmillan, 1969.

Harms, E., ed. DRUG ADDICTION IN YOUTH. New York: Pergamon Press, 1965.

The correspondents of TIME. THE HIPPIES, ed. Joe David Brown. New York: Time, Inc., 1967.

Hoffer, Abram, and Osmond, H. THE HALLUCINOGENS. New York: Academic Press, 1967.

41

Hopkins, Jerry. "Drugs: take tea and see; take LSD and be,"
THE HIPPIE PAPERS. New York: Signet, 1968, pp. 55-74.
Hyde, Margaret O., ed. MIND DRUGS. New York: McGraw-Hill,
1968.
International Conference on the Use of LSD in Psychotherapy
and Alcoholism, 2d, Amityville, New York, 1965. THE USE
OF LSD IN PSYCHOTHERAPY AND ALCOHOLISM, ed. Harold A.
Abramson, intro. Frank Fremont-Smith. Indianapolis:
Bobbs-Merrill, 1967.
Jacobsen, E. "The hallucinogens," PSYCHOPHARMACOLOGY: di-
mensions and perspectives, ed. C. Joyce. London: Tav-
istock, 1968, pp. 175-213.
Kluver, Heinrich. MESCAL THE DIVINE PLANT AND THE MECHAN-
ISM OF HALLUCINOGENS. Chicago: University of Chicago
Press, 1967.
Koella, W.P., and Bergen, J.R. CYCLIC RESPONSE TO REPEAT-
ED LSD ADMINISTRATION. Presented at the annual meeting
of the American College of Psychopharmacology, San Juan,
Puerto Rico, Jan., 1967.
Land, Herman W. WHAT YOU CAN DO ABOUT DRUGS AND YOUR CHILD.
New York: Hart Publications, 1969.
Laurie, Peter. DRUGS. Baltimore: Penguin Books, 1967.
Leary, Timothy. "American education as a narcotic addiction
and its cure," PSYCHEDELIC THEORY, by T. Leary. Mill-
brook, New York: Castalia Foundation, 1965. [Paper read
at Symposium of American Values, Eastern Washington
State College, 1963].
--"Art Kleps, mad Luther of psychedelia," EAST VILLAGE
OTHER, July, 1967. Reprinted in EX-STATIC ESSAYS, by
T. Leary. New York: Putnam, 1968.
--"The diagnosis of behavior and the diagnosis of exper-
ience," NEW APPROACHES TO PSYCHODIAGNOSTIC SYSTEMS, ed.
A. Mahrer. New York: Holt, 1968.
-- "The effects of test score feedback on creative per-
formance and of drugs on creative experience," WIDENING
HORIZONS IN CREATIVITY, ed. Calvin W. Taylor. New York:
Wiley, 1964. [Paper read at 1962 Utah Conference on
creativity].
--EX-STATIC ESSAYS. New York: Putnam, 1968.
--HIGH PRIEST. New York: World Publishing Company, 1968.
--"How to change behavior," PROCEEDINGS OF CONGRESS.
Copenhagen: Munksgaard Press, 1962. [Address presented
at 14th Congress of Applied Psychology, Copenhagen, 1962].
--HOW TO START YOUR OWN RELIGION. Millbrook, New York:
Kriya Press, 1967.
--"Interview," PLAYBOY INTERVIEWS. Chicago: Playboy Press,
1967, pp. 124-161.
--INTRODUCTION TO LSD - THE CONSCIOUSNESS EXPANDING DRUG,
ed. D. Solomon. New York: Putnam, 1964.
--THE POLITICS OF ECSTACY. New York: Putnam, 1968.
--PSYCHEDELIC PRAYERS AFTER THE TAO TE CHING. New Hyde
Park, New York: University Books, 1966
--"The religious experience: its interpretation and pro-
duction," PSYCHEDELIC REVIEW, no. 3. New York, 1965,

also THE PSYCHEDELIC READER, ed. G. Weil. New Hyde Park, New York: University Books, 1965. [Paper presented at the 1963 meeting of Lutheran psychologists and printed by the Lutheran Board of Higher Education].
--"The tribal family," WAYS OF GROWTH, ed. H. Otto and J. Mann. New York: Grossman, 1968.
Leary, Timothy, et al. THE PSYCHEDELIC EXPERIENCE. New Hyde Park, New York: University Books, 1965.
--THE PSYCHEDELIC MOMENT. Millbrook, New York: Castalia Foundation, 1965.
--PSYCHEDELIC THEORY. Millbrook, New York: Castalia Foundation, 1965.
Ling, Thomas M., and Buckman, J. LYSERGIC ACID (LSD-25) AND RITALIN IN THE TREATMENT OF NEUROSIS. London: The Lambarde Press, 1963.
McGlothlin, W. "Social and para-medical aspects of hallucinogenic drugs," THE USE OF LSD IN PSYCHOTHERAPY AND ALCOHOLISM, ed. H. Abramson. Indianapolis: Bobbs-Merrill, 1967, pp. 3-38.
-- "Toward a rational view of hallucinogenic drugs," BACKGROUND PAPERS ON STUDENT DRUG INVOLVEMENT, ed. C. Hollander. Washington: United States National Student Association, 1967, pp. 109-120.
McGlothlin, W., et al. "Discussion of McGlothlin's 'Social and para-medical aspects of hallucinogenic drugs'," THE USE OF LSD IN PSYCHOTHERAPY AND ALCOHOLISM , ed. H. Abramson. Indianapolis: Bobbs-Merrill, 1967, pp. 3-38.
Masters, Robert E.L., and Houston, J. PSYCHEDELIC ART. New York: Grove Press, 1968.
--THE VARIETIES OF PSYCHEDELIC EXPERIENCE. New York: Holt, Rinehart and Winston, 1966.
Metzner, R. THE ECSTATIC MOMENT. New York: Macmillan, 1968.
Michaux, Henry. LIGHT THROUGH DARKNESS. New York: Orion Press, 1963.
--MISERABLE MIRACLE (MESCALINE). Lowestoft, Suffolk: Scorpion Press, 1964.
Newland, Constance A. (pseud.). MY SELF AND I. New York: Coward-McCann, 1962.
Nowlis, Helen H. DRUGS ON THE COLLEGE CAMPUS. Garden City, New York: Doubleday, 1968.
Ostow, M. DRUGS IN PSYCHOANALYSIS AND PSYCHOTHERAPY. New York: Basic Books, 1962.
Perry, S.E. HUMAN NATURE OF SCIENCE; researchers at work in psychiatry. New York: Free Press, 1966.
Pollard, J.C., et al. DRUGS AND PHANTASY. The effects of LSD, psilocybin and sernyl on college students. Boston: Little, Brown and Company, 1967.
Princeton University. Student Committee on Mental Health. PSYCHEDELICS AND THE COLLEGE STUDENT. Princeton, New Jersey: Princeton University Press, 1967.

Roseman, Bernard. LSD: THE AGE OF MIND. Hollywood, California: Wilshire Book Company, 1967.
Smart, Reginald D., et al. LYSERGIC ACID DIETHYLAMIDE IN THE TREATMENT OF ALCOHOLISM. Toronto: University of Toronto Press, 1967.
Solomon, David, ed. LSD: THE CONSCIOUSNESS-EXPANDING DRUG. Intro. Timothy Leary. New York: Putnam, c1964.
Stafford, P.G., and Golightly, B.H. LSD: THE PROBLEM-SOLVING PSYCHEDELIC. New York: Award Books, 1967.
Ungerleider, J. Thomas, ed. THE PROBLEMS AND PROSPECTS OF LSD. Springfield, Illinois: C.C. Thomas, 1968.
U.S. Dept. of Health, Education and Welfare. LSD, SOME QUESTIONS AND ANSWERS. (Public Health Service publication no. 1828). Washington: U.S. Superintendent of Documents, Government Printing Office, 1969.
U.S. Senate. Committee on the Judiciary. JUVENILE DELINQUENCY: hearings pursuant to S. res. 240, pt. 19, March 4-6, 1968, LSD and marijuana among young people. 90th Congress, 2d session. Washington: U.S. Superintendent of Documents, Government Printing Office, 1968.
U.S. Senate. Judiciary Committee, 89th Congress. HEARINGS ON LSD AND MARIJUANA USE ON COLLEGE CAMPUSES. Washington: U.S. Superintendent of Documents, Government Printing Office, 1966.
Watts, Alan. THE JOYOUS COSMOLOGY. New York: Pantheon, 1962.
Weil, G.M., et al. THE PSYCHEDELIC READER. New Hyde Park, New York: University Books, 1965.
Williams, J.B. NARCOTICS AND HALLUCINOGENICS: a handbook. Revised Edition. New York: Glencoe Press, 1967.
Yablonsky, Lewis. THE HIPPIE TRIP. New York: Pegasus, 1968.
Yolles, Stanley F. RECENT RESEARCH ON LSD, MARIJUANA, AND OTHER DANGEROUS DRUGS. Statement before the Subcommittee on Juvenile Delinquency of the Committee on the Judiciary, U.S. Senate, March 6, 1968. Washington: Department of Health, Education and Welfare, 1968.

LYSERGIC ACID DIETHYLAMIDE: Doctoral Dissertations

Fadiman, James R. "Behavior change following psychedelic (LSD) therapy" (Thesis, unpublished, Stanford University). DISSERTATION ABSTRACTS. 26(11): 6843-6844, 1966.
Fiddleman, Paul Barry. "The prediction of behavior under lysergic acid diethylamide (LSD)" (Thesis, unpublished, University of North Carolina). DISSERTATION ABSTRACTS. 22(8):2873-2874, 1962.
LaRosa, Richard T. "A study of the pharmacological effects of substituted tryptamines and LSD and the investigation of the mechanism of action of these agents" (Thesis, unpublished, State University of New York at Buffalo).

44

DISSERTATION ABSTRACTS. 29(2-B):707, 1968.
Pahnke, W.N. "Drugs and mysticism: an analysis of the re-
lationship between psychedelic drugs and the mystical
consciousness" (Thesis, unpublished, Harvard University,
1963).
Peterson, E.A. "The effect of four psychotropic drugs on
sensitivity to electrically induced pain." DISSERTATION
ABSTRACTS. 23(8):2994-2995, 1963.
Schulman, Robert Emery. "Hypnosis and verbal learning"
(Thesis, unpublished, University of Illinois). DISSER-
TATION ABSTRACTS. 23(2):710-711, 1962.
Sjoberg, Bernard M., Jr. "The effects of lysergic acid diethylamide (LSD-25), mascaline, psilocybin and a combin-
ation of three drugs on primary suggestibility" (Thesis,
unpublished, Stanford University). DISSERTATION AB-
STRACTS. 26(8):4817-4818, 1966.

LYSERGIC ACID DIETHYLAMIDE: Periodical Literature

General Publications

"Abuse of barbiturates, stimulants, LSD, as great a danger
as illegal narcotics," by Braude A. AMERICAN ASSOCIA-
TION OF INDUSTRIAL NURSES JOURNAL. 15:40-41, Jan., 1967.
"Abuse of psychotomimetics," by Jorgensen, F. ACTA PSYCHI-
ATRICA SCANDINAVICA. suppl. 203: 205-216, 1968.
"Accidents and abuse of psychotropic drugs." BULLETIN ON
NARCOTICS. 21(1):40, Jan.-Mar., 1969.
"Addiction and the campus," by Lippincott, W.T. JOURNAL OF
CHEMICAL EDUCATION. 45:687, Nov., 1968.
"Adverse reactions from the use of lysergide in the United
Kingdom." BULLETIN ON NARCOTICS. 20(4):1, Oct.-Dec.,
1968.
"An analysis of the problems presented in the use of LSD,"
by Taylor, Graham C. BULLETIN ON NARCOTICS. 19(1):7-13,
Jan.-Mar., 1967.
"Another LSD hallucination; N. Yoder's fabricated story."
TIME. 91:66, Jan. 26, 1968.
"Another Session," by Leary, T. ORACLE. 1(10), Oct., 1967.
"Artificial paradises; Baudelaire and the psychedelic exper-
ience," by Baudelaire, C.P., tr. by Osborn, C.B. AMER-
ICAN SCHOLAR. 36:660-668, Aut., 1967.
"Aspirin, liquor and LSD," by Downs, H. SCIENCE DIGEST.
61:91-93, Jan., 1967.
"Assessment of LSD," by Davidoff, I.G. NEW ENGLAND JOURNAL
OF MEDICINE. 278:1022, May 2, 1968.
"Assessment of LSD," by Lane, J.M. NEW ENGLAND JOURNAL OF
MEDICINE. 278:1022, May 2, 1968.
"Assessment of LSD," by Miller, J.R. NEW ENGLAND JOURNAL
OF MEDICINE. 278:1022-1023, May 2, 1968.

"Ayahuasca drinkers among the Chama Indians of Northeast
Peru," by Kusel, Heinz. PSYCHEDELIC REVIEW. no. 6:
58-67, 1965.
"Basic aspects of psychotropic drug action," by Pletscher,
A. AMERICAN JOURNAL OF MENTAL DEFICIENCY. 67:238-244,
Sept., 1962.
"Before your kid tries drugs," by Yolles, S.F. NEW YORK
TIMES MAGAZINE. Nov. 17, 1968, p. 124 passim.
"Belladonna poisoning as a facet of psychedelia," by Cum-
mins, B.M., et al. JOURNAL OF THE AMERICAN MEDICAL
ASSOCIATION. 204:1011, June 10, 1968.
"Beyond LSD." TIME. 89:84-85, Feb. 10, 1967.
"Beyond the pleasure principle" [review article], by Coles,
R. PARTISAN REVIEW. 34:415-420, Summer, 1967.
"Big lies about mind-affecting drugs," by Larner, J. VOGUE.
151:88-89, Apr. 15, 1968.
"Bootlegged ecstasy," by Grinker, R.R. JOURNAL OF THE AMER-
ICAN MEDICAL ASSOCIATION. 187:768, 1964.
"The Buddha as drop out," by Leary, T. HORIZON. Spring,
1968.
"Campus drug craze: its dangers." U.S. NEWS AND WORLD RE-
PORT. 60:16-17, Apr. 18, 1966.
"Can this drug enlarge man's mind," by Heard, Gerald. PSY-
CHEDELIC REVIEW. 1:7-17, June, 1963.
"Case of the hypnotic hippie." NEWSWEEK. 74(24):30-37,
Dec. 15, 1969.
"Celebrating with Dr. Leary," by Trilling, D. ENCOUNTER.
28:36-46, June, 1967.
"A change program for adult offenders using psilocybin,"
by Leary, T., Metzner, R., Presnell, M., Weil, G.,
Schwitzgebel, R., and Kinne, S. PSYCHOTHERAPY. July,
1965.
"Chemical Mind Changers," by Coughlan, R. LIFE. 54:81-82+,
Mar. 15, 1963.
"Chemical salvation," AMERICA. 115:403, Oct. 8, 1966.
"Chronic LSD effect." BULLETIN ON NARCOTICS. 20(3):24,
July-Sept., 1968.
"Chronic users of LSD: The 'acidheads'," by Blacker, K.H.,
et al. AMERICAN JOURNAL OF PSYCHIATRY. 125(3):341-351,
1968.
"The circuits of the senses," by Campbell, R. LIFE. 54
(27):64-76, 1963.
"Clarifying the confusion regarding LSD-25," by Savage, C.,
and Stolaroff, M.J. JOURNAL OF NERVOUS AND MENTAL DIS-
EASES. 140(3):218-221, 1965.
"A classification of LSD complications," by Cohen, S. PSY-
CHOSOMATICS. 7:182-186, 1966.
"The clinical management of adverse effects of hallucino-
genic drugs," by Burgess, W.W. JOURNAL OF THE AMERICAN
COLLEGE HEALTH ASSOCIATION. 16:23-24, Oct., 1967.
"Congress: a new option for addicts; a look at LSD," by
Walsh, J. SCIENCE. 152:1728-1729, June 24, 1966.
"Cool talk about hot drugs; misconceptions about heroin,
LSD, and marijuana," by Louria, D.B. NEW YORK TIMES

MAGAZINE. pp. 12-13 passim, Aug. 6, 1967; also READER'S DIGEST. 91:111-117, Nov., 1967.
"A correctional dilemma: the narcotic addict," by Nahrendorf, R.O. SOCIOLOGY AND SOCIAL RESEARCH. 53:21-33, Oct., 1968.
"Correspondence: acid," by Sazbe, B. NEW REPUBLIC. 154: 35, May 7, 1966.
"Current concepts: Lysergic Acid Diethylamide," by Louria, D.B. NEW ENGLAND JOURNAL OF MEDICINE. 278:435, Feb. 22, 1968.
"Current status and future trends in psychedelic (LSD) research," by Mogar, Robert E. JOURNAL OF HUMANISTIC PSYCHOLOGY. 5(2):147-166, 1965.
"Current status of psychedelic research," by Savage, Charles. AMERICAN JOURNAL OF ORTHOPSYCHIATRY. 37(2):211-212, 1967.
"The cyclic psychedelics," by Cohen, Sidney. AMERICAN JOURNAL OF PSYCHIATRY. 125(3):393-394, Sept., 1968.
"Danger of LSD; Kessler case." TIME. 87:52, Apr. 22, 1966.
"Dangerous LSD?" SCIENTIFIC AMERICAN. 214:54, Feb., 1966.
"The dangerous magic of LSD," by Kobler, J. SATURDAY EVENING POST. 236(38): Nov. 2, 1963.
"Dangers of drug abuse," by Clark, M. PTA MAGAZINE. 62: 8-11, May, 1968.
"Dangers of LSD," by Glatt, M.M. LANCET. 2:1203, Dec. 2, 1967.
"The dangers of LSD," by Ungerleider, J.T., et al. JOURNAL OF THE AMERICAN MEDICAL ASSOCIATION. 197:389-392, Aug. 8, 1966.
"Dangers of the drug called LSD," by Sauer, L.W. PTA MAGAZINE. 61:31-32, Sept., 1966.
"Daru and Bhang: cultural factors in the choice of intoxicant," by Carstairs, G.M. PSYCHEDELIC REVIEW. no. 6: 67-83, 1965.
"De-automatization and the mystic experience," by Deikman, Arthur J. PSYCHIATRY. 29(4):324-338, 1966.
"Dependence on LSD and other hallucinogenic drugs." JOURNAL OF THE AMERICAN MEDICAL ASSOCIATION. 202:141-144, Oct. 2, 1967.
"Diethyltryptamine, a do-it-yourself hallucinogenic drug" (Letter to the Editor), by Rubin, D.R. JOURNAL OF THE AMERICAN MEDICAL ASSOCIATION. 201(2):143, 1967.
"Doctor Leary and Dr. Pusey." AMERICA. 115:440, Oct. 15, 1966.
"Donna and the sugar cube; increasing use of LSD." NEWSWEEK. 67:100, Apr. 18, 1966.
"Don't dodge the drug questions; hallucinogens," by Hawkins, M.E. SCIENCE TEACHER. 33:33, Nov., 1966.
"Does LSD really cause psychosis?" TRANSACTION. 5:6-7, Mar., 1968.
"Dosage levels of psychedelic compounds for psychotherapeutic experiences," by Fisher, G. PSYCHEDELIC REVIEW. no. 1, 1963.
"Do drugs have religious import?" by Smith, H. JOURNAL OF PHILOSOPHY. 61:517-530, Oct. 1, 1964.

47

"Drug abuse and the young," by Ledger, L. THE TEXAS OUT-
LOOK. 51:33-35, Dec., 1967.
"Drug abuse in the eyes of the law," by Ledger, L. THE
TEXAS OUTLOOK. 51:37-39, Nov., 1967.
"Drug dangers, the case gets stronger," by Snider, A.J.
SCIENCE DIGEST. 64:62-63, July, 1968.
"Drug movement," by Cooper, D. NEW STATESMAN. 71:305-306,
Mar. 4, 1966.
"Drug notes," by McClure, M. EVERGREEN REVIEW. 6:103-117,
July/Aug., 1962.
"The drug problem among young people: use of both LSD and
marijuana entails significant risk," by Farnsworth, D.
RHODE ISLAND MEDICAL JOURNAL. 51:179-182, 1968.
"Drug use on high school and college campuses," by Cwalina,
G.E. JOURNAL OF SCHOOL HEALTH. 38:638-646, Dec., 1968.
"Drugs; a student report," by Lake, A. SEVENTEEN. Sept.,
1966, p. 170.
"Drugs and mysticism," by Pahnke, Walter N. INTERNATIONAL
JOURNAL OF PARAPSYCHOLOGY. 8(2):295-314, 1966.
"Drugs on the campus," by Goldstein, R. SATURDAY EVENING
POST. 239:40-44 passim, May 21, 1966; 239:34-38 passim,
June 4, 1966.
"Drugs on campus: turned on and tuned out," by Freedman,
M.B., and Powelson, H. NATION. 202:125-127, Jan. 31,
1966.
"Dynamics of psychedelic drug abuse: a clinical study," by
Bowers, Malcolm, et al. ARCHIVES OF GENERAL PSYCHIATRY.
16(5):560-566, 1967.
"Early experience and LSD-25," by Caputo, Daniel V. JOURN-
AL OF GENETIC PSYCHOLOGY. 104(2):311-320, 1964.
"The ecstatic drop out," by Leary, T. SOL MAGAZINE, 1967.
"Effects of LSD." BRITISH MEDICAL JOURNAL. 5502:1495-
1496, June 18, 1966.
"The effects of love in prisoner rehabilitation," by Leary,
T., and Metzner, R. PSYCHEDELIC REVIEW. no. 11, 1967.
"The effects of psilocybin in a supportive environment,"
by Leary, T., Litwin, G., and Metzner, R. JOURNAL OF
NERVOUS AND MENTAL DISEASES. 137(6), 1963.
"The effects of psychotomimetic drugs on primary suggest-
ibility," by Sjoberg, B.M., Jr., and Hollister, L.E.
PSYCHOPHARMACOLOGIA. 8:251-262, Apr., 1965.
"Effects of STP." BULLETIN ON NARCOTICS. 20(4):7, Oct.-
Dec., 1968.
"The end of the trip," by Brackman, Jacob. ESQUIRE. Sept.,
1966
"Epidemic of acid heads; post-LSD symptoms after non-med-
ical use." TIME. 87:44 passim, Mar. 11, 1966.
"Expectation, mood and psilocybin," by Metzner, R., Litwin,
G., and Weil, G. PSYCHEDELIC REVIEW. no. 5, 1964.
"The experiential typewriter," by Leary, T. PSYCHEDELIC
REVIEW. no. 7, 1965.
"The exploding threat of the mind drug that got out of con-
trol, LSD." LIFE. Mar. 25, 1966, pp. 27-33.
"Fixed," by Hornick, N. 20TH CENTURY. 175(1033):16-18,
1967.

"Flight from violence: hippies and the green rebellion,"
by Allen, J.R., et al. AMERICAN JOURNAL OF PSYCHIATRY.
125(3):364-370, Sept., 1968.

"Four psilocybin experiences," by Swain, Frederick, et al.
PSYCHEDELIC REVIEW. no. 1:219-243, Fall, 1963.

"Four ways to go: the end of the trip," by Brackman, J.
ESQUIRE. 66:126 passim, Sept., 1966.

"Frequency of hallucinogenic drug use and its implications."
BULLETIN ON NARCOTICS. 20(4):2, Oct.-Dec., 1968.

"Frequency of hallucinogenic drug use and its implications,"
by Fisher, D.D. JOURNAL OF THE AMERICAN COLLEGE HEALTH
ASSOCIATION. 16:20-22, Oct., 1967.

"From opium to LSD," by Granier Doyeux, M. UNESCO COURIER.
21:12, May, 1968.

"A fundamental experiment," by Daumal, René. PSYCHEDELIC
REVIEW. no. 5:40-47, 1965.

"The god in the flowerpot," by Barnard, Mary. PSYCHEDELIC
REVIEW. no. 1:244-251, Fall, 1963.

"God's secret agent AUS$_3$," by Leary, T. ESQUIRE. Mar.,
1968.

"Grand mal seizures after LSD ingestion," by Fisher, D.,
and Ungerleider, J.T. CALIFORNIA MEDICINE. 106:210-
211, 1967.

"The great banana hoax," by Bozzetti, Louis, Jr., et al.
AMERICAN JOURNAL OF PSYCHIATRY. 124(5):678-679, 1967.

"The great prison break-out," by Leary, T., and Metzner, R.
PSYCHEDELIC REVIEW. no. 10, 1967.

"Growing peril: teenage use of drugs for kicks." GOOD HOUSE-
KEEPING. 162:168, May, 1966.

"Growth of a mystique," ed. J. Mitchell. NEWSWEEK. 67:60-
61, May 9, 1966.

"Hallucinogenic agents," by Farnswort, D.L. JOURNAL OF THE
AMERICAN MEDICAL ASSOCIATION. 185, 1963.

"Hallucinogenic drug abuse," by Solursh, L.P., and Clement,
W.R. CANADIAN MEDICAL ASSOCIATION JOURNAL. 98:407, 1968.

"Hallucinogenic drug abuse: manifestations and management,"
by Solursh, Lionel P., and Clement, Wilfred R. CANADIAN
MEDICAL ASSOCIATION JOURNAL. 98(8):407-410, 1968.

"The hallucinogenic drug cult," by Gordon, N. THE REPORTER.
29(3):35-43, 1963.

"The hallucinogenic drugs," by Barron, F., et al. SCIENTIF-
IC AMERICAN. 210:29-37, Apr., 1964.

"Hallucinogenic drugs: a perspective with special reference
to peyote and cannabis," by McGlothin, W.H. PSYCHEDELIC
REVIEW. no. 6:16-59, 1965.

"Hallucinogenic drugs: collision of values," by Jones, William H. YALE ALUMNI MAGAZINE. Nov., 1967, pp. 18-25.

"The hallucinogenic drugs: curse or blessing?" by Szara,
Stephen. AMERICAN JOURNAL OF PSYCHIATRY. 123(12):1513-
1518, 1967.

"Hallucinogenic drugs: influence of mental set and setting,"
by Faiblace, L.A., and Szara, S. DISEASES OF THE NER-
VOUS SYSTEM. 29(2):124-126, 1968.

"The hallucinogenic drugs: their use and abuse." MEDICAL
JOURNAL OF AUSTRALIA. 1:146-147, Jan. 27, 1968.

"The hallucinogenic drugs: their use and abuse," by Whitaker, L.H. MEDICAL JOURNAL OF AUSTRALIA. 1:370-371, Mar. 2, 1968.

"The hallucinogenic fungi of Mexico: an inquiry into the origins of the religious idea among primitive people," by Wasson, R. Gordon. PSYCHEDELIC REVIEW. no. 1:27-42, June, 1963.

"Hallucinogenic plants," by Farnsworth, N. SCIENCE. 162 (3858):1086-1092, 1968.

"Hallucinogenic plants: the morning glories," by Farnsworth, N.R. TILE AND TILL. 52(3):38-40, Sept., 1966.

"Hallucinogens," by Harrington, A. PLAYBOY. 10(11), Nov., 1963.

"Hallucinogens," by Sandison, R.A. PRACTITIONER. 192:30-36, 1964.

"Hallucinogens and psychosis." NATURE (London). 216:no. 5115, p. 538, 1967.

"Hallucinogens: the drugs and their effects on the user; the present legal response to the new drug problem and suggested alternate means of control." COLUMBIA LAW REVIEW. 68:521-560, Mar., 1968.

"Hang-loose ethic," by Simmons, J.L., and Winograd, B. NATIONAL EDUCATION ASSOCIATION JOURNAL. 56:18-20 passim, Oct., 1967.

"Harmful aspects of the LSD experience," by Ditman, Keith S., et al. JOURNAL OF NERVOUS AND MENTAL DISEASES. 145(6):464-474, 1967.

"Hazards of indiscriminate use of LSD getting across." NEW YORK JOURNAL OF MEDICINE. 68:1243-1244, May 15, 1968.

"Hazards of LSD." BULLETIN ON NARCOTICS. 21(1):45, Jan.-Mar., 1969.

"Heads and freaks: patterns and meanings of drug use among hippies," by Davis, Fred. and Munoz, Laura. JOURNAL OF HEALTH AND SOCIAL BEHAVIOR. 9(2):156-164, 1968.

"Heads and seekers; drugs on campus, counter-cultures and American society," by Kemiston, K. AMERICAN SCHOLAR. 38:97-112, Winter, 1968.

"The heaven or hell drugs," by Katz, S. MACLEAN'S. 77:9-13, June 20, 1964.

"Herman Hesse: poet of the interior journey," by Leary, T., and Metzner, R. PSYCHEDELIC REVIEW. no. 1:167-182, Fall, 1963.

"A high yogic experience achieved with mescaline," by Blofeld, John. PSYCHEDELIC REVIEW. no. 7:27-32, 1966.

"Hippies," TIME. 90:18-22, July 7, 1967; also READER'S DIGEST. 91:70-74, Oct., 1967.

"History, culture and subjective experience: an exploration of the social bases of drug-induced experience," by Becker, Howard S. JOURNAL OF HEALTH AND SOCIAL BEHAVIOR. 8(3):163-176, 1967.

"History of the psychedelic drug experience," by Mahabir, W. CANADIAN PSYCHIATRIC ASSOCIATION JOURNAL. 13(2):189-190, 1968.

"How to change behavior," by Leary, Timothy. CLINICAL PSYCHOLOGY. 4:211 ff, 1961.

"Hung on LSD; stuck on glue?" by Rich, L. AMERICAN EDUCA-
TION. 4:2-5, Feb., 1968.
"I tried LSD," by Michele, I. LADIES HOME JOURNAL. 83:
52 passim, Aug., 1966.
"The identification of some proscribed psychedelic drugs,"
by Clarke, E.G.C. JOURNAL OF THE FORENSIC SCIENCE SOC-
IETY. 7(1):46-50, Jan., 1967.
"If you want to know about LSD..." U.S. NEWS AND WORLD RE-
PORT. 61:82, July 18, 1966.
"Illicit drug use among Canadian youth," by Unwin, J. Ro-
bertson. CANADIAN MEDICAL ASSOCIATION JOURNAL. 98(8):
402-407, 1968.
"Illicit LSD traffic hurts research efforts." SCIENCE NEWS.
89:327, Apr. 30, 1966.
"Implication of LSD and experimental mysticism," by Pahnke,
Walter N., and Richards, William A. JOURNAL OF RELIGION
AND HEALTH. 5(3):175-208, 1966.
"In the beginning, Leary turned on Ginsberg and saw that
it was good," by Leary, T. ESQUIRE. 70:83-87 passim,
July, 1968.
"Inn of synthetic dreams," by Jacole, Andreas. ATLAS.
16:35-38, Nov., 1968.
"Instant ecstasy," by Muggeridge, M. NEW STATESMAN. 72:
387, Sept. 16, 1966.
"Is the trip over for LSD? journey into the human sub-
conscious with unknown consequences." BUSINESS WEEK.
pp. 141-142, Apr. 23, 1966.
"The issues of the consciousness-expanding drugs," by Har-
man, W.W. MAIN CURRENTS IN MODERN THOUGHT. 20(1):5-14,
1963.
"It's psychedelic!" by Sayre, N. NEW STATESMAN. 72:902,
Dec. 16, 1966.
"LSD." MEDICAL LETTER ON DRUGS AND THERAPEUTICS. 9:1-2,
1967.
"LSD - a dangerous drug." NEW ENGLAND JOURNAL OF MEDICINE.
273:1280, 1965.
"LSD: a meaningful approach to drug education," by Harmon,
S. JOURNAL OF SCHOOL HEALTH. 38:386-391, June, 1968.
"LSD abuse in the United Kingdom." BULLETIN ON NARCOTICS.
20(2):55, Apr.-June, 1968.
"LSD; an historical reevaluation," by Nunes, F. JOURNAL
OF CHEMICAL EDUCATION. 45:688-691, Nov., 1968.
"LSD - An outsider's viewpoint," by Alexander, E.J. HENRY
FORD HOSPITAL MEDICAL BULLETIN. 15(1):23-26, 1967.
"LSD analysis in seizures," by Lerner, Melvin. BULLETIN ON
NARCOTICS. 19(3):39-45, July-Sept., 1967.
"LSD and amphetamines." BULLETIN ON NARCOTICS. 20(3):17,
July-Sept., 1968.
"LSD and broken chromosomes." SCIENCE DIGEST. 63:18-21,
Apr., 1968
"LSD and chromosomes," by Prince, Alfred M. PSYCHEDELIC
REVIEW. no. 9:38-40, 1967.
"LSD and marijuana," by Abelson, P.H. SCIENCE. 159(3820):
1189, Mar. 15, 1968.

"LSD and marihuana: where are the answers?" by Myers, W.A.
SCIENCE. 160(3832):1062, 1968.
"LSD and marihuana: where are the answers?" by Wertlake,
Paul T. SCIENCE. 160(3832):1064-1065, June 7, 1968.
"LSD and marijuana," by Abelson, P.H. SCIENCE. 159(3820):
1189, Mar. 15, 1968.
"LSD and psychiatric inpatients," by Hensala, J.D., et al.
ARCHIVES OF GENERAL PSYCHIATRY. 16(5):554-559, 1967.
"LSD and the anguish of dying," by Cohen, Sidney. HARPER'S
MAGAZINE. 231:69-78, Sept., 1965.
"LSD and the creative experience," by Korngold, M. PSYCHO-
ANALYTIC REVIEW. 50(4):152-155, 1963.
"LSD and the drugs of the mind; uses, abuses, promise and
perils." NEWSWEEK. 67:59-60 passim, May 9, 1966.
"LSD and the dying patient," by Kast, E. CHICAGO MEDICAL
SCHOOL QUARTERLY. 26:80-87, Feb., 1966.
"LSD and the enlightenment of Zen," by VanDusen, Wilson.
PSYCHOLOGIA: AN INTERNATIONAL JOURNAL OF PSYCHOLOGY IN
THE ORIENT. 4(1):11-16, 1961.
"LSD and the law," by Trout, M.E. HOSPITAL FORMULARY MAN-
AGEMENT. 2:71, 1967.
"LSD and the third eye; theories on the role of the pineal
organ and its chemicals," by Bleibtreu, J.N. ATLANTIC
MONTHLY. 218:64-69, Sept., 1966.
"LSD; avant-garde cult or reversion to savagery?" by Wid-
ener, A. BARRON'S. 46:8, Sept. 12, 1966.
"LSD: control, not prohibition." LIFE. 60:4, Apr. 29, 1966.
"The LSD controversy," by Levine, Jerome, and Ludwig, Arnold.
COMPREHENSIVE PSYCHIATRY. 5(5):314-319, 1964.
"LSD crackdown," by Sanford, D. NEW REPUBLIC. 158:11-12,
Mar. 16, 1968.
"LSD: Experimental findings," by Aaronson, Bernard S. IN-
TERNATIONAL JOURNAL OF PARAPSYCHOLOGY. 9(2):86-90, 1967.
"LSD: Fact and fantasy," by Ungerleider, J.T., and Fisher,
D. ARTS AND ARCHITECTURE. 83:18-20, 1966.
"LSD: false illusion," by Smith, J.P. FOOD AND DRUG ADMIN-
ISTRATION PAPERS. 1:10-18, 1967.
"LSD: far-reaching peril," by Leffler, L., and Augenstein,
L. MICHIGAN EDUCATION JOURNAL. 45:20-21, May, 1968.
"LSD helps alcoholics." SCIENCE NEWS. 90:22, July 9, 1966.
"LSD helps severely disturbed children." SCIENCE NEWS.
89:378, May 14, 1966.
"LSD is no problem for us, public schoolmen report; school
administrators poll. NATION'S SCHOOLS. 78:55, Aug.,
1966.
"LSD is not a tonic," by McBroom, P. SCIENCE NEWS. 89:433,
June 4, 1966.
"LSD is seen needing no new control laws." OIL, PAINT AND
DRUG REPORT. 189:4 passim, May 30, 1966.
"LSD, law and society," by Leary, T. THE REALIST. no. 69,
Sept., 1966.
"LSD lion loses to M?I?T? mauler," by Collins, Bud. PSY-
CHIATRIC QUARTERLY. 42(1):104-106, 1968.
"LSD may become legal if it gets religion." SCIENCE NEWS.

90:22, July 9, 1966.
"LSD: maybe fetal deformities from a bad trip." OIL, PAINT AND DRUG REPORT. 192:5 passim, Aug. 7, 1967.
"LSD - medical overview," by Louria, D.B. SATURDAY REVIEW. 50:91-92, Apr. 22, 1967.
"LSD new menace to youth," by Evang, K. UNESCO COURIER. 21:18-20, May, 1968.
"LSD: 1967," by Bennet, Glin. BRITISH JOURNAL OF PSYCHIATRY. 114(515):1219-1222, 1968.
"LSD possession measure gets Goddard's hesitant ok." OIL, PAINT AND DRUG REPORT. 193:4 passim, Mar. 4, 1968.
"LSD pother." AMERICA. 115:377, Oct. 1, 1966.
"LSD; problems and promise," by Smart, Reginald D. CANADA'S MENTAL HEALTH SUPPLEMENT. no. 57, May/Aug., 1968.
"LSD psychosis," by Rosenberg, C.M., et al. MEDICAL JOURNAL OF AUSTRALIA. 1:129-131, Jan. 27, 1968.
"LSD: research and joyride," by Ungerleider, J.T., and Fisher, D.D. THE NATION. 202:574-576, May 16, 1966.
"LSD research: the impact of lay publicity," by Dahlberg, Charles C., et al. AMERICAN JOURNAL OF PSYCHIATRY. 125(5):685-689, 1968.
"LSD side effects and complications," by Cohen, S. JOURNAL OF NERVOUS AND MENTAL DISEASES. 130:1960.
"LSD spelled out," by Lerner, M., and Abramson, H.A. MADEMOISELLE. 64:52-53 passim, Jan., 1967.
"LSD state." THE AMERICAN BIOLOGY TEACHER. 30:656, Oct., 1968.
"LSD subcultures: acidoxy versus orthodoxy," by Gioscia, Victor. AMERICAN JOURNAL OF ORTHOPSYCHIATRY. 39:428-436, Apr., 1969.
"LSD: tamed for research," by Dahlberg, C.C. SCIENCE. 153:1595, Sept. 30, 1966.
"LSD: Therapeutic effects of the psychedelic experience," by Savage, Charles, et al. PSYCHOLOGICAL REPORTS. 14(1):111-120, 1964.
"LSD; time essay." TIME. 87:30-31, June 17, 1966.
"LSD tough laws: move is on in Congress." OIL, PAINT AND DRUG REPORT. 192:7 passim, Nov. 27, 1967.
"LSD, transcendence, and the new beginning," by Savage, C., et al. JOURNAL OF NERVOUS AND MENTAL DISEASES. 135:425-439, 1962.
"LSD trigger; crystal palaces and absolute horror," by Buckley, T. NEW REPUBLIC. 154:15-21, May 14, 1966.
"LSD versus pot: effects compared." THE ATTACK ON NARCOTIC ADDICTION AND DRUG ABUSE. 2(4):6, Nov., 1968.
"LSD warning," by Glew, D.H., Jr. MILITARY MEDICINE. 131:1340-1341, 1966.
"Law and LSD." TIME. 87:34, June 10, 1966.
"Law-medicine notes: Law, medicine, and LSD," by Chayet, Neil L. NEW ENGLAND JOURNAL OF MEDICINE. 277(5):253--254, 1967.
"Long lasting effects of LSD on normals," by McGlothlin, William, et al. ARCHIVES OF GENERAL PSYCHIATRY. 17(5):521-532, 1967.

"Love needs care; clinic devoted exclusively to helping hippies with health problems." NEWSWEEK. 70:98, July 17, 1967.

"Love potions of the East," by Vijayatunga, J. NEW STATESMAN. 67:517-518, Apr. 3, 1964.

"Lumps for LSD." ECONOMIST. 219:366, Apr. 23, 1966.

"Lysergic acid and the alcoholic," by O'Rilly, P., and Reich, G. DISEASES OF THE NERVOUS SYSTEM. 23:331-334, 1962.

"Lysergic acid diethylamide." BRITISH MEDICAL JOURNAL. 5504:48-49, July 2, 1966.

"Lysergic acid diethylamide," by Ledger, L. THE TEXAS OUTLOOK. 51:40-43, Oct., 1967.

"Lysergic acid diethylamide: side effects and complications," by Cohen, S. JOURNAL OF NERVOUS AND MENTAL DISEASES. 130:35-36, 1960.

"Marihuana and LSD usage among male college students: Prevalence rate, frequency, and self-estimates of future use," by King, Francis W. PSYCHIATRY. 32:265-276, Aug., 1969.

"Marijuana and LSD: a survey of one college campus," by Eebbs, K. JOURNAL OF COUNSELING PSYCHOLOGY. 15(5, pt.1): 459-467, 1968.

"Marijuana, LSD, and other dangerous substances," by Quinn, W. BULLETIN OF THE LOS ANGELES COUNTY MEDICAL ASSOCIATION. 97:20-21, 1967.

"Matter over mind; mind-control drugs." NEWSWEEK. 71:113, Apr. 15, 1968.

"Meaning and the mind-drugs," by Marsh, Richard P. ETC: A REVIEW OF GENERAL SEMANTICS. 22(4):408-425, 1965.

"Memo on the religious implications of the consciousness-changing drugs," by Havens, Joseph. JOURNAL FOR THE SCIENTIFIC STUDY OF RELIGION. 3(2):216-226, 1964.

"Mental age regression induced by lysergic acid diethylamide," by Lienert, G.A. JOURNAL OF PSYCHOLOGY. 63(1): 3-11, 1966.

"Mental drugs; the big draw. Hallucinogens are in their infancy." CHEMICAL WEEK. 98:47, May 28, 1966.

"Mescaline, LSD, psilocybin, and personality change," by Unger, Sanford M. PSYCHIATRY. 26(2):111-125, 1963.

"Mescaline, madness and mysticism," by Moraczewski, A.S. THOUGHT. 42:358-382, Autumn, 1967.

"Mind drugs puzzling," by McBroom, P. SCIENCE NEWS. 90: 196, Sept. 17, 1966.

"Mind-altering drugs, LSD, marijuana, hashish, etc., a scientific appraisal," by Blum R.H. UNESCO COURIER. 21:13-17, May, 1968.

"Moire patterns and visual hallucinations," by Oster, Gerald. PSYCHEDELIC REVIEW. no. 1:33-40, 1966.

"More light, less heat over LSD." BUSINESS WEEK. p. 78 passim, June 25, 1966.

"Morning glory seed reaction," by Ingram, A.L. JOURNAL OF THE AMERICAN MEDICAL ASSOCIATION. 190:1133-1134, 1964.

"Motivation and the behavioral effects of LSD," by Appel, J.B., and Whitehead, W.E. PSYCHONOMIC SCIENCE. 12(7):

305-306, 1968
"Motivation for self-administration of LSD," by Frosch, W., et al. PSYCHONOMIC SCIENCE. 9(7-B):425-426, 1967.
"Motivational factors in psychedelic drug use by male college students," by Lipinski, E., et al. JOURNAL OF THE AMERICAN COLLEGE HEALTH ASSOCIATION. 16:145-149, Dec., 1967.
"Multiple-drug addiction in New York City in a selected population group," by Abeles, Hans, et al. PUBLIC HEALTH REPORTS. 81:685-690, Aug., 1966.
"Murder by LSD? Kessler case." NEWSWEEK. 67:29, Apr. 25, 1966.
"My son is on LSD," by Roberts, M. LADIES HOME JOURNAL. 85:38 passim, Jan., 1968.
"Mysticism in the lab: drug-induced mysticism." TIME. 88:62, Sept. 23, 1966.
"Native hallucinogenic drugs piptadenias," by Granier-Doyeux, Marcel. BULLETIN ON NARCOTICS. 17(2):29-38, Apr.-June, 1965.
"Non-communications: concerning Northwestern University's symposium," by Michelson, P. NEW REPUBLIC. 156:35-38, Mar. 4, 1967.
"Notes and comment: effects of consciousness-expanding drugs." NEW YORKER. 42:41-42, Oct. 1, 1966.
"Notes on current psychedelic research," by Metzner, R. PSYCHEDELIC REVIEW. no. 9:80-82, 1967.
"Notes on Soma," by Sampurnanand. PSYCHEDELIC REVIEW. no. 9:67-70, 1967.
"Notes on the present status of ololiuhqui and other hallucinogens of Mexico," by Wasson, R. Gordon. PSYCHEDELIC REVIEW. no. 1:275-301, 1964.
"Offerings at the psychedelicatessen," by Lingeman, R.R. NEW YORK TIMES MAGAZINE. pp. 6-7 passim, July 10, 1966.
"On and off: T. Leary and guests arrested." NEWSWEEK. 67: 21-22, May 2, 1966.
"On programming psychedelic experiences," by Metzner, R., and Leary, T. PSYCHEDELIC REVIEW. no. 9:5-19, 1967.
"On the use and abuse of LSD," by Freedman, Daniel X. ARCHIVES OF GENERAL PSYCHIATRY. 18(3):330-347, 1968.
"The 100 minute hour," by Dahlberg, Charles C. CONTEMPORARY PSYCHOANALYSIS. 4(1):1-18, 1968.
"Organic hyperkinetic syndrome," by Doyle, P.J. JOURNAL OF SCHOOL HEALTH. 32:299-306, Oct., 1962.
"Other side: excerpts, ed. by D. Kennedy," by Pike, J.A. LOOK. 32:43-48 passim, Oct. 29, 1968.
"Other side of LSD: the promise and the peril," by Osmundsen, J.A. LOOK. 30:78, July 26, 1966.
"Overdosage of psychotropic drugs and minor tranquilizers," by Davis, J.M., et al. DISEASES OF THE NERVOUS SYSTEM. 29:157-164, Mar., 1968.
"Overdosage of psychotropic drugs: antidepressants and other psychotropic agents," by Davis, J.M., et al. DISEASES OF THE NERVOUS SYSTEM. 29:246-256, Apr., 1968.
"Painting under LSD." TIME. 94(23):88, Dec. 5, 1969.

"Parnassus revisited; letter," by Cherkin, A. SCIENCE. 155:266 passim, Jan. 20, 1967.

"Patterns and profiles of addiction and drug abuse," by Scher, Jordan. INTERNATIONAL JOURNAL OF ADDICTIONS. 2:171-190, Fall, 1967; also: ARCHIVES OF GENERAL PSYCHIATRY. 15(5):539-551, 1966.

"Patterns of hallucinogenic drug abuse," by Ludwig, A., and Levine, J. JOURNAL OF THE AMERICAN MEDICAL ASSOCIATION. 191(2):92-96, Jan. 11, 1965.

"Paul Krassner on LSD," by Krassner, P. REALIST. pp. 1-2, June 6, 1965.

"Penalties for LSD." TIME. 91:53, Mar. 8, 1968.

"Performance as a function of drug, dose, and level of training," by Ray, O.S., and Bivens, L.W. PSYCHOPHARMACOLOGIA. 10(8):103-109, 1966.

"Personality differences between psychedelic drug users and nonusers," by Kleckner, J.H. PSYCHOLOGY. 5(2):66-71, 1968.

"Peyote." UNITED NATIONS BULLETIN ON NARCOTICS. v. 11, 1959.

"Peyote night," by Osmond, H. TOMORROW MAGAZINE. 9:112, Feb., 1961.

"A physician's guide to LSD," by Fox, R.P. GP. 35:95-100, Jun., 1967.

"Pills that make you feel good," by Blum, S. REDBOOK. 131:70-71 passim, Aug., 1968.

"The plant kingdom and hallucinogens (part I)," by Schultes, R.E. BULLETIN ON NARCOTICS. 21(3):3-16, July-Sept., 1969.

"Politics and ethics of ecstacy," by Leary, T. CAVALIER MAGAZINE. July, 1966.

"The politics of the nervous system," by Leary, T., Litwin, G., et al. THE BULLETIN OF ATOMIC SCIENCE. Mar., 1962.

"The present and rather curious state of the psychedelic art," by Sagehorn, R. WESTERN WORLD REVIEW. 1:18-32, 1966.

"Problems associated with LSD," by Tylden, E. BRITISH MEDICAL JOURNAL. 1:704-705, Mar. 16, 1968.

"Problems in an unconscious patient who had taken lysergic acid diethylamide," by Clayton, Roger. BRITISH MEDICAL JOURNAL. 1(5585):163, 1968.

"Problems in getting patients off psychotropic drugs," by Arneson, G.A., et al. SOUTHERN MEDICAL JOURNAL. 61:134-138, Feb., 1968.

"The problems of LSD-25 and emotional disorder," by Ungerleider, J.T., et al. CALIFORNIA MEDICINE. 106:49-55, Jan., 1967.

"Programmed communication during experience with DMT," by Leary, Timothy. PSYCHEDELIC REVIEW. no. 8:83-95, 1966.

"Programmed communication during the psychedelic session," by Leary, Timothy. PSYCHEDELIC REVIEW. no. 8, 1965.

"Prolonged adverse reactions from unsupervised use of hallucinogenic drugs," by Kleber, Herbert D. JOURNAL OF NERVOUS AND MENTAL DISEASES. 144(4):308-319, 1967.

56

"Prolonged adverse reactions to LSD." JOURNAL OF THE AMER-
ICAN MEDICAL ASSOCIATION. 198(6):658, 1966.
"Prolonged adverse reactions to LSD in psychotic subjects,"
by Fink, M., et al. ARCHIVES OF GENERAL PSYCHIATRY.
15(5):450-454, 1966.
"Prolonged adverse reactions to lysergic acid diethylamide,"
by Cohen, S., and Ditman, K. ARCHIVES OF GENERAL PSY-
CHIATRY. 8:475-480, 1963.
— "Psychedelic agents in creative problem-solving: A pilot
study," by Harman, Willis, W., et al. PSYCHOLOGICAL RE-
PORTS. 19(1):211-227, 1966.
"Psychedelic drug use by adolescents," by Shachter, Burt.
SOCIAL WORK. 13:33-39, July, 1968.
"Psychedelic drugs," by Nahum, L.H. CONNECTICUTT MEDICINE.
30:162-165, 1966.
"Psychedelic drugs," by Rinkel. M. AMERICAN JOURNAL OF PSY-
CHIATRY. 122:1415-1416, 1966.
"Psychedelic drugs: cannabis and LSD." NURSING TIMES. 64:
326-327, Mar. 8, 1968.
"Psychedelic game; excerpt from psychedelic reader," by
Hoffmann, R. MADEMOISELLE. 62:179 passim, Mar., 1966.
"The psychedelic 'Hip scene': return of the death instinct,"
by Brickman, H.R. AMERICAN JOURNAL OF PSYCHIATRY. 125:
766-772, Dec., 1968.
"Psychedelic metaphysics," by Drake, David. PSYCHEDELIC
REVIEW. no. 5:56-58, 1965.
"Psychedelic research in the context of contemporary psy-
chology," by Mogar, Robert E. PSYCHEDELIC REVIEW.
no. 8:96-104, 1966.
"Psychedelic sentence; T.F.Leary and daughter." NEWSWEEK.
67:35, Mar 20, 1966.
"Psychedelic state fluid." SCIENCE NEWS. 90:238, Sept.
24, 1966.
"Psychedelicoanalysis," by Hermon, H. JOURNAL OF THE TRAVIS
COUNTY MEDICAL SOCIETY. v. 13(3), Mar., 1968.
"Psychedelics and the Law: a prelude in question marks,"
by Bates, R. PSYCHEDELIC REVIEW. no. 1:379-393, 1964.
"A psychiatrist looks at LSD," by Freedman, Daniel X. FED-
ERAL PROBATION. 32:16-24, June, 1968.
"Psycho-chemistry and the religious consciousness," by
Houston, J. INTERNATIONAL PHILOSOPHICAL QUARTERLY.
5:397-413, Sept., 1965.
"Psychodelphic oracles," by Jones, D.A.N. NEW STATESMAN.
73:234-235, Feb. 17, 1967.
"Psychological determinants of LSD reactions," by Glickman,
L., and Blumenfield, M. JOURNAL OF NERVOUS AND MENTAL
DISEASES. 145(1):79-83, 1967.
"The psychology of religious experience," by Clark, W.H.
PSYCHOLOGY TODAY. 1(9):42-47, Feb., 1968.
"The psychotomimetic drugs: an overview," by Cole, J.O.,
and Katz, M.M. JOURNAL OF THE AMERICAN MEDICAL ASSOCIA-
TION. 187:758-761, Oct., 1964.
"Psychotomimetics and their abuse," by Der Marderosian, A.
AMERICAN JOURNAL OF PHARMACOLOGY. 140:83-96, May/June,
1968.

"Psychotropic preparations and suicides in France." BUL-
LETIN ON NARCOTICS. 20(4):7, Oct.-Dec., 1968.
"Radiomimetic properties of LSD." NEW ENGLAND JOURNAL OF
MEDICINE. 277(20):1090-1091, 1967.
"Raid on Castalia," by Mannes, M. REPORTER. 34:27-28 pas-
sim, May 19, 1966.
"Real STP." SCIENCE NEWS. 92:80-81, July 22, 1967.
"Recent trends in substance abuse - Morning glory seed psy-
chosis," by Fink, P.J., et al. INTERNATIONAL JOURNAL
OF THE ADDICTIONS. 2(1):143-151, 1967.
"The regulation of psychedelic drugs," by Barrigar, Robert
H. PSYCHEDELIC REVIEW. no. 1:394-441, 1964.
"The relative potencies of psychotomimetic drugs," by Appel,
J.B., and Freedman, D.X. LIFE SCIENCES. 4:2181-2186,
1965.
"The religious experience: its production and interpreta-
tion," by Leary, T. PSYCHEDELIC REVIEW. no. 1:324-346,
1964.
"The religious implications of consciousness expanding
drugs," by Leary, T., and Clark, W.H. RELIGIOUS EDUCA-
TION. 58(2):251-256, 1963.
"Religious significance of psychedelic substances," by Clark,
W.H. RELIGION IN LIFE. 36:393-403, Aut., 1967.
"Reports of wives of alcoholics of effects of LSD-25 treat-
ment of their husbands," by Sarett, M., et al. ARCHIVES
OF GENERAL PSYCHIATRY. 14:171-178, 1966.
"Research issues in the use and abuse of psychedelic drugs,"
by Elkin, E., et al. PROCEEDINGS OF THE 76TH ANNUAL CON-
VENTION OF THE AMERICAN PSYCHOLOGICAL ASSOCIATION. v.3:
716, 1968.
"STP under abuse control: that's a proposal of FDA." OIL,
PAINT AND DRUG REPORT. 192:7 passim, Nov. 27, 1967.
"Seeds of glory," by Wolff, Robert. PSYCHEDELIC REVIEW.
no. 8:111-122, 1966.
"Sex and psychedelics," by Leary, T. PLAYBOY. Sept., 1966.
"Short-term effects of LSD on anxiety, attitudes and per-
formance," by McGlothlin, William H., et al. JOURNAL OF
NERVOUS AND MENTAL DISEASES. 139(3):266-273, 1964.
"Shouted from the housetops: a peyote awakening," by James,
Joyce. PSYCHEDELIC REVIEW. no. 1:459-482, 1964.
"Shrouds around LSD," by Pollard, J.C. SCIENCE. 154:844,
Nov. 18, 1966.
"Some aspects of an office utilizing LSD 25," by Butter-
worth, A.T. THE PSYCHIATRIC QUARTERLY. 36(4):734-753,
1962.
"Some consequences of the LSD revolution," by Schneider,
Walter L. PSYCHEDELIC REVIEW. no. 9:51-57, 1967.
"Some cool thoughts on a hot issue," by Leary, T., and Al-
pert, R. ESQUIRE. Dec., 1963.
"Some effects of LSD-25 on verbal communication," by Amarel,
Marianne, and Cheek, Frances E. JOURNAL OF ABNORMAL
PSYCHOLOGY. 70(6):453-456, 1965.
"Some less-known hallucinogens." BULLETIN ON NARCOTICS.
20(1):38, Jan.-Mar., 1968.
"Sound of rushing water," by Harner, M.J. NATURAL HISTORY.

77:28-33 passim, June, 1968.
"Spiders, webs, and LSD." CHEMISTRY. 41:27, Mar., 1968.
"Spread and perils of LSD; with reports by Rosenfeld, A.,
and Farrell, B." LIFE. 60:28-33, Mar. 25, 1966.
"Statement of purposes," by Metzner, R., and editors of
Psychedelic Review." PSYCHEDELIC REVIEW. no. 1, 1963.
"A statistical survey of adverse reactions to LSD in Los
Angeles County," by Ungerleider, J.Thomas, et al. AMER-
ICAN JOURNAL OF PSYCHIATRY. 125(3):352-357, 1968.
"Student use of hallucinogens," by Kleber, H. JOURNAL OF
THE AMERICAN COLLEGE HEALTH ASSOCIATION. 14:109-117,
Dec., 1965.
"The subjective aftereffects of psychedelic experiences,"
by Metzner, R., and editors of Psychedelic Review. PSY-
CHEDELIC REVIEW. no. 1:18-26, June, 1963.
"Subjective reactions to lysergic acid diethylamide (LSD-
25): measured by a questionnaire," by Linton, H.B., and
Langs, R.J. ARCHIVES OF GENERAL PSYCHIATRY. 6(5):352-
368, 1962.
"Suggestions for LSD treatment." THE AMERICAN BIOLOGY TEACH-
ER. 31:173, Mar., 1969.
"Suicide during an LSD reaction" by Keeler, M.H., and Reif-
ler, C.B. AMERICAN JOURNAL OF PSYCHIATRY. 123(7):884-
885, 1967.
"Suicide following morning glory seed ingestion," by Cohen,
S. AMERICAN JOURNAL OF PSYCHIATRY. 120:1024-1025, 1964.
"Symposium: psychedelic drugs and religion (2nd semi-annual
conference, psychopharmacological study group)," by
Smith, D., et al. JOURNAL OF PSYCHEDELIC DRUGS. 1:45-
71, 1967.
"Ten months experience with LSD users admitted to county
psychiatric receiving hospital," by Blumenfield, Michael,
and Glickman, Lewis. NEW YORK STATE JOURNAL OF MEDICINE.
67(13):1849-1853, 1967.
"There's no hiding place down there," by Janowitz, Julian F.
AMERICAN JOURNAL OF ORTHOPSYCHIATRY. 37(2):296, 1967.
"They split my personality," by Asher, Harry. SATURDAY
REVIEW. June 1, 1963.
"Three motives for good behavior: youthful experimentation
with LSD. AMERICA. 114:579, Apr. 23, 1966.
"Time to mutate," by Leary, T. TIME. 87:30-31, Apr. 29,
1966.
"Town that went mad; excerpts from 'The day of St. Anthony's
fire'," by Fuller, J.G. LOOK. 32:41-46 passim, June 25,
1968.
"Tranquil society, or why LSD?" by Schwieder, R.M., and Koh-
lan, R.G. THE RECORD. 70:627-633, Apr., 1969.
"Transcendental experience in relation to religion and psychosis," by Laing, R.D. PSYCHEDELIC REVIEW. no. 6:7-15,
1965.
"Trippers can't follow maps." SCIENCE NEWS. 93:400, Apr.
27, 1968.
"Truth about LSD," by Young, W.R. READER'S DIGEST. 89:
56-59, Sept., 1966.
"Turn-on, tune-in, drop-out," by Leary, T. EAST VILLAGE

OTHER. May-June, 1966.

"Turned-on and super-sincere in California," by Todd, R. HARPERS. 234:42-47, Jan., 1967.

"Turned on, turned off; researchers meeting, San Francisco." NEWSWEEK. 67:63, June 27, 1966.

"Turned-on way of life. NEWSWEEK. 68:72 passim, Nov. 28, 1966.

"Turning it on with LSD; doses to mental patients." TIME. 88:58, Nov. 25, 1966.

"UCLA treats large number of LSD cases." SCIENCE NEWS. 90:117, Aug. 20, 1966.

"Unfavourable reactions to LSD." BULLETIN ON NARCOTICS. 20(4):2, Oct.-Dec., 1968.

"Unfavourable reactions to LSD: a review and analysis of the available case reports," by Smart, R.G., and Bateman, K. CANADIAN MEDICAL ASSOCIATION JOURNAL. 97(20): 1214-1221, 1967.

"An untoward reaction to accidental ingestion of LSD in a 5-year-old girl," by Milman, Doris H. JOURNAL OF THE AMERICAN MEDICAL ASSOCIATION. 201(11):821-824, 1967.

"Untoward reactions to lysergic acid diethylamide (LSD) resulting in hospitalization," by Frosch, W.A., et al. NEW ENGLAND JOURNAL OF MEDICINE. 273:1235-1239, 1965.

"The use and abuse of LSD in Haight-Ashbury (Observations by the Haight-Ashbury Medical Clinics)," by Smith, D.E., et al. CLINICAL PEDIATRICS. 7:317-322, June, 1968.

"Use and abuse of psychedelic drugs; excerpts from address," by Freedman, D.X. BULLETIN OF THE ATOMIC SCIENTISTS. 24:6-14, Apr., 1968.

"Use of amphetamines, marihuana and LSD by students," by Blachly, P. NEW PHYSICIAN. 15:88-93, 1966.

"Use of diazepam in hallucinogenic drug crisis," by Solirsh, Lionel P., and Clement, Wilfrid R. JOURNAL OF THE AMERICAN MEDICAL ASSOCIATION. 205(9):644-655, 1968.

"The use of hallucinogenic drugs among college students," by McGlothlin, W.H., and Cohen, S. AMERICAN JOURNAL OF PSYCHIATRY. 122:572-574, May, 1965.

"Use of hallucinogenic drugs on campus," by Imperi, Lilian L., et al. JOURNAL OF THE AMERICAN MEDICAL ASSOCIATION. 204:1021-1024, June 17, 1968.

"The use of hallucinogenic, psychotomimetic, psychedelic drugs in North Carolina," by Keeler, M.H. NORTH CAROLINA MEDICAL JOURNAL. 24:555-557, 1963.

"The use of hyoscyamine as a hallucinogen and intoxicant," by Keeler, Martin H., and Kane, Francis J. AMERICAN JOURNAL OF PSYCHIATRY. 124:852-854, Dec., 1967.

"The use of marijuana and LSD on the college campus," by Kurtz, R.S. JOURNAL OF THE NATIONAL ASSOCIATION OF WOMEN'S DEANS AND COUNSELORS. 30:124-128, Spring, 1967.

"The use of nutmeg as a psychotropic agent," by Weil, Andrew T. BULLETIN ON NARCOTICS. 18(4):15-23, Oct.-Dec., 1966.

"Use of psychotropic drugs by employed persons," by Rogg, S.G., and Pell, S. INDUSTRIAL MEDICINE AND SURGERY. 32(7):255-260, 1963.

"What is LSD?" TODAY'S EDUCATION. 58:45-47, Mar., 1969.

"What is the clinical evidence?" by Ochota, L. NEW REPUB-
LIC. 154:21-22, May 14, 1966.
"What the minister ought to know about LSD," by Becker, A.H.
PASTORAL PSYCHOLOGY. 16(157):37-47, 1965.
"World's most controversial drug: LSD." AMERICAN DRUGGIST.
156:41-42, Oct. 9, 1967.
"You can't even step in the same river once," by Lettvin, J.
NATURAL HISTORY. 76:6-12 passim, Oct., 1967.
"Young people and LSD: a talk with Susan Leary," ed. by M.
Mannes. MCCALLS. 93:14 passim, July, 1966.
"Your adolescent health; dangers of the drug called LSD,"
by Sauer, L.W. PTA MAGAZINE. 61:31-32, Sept., 1966.

LYSERGIC ACID DIETHYLAMIDE: Periodical Literature

Scientific Publications

"Accentuation of the psychological effects of LSD-25 in
normal subjects treated with reserpine," by Resnick,
Oscar, et al. LIFE SCIENCES. 4(14):1433-1437, 1965.
"The action of LSD in psychotherapy," by Roubicek. ACTI-
VITAS NERVOSA SUPERIOR. 4(2):240-241, 1962.
"The active principles of the seeds of rivea corymbosa and
ipomoea violacea," by Hofmann, Albert. PSYCHEDELIC RE-
VIEW. no. 1:302-316, 1964.
"Acute leukemia with PH[1]-like chromosome in an LSD user,"
by Grossbard, L., et al. JOURNAL OF THE AMERICAN MEDI-
CAL ASSOCIATION. 205(11):791-793, 1968.
"Abuse characteristics of psychotoxic drugs." SOUTH DAKOTA
JOURNAL OF MEDICINE AND PHARMACY. 16:36-39, 1963.
"Alicyclic analogue of mescaline," by Walters, C.C., and
Cooper, P.D. NATURE. 218(5138):298-300, 1968.
"Alterations in consciousness produced by combinations of
LSD, hypnosis and psychotherapy," by Levine, J., and
Ludwig, A.M. PSYCHOPHARMACOLOGIA. 7(2):123-137, 1965.
"Alterations in the nocturnal sleep cycle resulting from
LSD," by Munzio, J.N., et al. ELECTROENCEPHALOGRAPHY
AND CLINICAL NEUROPHYSIOLOGY. 21:313-324, 1966.
"The analgesic action of lysergic acid compared with dihy-
dromorphinome and meperidine," by Kast, E.C. BULLETIN
OF DRUG ADDICTION AND NARCOTICS. appendix 27:3517, 1963.
"Analytic and integrative therapy with the help of LSD-25,"
by Holzinger, Rudolf. JOURNAL OF EXISTENTIAL PSYCHIATRY.
4(15):225-236, 1964.
"Analytical separations of mixtures of hallucinogenic drugs,"
by Lerner, Melvin, and Katsiafics, Mary Diane. BULLETIN
ON NARCOTICS. 21(1):47-51, Jan.-Mar., 1969.
"Annihilating illumination," by Andrews, George. PSYCHEDEL-
IC REVIEW. no. 1:66-68, June, 1963.
"The application of gas-chromatography to the examination
of the constituents of cannabis sativa 1," by Heaysman,

61

L., et al. ANALYST. 92:450-455, 1967.
"Approaches to the pharmacology of LSD-25," by Freedman,
D.X., and Aghajanian, G.K. LLOYDIA. 29:309, 1966.
"Aspects of biochemical pharmacology of psychotropic drugs,"
by Freedman, David K. PSYCHEDELIC REVIEW. no. 8:33-
58, 1966.
"Attenuation of anticipation: a therapeutic use of lysergic
acid diethylamide," by Kast, Eric. PSYCHIATRIC QUARTER-
LY. 41(4):646-657, 1967.
"The bad trip: the etiology of the adverse LSD reaction,"
by Ungerleider, J. Thomas, et al. AMERICAN JOURNAL OF
PSYCHIATRY. 124(11):1483-1490, 1968.
"Barbiturates, lysergic acid diethylamide, and the social
behavior of rats," by Silverman, A.P. PSYCHOPHARMACO-
LOGIA. 10(2):155-171, 1966.
"Behavioral reaction of rats pretreated with reserpine to
LSD-25," by Votava, Z., et al. INTERNATIONAL JOURNAL
OF NEUROPHARMACOLOGY. 6(6):543-547, 1967.
"The behavioural effects of some derivatives of mescaline
and N,N-dimethyltryptamine in the rat," by Smythies,
J.R., et al. LIFE SCIENCES. 6(17):1887-1893, 1967.
"Biochemical observations on LSD-25 and deseril," by Doepf-
ner, W. EXPERIENTIA. 18:256, 1962.
"Botanical sources of the New World narcotics," by Schultes,
Richard Evans. PSYCHEDELIC REVIEW. no. 1:145-166, Fall,
1963.
"A case of early paranoiac psychosis treated by lysergic
acid diethylamide (LSD)," by Martin, A. Joyce. ACTA
PSYCHOTHERAPEUTICA ET PSYCHOSOMATICA. 12(2):119-130,
1964.
"A case of homosexuality and personality disorder in a man
of 36 treated by LSD and resolved within two months,"
by Martin, A.J. PSYCHOTHERAPY AND PSYCHOSOMATICS. 15
(1):44, 1967.
"Cerebral synaptic transmission and behavioral effects of
dimethoxyphenylethylamine: a potential psychotogen," by
Vacca, Lucio, et al. SCIENCE. 160(3823):95-96, 1968.
"Changes in correlation between responses to items of the
Addiction Research Center Inventory produced by LSD-25,"
by Haertzen, Charles A. JOURNAL OF PSYCHOPHARMACOLOGY.
1(1):27-36, 1966.
"Changes in locomotor activity and brain chemistry follow-
ing LSD-25 administration in mice," by Essman, Walter B.
PSYCHOLOGICAL REPORTS. 20(1):124-126, 1967.
"Characterizing the psychological state produced by LSD,"
by Katz, M.M., et al. JOURNAL OF ABNORMAL PSYCHOLOGY.
73(1):1-14, 1968.
"Chemical constituents of the morning glory seed." BUL-
LETIN ON NARCOTICS. 20(4):7, Oct.-Dec., 1968.
"Chemical pharmacology and medical aspects of psychotomi-
metics," by Hofmann, A. JOURNAL OF EXPERIMENTAL MEDICAL
SCIENCES. 5:31, 1961.
"Chemically-induced alterations in the behavioral effects
of LSD-25," by Appel, J.B. and Freedman, D.X. BIOCHEM-
ICAL PHARMACOLOGY. 13:861, 1964.

"Chlorpromazine antagonism of psilocybin effect," by Keeler, Martin H. INTERNATIONAL JOURNAL OF NEUROPSYCHIATRY. 3(1):66-71, 1967.

"Chromosomal abnormalities in leukocytes from LSD users," by Irwin, S., and Egozcue, J. SCIENCE. 157:313, 1967.

"The chromosomal and teratogenic effects of lysergic acid diethylamide: a review of current literature," by Smart, Reginald G., and Bateman, Karen. CANADIAN MEDICAL ASSOCIATION JOURNAL. 99(16):805-810, 1968.

"Chromosomal damage in human leukocytes induced by lysergic acid diethylamide," by Cohen, M.M., et al. SCIENCE. 155:1417-1419, 1967.

"Chromosomal damage in LSD users," by Egozcue, José, et al. JOURNAL OF THE AMERICAN MEDICAL ASSOCIATION. 204(3):214-218, Apr. 15, 1968.

"Chromosomal effect in vivo of exposure to lysergic acid diethylamide," by Sparkes, R., et al. SCIENCE. 160 (3834):1343-1345, 1968.

"Chromosome abnormalities and psychotropic drugs," by Nielsen, J., et al. NATURE. 218(5140):488-489, 1968.

"Chromosome damage not found in leukocytes of children treated with LSD-25," by Bender, L., and Sankar, D.V. SCIENCE. 159(3816):749, 1968.

"Clarifying the confusion regarding LSD-25," by Savage, Charles, and Stolaroff, Myron J. JOURNAL OF NERVOUS AND MENTAL DISEASES. 140(3):218-221, 1965.

"The clinical effects of psychedelic agents," by Ludwig, A.M., and Levine, J. CLINICAL MEDICINE. 73(6):21-24, 1966.

"Clinical evaluation of some hallucinogenic tryptamine derivatives," by Faillace, L.A., et al. JOURNAL OF NERVOUS AND MENTAL DISEASES. 145(4):306-313, 1968.

"The clinical pharmacology of the hallucinogens," by Jacobsen, E. CLINICAL PHARMACOLOGY AND THERAPEUTICS. 4:480-503, Apr., 1963.

"Clinical prediction of insightful response to a single large dose of LSD," by Eggert, D.C., and Shagass, C. PSYCHOPHARMACOLOGIA. 9(4):340-346, 1966.

"Clinical syndromes and biochemical alterations following mescaline, lysergic acid diethylamide, psilocybin and a combination of the three psychotomimetic drugs," by Hollister, L.E., and Sjoberg, B.M. COMPREHENSIVE PSYCHIATRY. 5(3):170-178, 1964.

"Cognitive test performance under LSD-25, placebo and isolation," by Goldberger, L. JOURNAL OF NERVOUS AND MENTAL DISEASES. 142(1):4-9, 1966.

"Comparison of effects of dexamphetamine and LSD-25 on perceptual and autonomic function," by Claridge, G.S., and Hume, W.I. PERCEPTUAL AND MOTOR SKILLS. 23(2):456-458, 1966.

"A comparison of LSD-25 with (....)-Δ^9-transtetrahydrocannabinol (THC) and attempted cross tolerance between LSD and THC," by Isbell, H., and Jasinski, D.R. PSYCHOPHARMACOLOGIA. 14(2):115-123, 1969.

"Comparison of the reaction induced by psilocybin and LSD-25 in man," by Isbell, Harris. PSYCHOPHARMACOLOGIA. 1(1):29-38, 1959.

"Comparison of two drugs with psychotomimetic effects (LSD and DITRAN)," by Wilson, Roy Edward and Shagass, Charles. JOURNAL OF NERVOUS AND MENTAL DISEASES. 138(3):277-286, 1964.

"Complications associated with lysergic acid diethylamide (LSD-25)," by Cohen, S., and Ditman, K.S. JOURNAL OF THE AMERICAN MEDICAL ASSOCIATION. 181:161-162, Feb., 1962.

"The complications of LSD: a review of the literature," by Schwarz, Conrad J. JOURNAL OF NERVOUS AND MENTAL DISEASES. 146(2):174-186, 1968.

"Congenital malformations induced by mescaline, LSD, and bromolysergic acid in the hamster," by Geber, V. SCIENCE. 158:265-266, 1967.

"'Consciousness-limiting' side effects of 'consciousness-expanding' drugs," by Mamlet, Lawrence N. AMERICAN JOURNAL OF ORTHOPSYCHIATRY. 37:296-297, Mar. 1967.

"Considerations for the pre-clinical evaluation of new psychiatric drugs: a case study with phenothiazine-like tranquillizers," by Irwin, S. PSYCHOPHARMACOLOGIA. 9(4):259-287, 1966.

"Contribution to serotonin theory of dreaming (LSD infusion)," by Torda, Clara. NEW YORK STATE JOURNAL OF MEDICINE. 68(9):1135-1138, 1968.

"A controlled comparison of five brief treatment techniques employing LSD, hypnosis, and psychotherapy," by Levine, J., and Ludwig, A.M. AMERICAN JOURNAL OF PSYCHOTHERAPY. 19(3):417-435, 1965.

"The controlled psychedelic state," by Levine, J., et al. AMERICAN JOURNAL OF CLINICAL HYPNOSIS. 6:163-164, 1963.

"A controlled study of lysergide in the treatment of alcoholism. 1. The effects on drinking behavior," by Smart, R.G., et al. QUARTERLY JOURNAL OF STUDIES ON ALCOHOL. 27:469-482, 1966.

"Cross tolerance between LSD and psilocybin," by Isbell, H., et al. PSYCHOPHARMACOLOGIA. 1:147, 1961.

"D-lysergic acid diethylamide (LSD): a review of its present status," by Hoffer, A. CLINICAL PHARMACOLOGY AND THERAPEUTICS. 6:183-255, Feb., 1965.

"D-lysergic acid in the treatment of the biological features of childhood schizophrenia," by Bender, L. DISEASES OF THE NERVOUS SYSTEM. 27(7, pt.2):43-46, 1966.

"D-lysergic acid diethylamide (LSD-25): a survey of the literature," by Schwartz, Melvin. MILITARY MEDICINE. 132 (9):667-673, 1967.

"DOM (STP), a new hallucinogenic drug, and DOET: effects in normal subjects," by Snyder, Solomon H., et al. AMERICAN JOURNAL OF PSYCHIATRY. 125(3):357-364, 1968.

"The dangers of LSD. Analysis of seven months' experience in a university hospital's psychiatric service," by Ungerleider, J.T., et al. JOURNAL OF THE AMERICAN MEDICAL ASSOCIATION. 197:389-392, Aug. 8, 1966.

"Detection of trace amounts of lysergic acid diethylamide in sugar cubes," by Radecka, C., and Nigam, I.C. JOURNAL OF PHARMACEUTICAL SCIENCES. 55:861-862, 1966.

"Development of scales based on patterns of drug effects, using the Addiction Research Center Inventory (ARCI)," by Haertzen, Charles A. PSYCHOLOGICAL REPORTS. 18(1): 163-194, 1966.

"Discussion of 'Abuse of psychotomimetics'," by Geert-Jorgensen, E., et al. ACTA PSYCHIATRICA SCANDINAVICA. (Suppl. 203):215-216, 1968.

"Disruption of size discrimination in squirrel monkeys (Saimiri sciureus) by LSD-25," by Sharpe, Lawrence G., et al. PSYCHONOMIC SCIENCE. 7(3):103-104, 1967.

"Dissociative delirium after treatment with lysergide," by Denson, R. CANADIAN MEDICAL ASSOCIATION JOURNAL. 97 (20):1222-1224, 1967.

"Distribution and metabolism of mescaline-C^{14} in cat brain," by Neff, N., et al. JOURNAL OF PHARMACOLOGY AND EXPERIMENTAL THERAPEUTICS. 144:1, 1964.

"Drosophila Melanogaster treated with LSD: absence of mutation and chromosomal breakage," by Grace, D., et al. SCIENCE. 161:694-696, 1968.

"A drug-induced ecstatic experience," by Bergman, Paul. PSYCHOTHERAPY: THEORY, RESEARCH AND PRACTICE. 1(1): 44-48, 1963.

"Dynamics of psychedelic drug abuse: clinical study," by Bowers, M.B., et al. ARCHIVES OF GENERAL PSYCHIATRY. 16:560-566, 1967.

"The dysleptics: note on a no man's land," by Elkes, Joel. COMPREHENSIVE PSYCHIATRY. 4:195-198, June, 1963.

"The EEG effects of LSD-25 in epileptic patients before and after temporal lobectomy," by Serafetinides, E.A. PSYCHOPHARMACOLOGIA. 7(6):453-460, 1965.

"The EEG of the olfactory bulb of the rabbit and its reaction to psychopharmacological agents," by Khazan, N., et al. PSYCHOPHARMACOLOGIA. 10(3):226-236, 1967.

"ESP experiments with LSD and psilocybin: a methodological approach," by Cavanna, Roberto, and Servadio, Emilio. PARAPSYCHOLOGICAL MONOGRAPHS. no. 5:1-123, 1964.

"Effect of an hallucinogenic agent on verbal behavior," by Honigfeld, Gilbert. PSYCHOLOGICAL REPORTS. 13(2): 383-385, 1963.

"The effect of LSD and L-tryptophane on the sleepdream cycle in the rat," by Hartmann, Ernest. PSYCHOPHYSIOLOGY. 4(3):390, 1968.

"Effect of LSD-25 in the rat on operant approach to a visual or auditory conditioned stimulus," by Caldwell, Donald F., and Domino, Edward F. PSYCHOLOGICAL REPORTS. 20(1):199-205, 1967.

"Effect of LSD-25 on activity level of the hooded rat," by Slivka, Robert M., et al. PSYCHOLOGICAL REPORTS. 20(1): 158, 1967.

"Effect of LSD on pace of performing a variety of tasks," by Krus, D.M., and Wapner, S. PERCEPTUAL AND MOTOR SKILLS. 14:255-259, 1962.

"The effect of LSD-25 on perseverative tendencies in rats," by Butters, Nelson. PROCEEDINGS OF THE 73RD ANNUAL CONVENTION OF THE AMERICAN PSYCHOLOGICAL ASSOCIATION. pp. 125-126, 1965.

"The effect of LSD-25 on potentials evoked in specific sensory pathways," by Key, B.J. BRITISH MEDICAL JOURNAL. 21(1):30-35, 1965.

"Effect of LSD on responses to colored photic stimuli as related to visual imagery ability in man," by Shryne, J.E., Jr., and Brown, B.B. PROCEEDINGS OF THE WESTERN PHARMACOLOGY SERIES. 8:42-46, 1965.

"The effect of LSD-25 on spatial and stimulus perseverative tendencies in rats," by Butters, N. PSYCHOPHARMACOLOGIA. 8(6):454-460, 1966.

"The effect of LSD on the sleep cycle of the cat," by Hobson, J.A. ELECTROENCEPHALOGRAPHY AND CLINICAL NEUROPHYSIOLOGY. 17(1):52-56, 1964.

"The effect of LSD on the sleep-dream cycle. An exploratory study," by Green, W.J. JOURNAL OF NERVOUS AND MENTAL DISEASES. 140(6):417-426, 1965.

"Effect of LSD on the tonic activity of the visual pathways of the cat," by Schwartz, Arthur S., and Cheney, Carl. LIFE SCIENCES. 4(7):771-778, 1965.

"Effect of lysergic acid diethylamide (LSD-25) on perception with stabilized images," by Kohn, B., and Bryden, M.P. PSYCHOPHARMACOLOGIA. 7:311, 1965.

"The effect of lysergic acid diethylamide on swimming time in albino mice," by Wilber, C.G., and Burke, J.A. LIFE SCIENCES. 2:134-138, 1963.

"The effect of methysergide (an antiserotonin agent) on schizophrenia," by Mendels, Joe. AMERICAN JOURNAL OF PSYCHIATRY. 124:849-852, Dec., 1967.

"Effect of psilocybin, LSD, and mescaline on small, involuntary eye movements," by Hebbard, F.W., and Fischer, R. PSYCHOPHARMACOLOGIA. 9(2):146-156, 1966.

"Effects of chlorpromazine and d-lysergic acid diethylamide on sex behavior of male rats," by Gillett, E. PROCEEDINGS OF THE SOCIETY FOR EXPERIMENTAL BIOLOGY AND MEDICINE. 103:392, 1960.

"Effects of d-lysergic acid diethylamide and 2-brom-lysergic acid diethylamide on dominance behavior of the rat," by Uyeno, E.T. INTERNATIONAL JOURNAL OF NEUROPHARMACOLOGY. 5(4):317-322, 1966.

"The effects of d-lysergic acid diethylamide tartrate (LSD-25) on the cholinesterases and momoamine oxidase in the spinal cord: a possible factor in the mechanism of hallucination," by Nandy, K., and Bourne, G.H. JOURNAL OF NEUROLOGY, NEUROSURGERY AND PSYCHIATRY. 27(3):259-267, 1964.

"Effects of LSD-25 and amphetamine on a running response in the rat," by Hamilton, C.L. ARCHIVES OF GENERAL PSYCHIATRY. 2:104, 1960.

"Effects of LSD-25 and JB318 on tests of visual and perceptual function in man," by Ostfeld, A.M. FEDERATION

PROCEEDINGS. 20:876, 1961.
"The effects of LSD-25 on alpha blocking and conditioning in epileptic patients before and after temporal lobectomy," by Serafetinides, E.A. CORTEX. 1(4):485-492, 1965.
"Effects of LSD-25 on bar-pressing behavior in the hooded rat," by Gardner, Eliot L. PSYCHONOMIC SCIENCE. 3(11): 507-508, 1965.
"The effects of LSD-25 on brain serotonin," by Friedman, D.X. JOURNAL OF PHARMACOLOGY AND EXPERIMENTAL THERAPEUTICS. 134:160, 1961.
"The effects of LSD-25 on creativity and tolerance to regression," by Zegans, Leonard S., et al. ARCHIVES OF GENERAL PSYCHIATRY. 16(6):740-749, 1967.
"Effects of LSD-25 on potentials in specific sensory pathways," by Key, B.J. BRITISH MEDICAL BULLETIN. 21:30, 1965.
"The effects of LSD-25 on the amplitudes of evoked potentials in the hippocampus of the cat," by Revzin, Alvin M., and Armstrong, Alvin. LIFE SCIENCES. 5(3):259-266, 1966.
"Effects of LSD-25 on the EEG and photic evoked responses," by Rodin, E., and Luby, E. ARCHIVES OF GENERAL PSYCHIATRY. 14(4):435-441, 1966.
"Effects of LSD-25, psilocybin and psilocin on temporal lobe EEG patterns and learned behavior in the cat," by Adey, W.R., et al. NEUROLOGY. 12:591, 1962.
"The effects of lysergic acid diethylamide. I: critical flicker frequency," by Holliday, A.R., et al. PROCEEDINGS OF THE WESTERN PHARMACOLOGY SOCIETY. 8:48-50, 1965.
"The effects of lysergic acid diethylamide. II: intraocular pressure," by Holliday, A.R., and Sigurdson T. PROCEEDINGS OF THE WESTERN PHARMACOLOGY SOCIETY. 8:51-54, 1965.
"The effects of mescaline, amphetamine, and four-ring substituted amphetamine derivatives on spontaneous brain electrical activity in the cat," by Fairchild, M.D., et al. INTERNATIONAL JOURNAL OF NEUROPHARMACOLOGY. 6(3): 151-167, 1967.
"The effects of psychedelic (LSD) therapy on values, personality, and behavior," by Savage, C., et al. INTERNATIONAL JOURNAL OF NEUROPSYCHIATRY. 2(3):241-254, 1966.
"Effects of psychoactive agents on acquisition of conditioned pole jumping in rats," by Domino, Edward F., et al. PSYCHOPHARMACOLOGIA. 8(4):285-298, 1965.
"The effects of psychotomimetic drugs on primary suggestibility," by Sjoberg, B.M., Jr., and Hollister, L.E. PSYCHOPHARMACOLOGIA. 8(4):251-262, 1965.
"The effects of scopolamine and atropine on the performance of an exercise-avoidance test in dogs," by Mennear, J.H., et al. PSYCHOPHARMACOLOGIA. 9(4):347-350, 1966.
"Electroencephalographic study of mental disturbances experimentally induced by LSD-25," by Shirahashi, Koichiro. FOLIA PSYCHIATRICA ET NEUROLOGICA JAPONICA. 14:140-155, 1960.

"Elixir of anguish: the phenomenology of the alcoholic's quest," by Curry, A.E. PSYCHIATRIC QUARTERLY SUPPLEMENT. 38(1):13-20, 1964.

"Empirical dimensions of LSD-25 reaction," by Linton, Harriet B., and Langs, Robert J. ARCHIVES OF GENERAL PSYCHIATRY. 10(5):469-485, 1964.

"Enzymatic formation of a phenolic metabolite from LSD by rat liver microsomes," by Szara, S. LIFE SCIENCES. 1: 662, 1963.

"Experimental investigation of LSD as a psychotherapeutic adjunct," by Mechaneck, Ruth S., et al. AMERICAN JOURNAL OF ORTHOPSYCHIATRY. 37(2):210-211, 1967.

"Exploratory study of drugs and social interaction," by Cheek, Frances E. ARCHIVES OF GENERAL PSYCHIATRY. 9(6): 566-574, 1963.

"Hallucination of geometric forms associated with the use of sympatho-mimetic agents," by Kane, Francis J., et al. DISEASES OF THE NERVOUS SYSTEM. 30(1):28-30, 1969.

"Hallucinogenic drugs and hypnosis in psychotherapy," by Gubel, Isaac. AMERICAN JOURNAL OF CLINICAL HYPNOSIS. 4:169-173, 1962.

"Hallucinogenic spatial disorientation," by Cohen, L.A. INTERNATIONAL JOURNAL OF NEUROPSYCHIATRY. 1:347-351, 1965.

"The hypnodelic treatment technique," by Levine, Jerome, and Ludwig, Arnold M. INTERNATIONAL JOURNAL OF CLINICAL AND EXPERIMENTAL HYPNOSIS. 14(3):207-215, 1966.

"The hypnotic trance, the psychedelic experience, and the creative act," by Kreppner, Stanley. AMERICAN JOURNAL OF CLINICAL HYPNOSIS. 7(2):140-147, 1964.

"The identification and determination of lysergic acid diethylamide in narcotic seizures," by Genest, K., and Farmilo, C.G. JOURNAL OF PHARMACY AND PHARMACOLOGY. 16(4): 250-257, 1964.

"Impairment by lysergic acid diethylamide of accuracy in performance of a delayed alternation test in monkeys," by Jarvik, M.E., and Chorover, S. PSYCHOPHARMACOLOGIA. 1:221, 1960.

"Implication of untoward reactions to hallucinogens," by Robbins, E., et al. BULLETIN OF THE NEW YORK ACADEMY OF MEDICINE. 43:985-999, 1967.

"Individual differences in the recall of drug experience," by Paul, I.H., et al. JOURNAL OF NERVOUS AND MENTAL DISEASE 140(2):132-145, 1965.

"Inhibitory effect of chlorpromazine on alterations in electroencephalograms induced by lysergic acid diethylamide in dogs," by Djahanguiri, B., and Guiti, N. NATURE. 212(5057):87-88, 1966.

"Inhibitory effects of steroids on LSD-25 action in man," by Krus, D.M., et al. LIFE SCIENCES. 6(7):691-701, 1967.

"The interaction of high altitude and psychotropic drug action," by Evans, W.C., and Witt, N.F. PSYCHOPHARMACOLOGIA. 10:184-188, 1966.

"Interaction of LSD and quantity of encoded visual data upon size estimation," by Edwards, Allen E., and Cohen, Sidney.

JOURNAL OF PSYCHOPHARMACOLOGY. 1(3):96-100, 1966. "Interrelations of the effects of psilocybin on subjective sensation, photopic critical frequency of fusion and circulating non-esterified fatty acids," by Keeler, M.H. EXPERIEMTIA. 19:37, 1963.

"The investigation and treatment of a power syndrome in alcoholics by means of LSD-25," by Belden, Ernest. CALIFORNIA MENTAL HEALTH RESEARCH DIGEST. 3(3-4):100-102, 1965.

"LSD-25 action in normal subjects treated with a monoamine oxidase inhibitor," by Resnick, Oscar, et al. LIFE SCIENCES. 3(11):1207-1214, 1964.

"LSD and chromosomes." BRITISH MEDICAL JOURNAL. 2(5608): 778-779, 1968.

"LSD-25 and genetic damage," by Kato, Takashi, and Jarvik, Lissy F. DISEASES OF THE NERVOUS SYSTEM. 30(1):42-46, 1969.

"LSD and JB318: a comparison of two hallucinogens. III. Qualitative analysis and summary of findings," by Lebovits, Binyamin Z., et al. ARCHIVES OF GENERAL PSYCHIATRY. 7(7):39-45, 1962.

"LSD and psychiatric inpatients," by Hensala, J.D., et al. ARCHIVES OF GENERAL PSYCHIATRY (Chicago). 16:554-559, May, 1967.

"LSD and psychotherapy: a bibliography of the English-language literature," by Unger, Sanford M. PSYCHEDELIC REVIEW. no. 1:442-449, 1964.

"LSD-25 and the status and level of brain serotonin," by Freedman, D.X., and Giarman, N.J. ANNALS OF THE NEW YORK ACADEMY OF SCIENCES. 96:98, 1962.

"LSD and UML treatment of hospitalized disturbed children," by Bender, L., et al. RECENT ADVANCES IN BIOLOGICAL PSYCHIATRY. 5:84, 1963.

"LSD as an adjunct to psychotherapy with alcoholics," by Rolo, A., et al. JOURNAL OF PSYCHOLOGY. 50:85-104, 1960.

"LSD, effect on embryos," by Auerbach, R., et al. SCIENCE. 157:1325-1326, 1967.

"LSD: effects on offspring," by DiPaolo, Joseph A. SCIENCE. 158(3800):522, 1967.

"LSD in mice: abnormalities in meiotic chromosomes," by Skakkeback, N.E., et al. SCIENCE. 160(3833):1246-1248, 1968.

"LSD in psychotherapy and alcoholism," by Abramson, H.A. AMERICAN JOURNAL OF PSYCHOTHERAPY. 20(3):415-438, 1966.

"LSD injection in early pregnancy produces abnormalities in offspring in rats," by Alexander, G., et al. SCIENCE. 157(3787):459-460, 1967.

"LSD 'mainlining' - a new hazard to health," by Materson, B.J., and Barrett-Connor, E. JOURNAL OF THE AMERICAN MEDICAL ASSOCIATION. 200(12):1126-1127, 1967.

"LSD: the search for definite conclusions." JOURNAL OF THE AMERICAN MEDICAL ASSOCIATION. 196(suppl.):32-33, 1966.

"LSD used as an analgesic," by Kast, E.C. JOURNAL OF THE AMERICAN MEDICAL ASSOCIATION. 187:33, Jan. 4, 1964.

"Lack of cross-tolerance in rats among (-)Δ^9-trans-tetra-hydrocannabinol (Δ^9-THC), cannabis extract, mescaline and lysergic acid diethylamide (LSD-25)," by Silva, M.T., et al. PSYCHOPHARMACOLOGIA. 13(4):332-340, 1968.

"Leukocytes of human exposed to lysergic acid diethylamide: lack of chromosomal damage," by Loughman, W.D., et al. SCIENCE. 158:508-510, Oct., 1967.

"Liver function and pyrexia caused by a pyrogen from Escherichia coli, lysergic acid dirthylamide and dinitrophenol," by Venulet, J., and Desperak-Naciazek, A. JOURNAL OF PHARMACY AND PHARMACOLOGY. 18:38-40, 1966.

"Long-lasting effects of LSD on normals," by McGlothlin, W.H., et al. ARCHIVES OF GENERAL PSYCHIATRY. 17:521-532, 1967.

"Lysergic acid diethylamide (LSD-25) and ego functions," by Klee, Gerald D. ARCHIVES OF GENERAL PSYCHIATRY. 8(5):461-474, May, 1963.

"Lysergic acid diethylamide (LSD-25) and schizophrenic reactions," by Langs, R.J., and Barr, H.L. JOURNAL OF NERVOUS AND MENTAL DISEASE. 147(2):163-172, 1968.

"Lysergic acid diethylamide and sexual dominance behavior of the male rat," by Uyeno, Edward T. INTERNATIONAL JOURNAL OF NEUROPSYCHIATRY. 3(2):188-190, 1967.

"Lysergic acid diethylamide (LSD-25) as a facilitating agent in psychotherapy," by Chandler, Arthur L., and Hartman, Mortimer A. AMERICAN MEDICAL ASSOCIATION ARCHIVES OF GENERAL PSYCHIATRY. 2:286-299, 1960.

"Lysergic acid diethylamide (LSD-25): comparison by questionnaire of psychotomimetic activities of congeners on normal subjects and drug addicts." JOURNAL OF MENTAL SCIENCE. 106:1120, 1960.

"Lysergic acid diethylamide (LSD-25): XXXVI. Comparison of effect of methysergide (UML491) on goldfish and Siamese fighting fish," by Gettner, H.H., et al. JOURNAL OF PSYCHOLOGY. 61(1):87-92, 1965.

"Lysergic acid diethylamide (LSD-25): XXXIV. Comparison with effect of psilocybin on the Siamese fighting fish," by Abramson, Harold A. JOURNAL OF PSYCHOLOGY. 56(2):363-374, 1963.

"Lysergic acid diethylamide: its effects on a male Asiatic elephant," by West, L.J., and Pierce, C.M. SCIENCE. 138:1100, 1962.

"Lysergic acid diethylamide: mutagenic effects in drosophila," by Browning, L.S. SCIENCE. 161:1022-1023, 1968.

"Lysergic acid diethylamide (LSD): no teratogenicity in rats," by Warkang, J., and Takacs, E. SCIENCE. 159 (3816):731-732, 1968.

"Lysergide in the treatment of neurosis (a report of two cases)," by Denson, R. DISEASES OF THE NERVOUS SYSTEM. 27(8):511-514, 1966

"Mental age regression induced by lysergic acid diethylamide," by Lienert, G. JOURNAL OF PSYCHOLOGY. 63:3-11, 1966.

"Modification of aggressive behavior of green sunfish with

70

d-lysergic acid diethylamide," by McDonald, Arthur L., and Heimstra, Norman W. JOURNAL OF PSYCHOLOGY. 57(1): 19-23, 1964.
"Modification of autistic behavior with LSD-25," by Simmons, James Q., et al. AMERICAN JOURNAL OF PSYCHIATRY. 122 (11):1201-1211, 1966.
"Modification of the effect of some central stimulants in mice pretreated with a-methyl-1-tyrosine," by Menon, M.K., et al. PSYCHOPHARMACOLOGIA. 10(5):437-444, 1967.
"Modifications in the technique of LSD therapy," by Spencer, A.M. COMPREHENSIVE PSYCHIATRY. 5(4):232-252,1964.
"Nature and frequency of claims following LSD," by Ditman, K.S., et al. JOURNAL OF NERVOUS AND MENTAL DISEASE. 134:346-352, 1962.
"New developments in metabolism of mescaline and related amines," by Friedhoff, A.J., and Goldstein, M. ANNALS OF THE NEW YORK ACADEMY OF SCIENCE. 96:5-13, 1962.
"New psychotropic agents. Analogs of amitriptyline containing the normeperidine group," by Davis, M.A., et al. JOURNAL OF MEDICINAL CHEMISTRY. 10(4):627-635, 1967.
"Nitrous oxide inhalation as a fad. Dangers in uncontrolled sniffing for psychedelic effect," by Dillon, J.B. CALIFORNIA MEDICINE. 106:444-446, June, 1967.
"Observations on direct and cross-tolerance with LSD and d-amphetamine in man," by Rosenberg, D.E., et al. PSYCHOPHARMACOLOGIA. 5:1, 1963.
"Observations regarding the use of LSD-25 in the treatment of alcoholism," by Cheek, Frances E., et al. JOURNAL OF PSYCHOPHARMACOLOGY. 1(2):56-74, 1966.
"On addiction research center inventory scores of former addicts receiving LSD and untreated schizophrenics, by Haertzen, C.A. PSYCHOLOGICAL REPORTS. 14(2):483, 1964.
"On the similarity between hypnotic and mescaline hallucinations," by Halpern, Seymour. INTERNATIONAL JOURNAL OF CLINICAL AND EXPERIMENTAL HYPNOSIS. 9:139-149, 1961.
"Our experiences with individual and group psychotherapy with the aid of LSD," by Dolezal, V., and Hausner, M. ACTIVITAS NERVOSA SUPERIOR. 4(2):241-242, 1962.
"Paradoxical responses to chlorpromazine after LSD," by Schwarz, Conrad J. PSYCHOSOMATICS. 8(4, pt.1):210-211, 1967.
"Peak experiences: investigation of their relationship to psychedelic therapy and self-actualization," by Klavetter, R.E., and Mogar, R.E. JOURNAL OF HUMANISTIC PSYCHOLOGY. 7(2):171-177, 1967.
"Persistence of lysergic acid diethylamide in the plasma of human subjects," by Aghajanian, G.K., and Bing, O.H.L. CLINICAL PHARMACOLOGY AND THERAPEUTICS. 5:611, 1964.
"Persistent hallucinosis following repeated administration of hallucinogenic drugs," by Rosenthal, Saul H. AMERICAN JOURNAL OF PSYCHIATRY. 121(3):238-244, 1964.
"Personality and psychodysleptic experience: an experimental study," by Dolezal, V., and Hausner, M. PSYCHOTHERAPY AND PSYCHOSOMATICS. 15(1):17, 1967.

"Personality change associated with psychedelic (LSD) therapy: a preliminary report," by Mogar, Robert E., and Savage, Charles. PSYCHOTHERAPY: THEORY, RESEARCH AND PRACTICE. 1(4):154-162, 1964.
"Perspectives in psychedelic research," by Metzner, R., Alpert, R., and Weil, G. PSYCHIATRIC OPINION. v.1, no.1, 1964.
"Pharmacologic influences on mating behavior in the male rat," by Bignami, G. PSYCHOPHARMACOLOGIA. 10(1):44-58, 1966.
"Pharmacological characterization and detection of hallucinogenic substances. I. Hyperthermic action in the rabbit," by Jacob, J. ARCHIVES INTERNATIONALES DE PHARMACODYNAMIE ET DE THERAPIE. 145:528-545, 1963.
"The pharmacology of psychedelic drugs," by Metzner, R. PSYCHEDELIC REVIEW. no. 1:69-100, June, 1963.
"The pharmacology of the psychoactive drugs," by Cohen, S. NORTHWEST MEDICINE. 65:197-203, 1966.
"Placebo reactions in a study of lysergic acid diethylamide (LSD-25)," by Linton, H.B., and Langs, R.J. ARCHIVES OF GENERAL PSYCHIATRY. 6(5):369-383, 1962.
"A possible correlation between drug-induced hallucinations in man and a behavioural response in mice," by Corne, S.J., and Pickering, R.W. PSYCHOPHARMACOLOGIA. 11(1): 67-78, 1967
"Practical experiences with hallucinogens in psychotherapy," by Hausner, M., and Dolezal, V. CESKOSLOVENSKA PSYCHIATRIE. 59(5):328-335, 1963.
"Preliminary method for study of LSD with children," by Rolo, Andre., et al. INTERNATIONAL JOURNAL OF NEUROPSYCHIATRY. 1(6):552-555, 1965.
"Prolonged adverse reactions from unsupervised use of hallucinogenic drugs," by Kleber, H.D. JOURNAL OF NERVOUS AND MENTAL DISEASE. 144:308-319, 1967.
"Prolonged effects of LSD on EEG records during discriminative performance in cat; evaluation by computer analysis," by Adey, W.R., et al. ELECTROENCEPHALOGRAPHY AND CLINICAL NEUROPHYSIOLOGY. 18(1):25-35, 1965.
"Psychedelic agents in creative problem-solving : a pilot study," by Harman, W.W., et al. PSYCHOLOGICAL REPORTS. 19:211-227, 1966.
"Psychedelic research in the context of contemporary psychology," by Mogar, Robert E. PSYCHEDELIC REVIEW. no. 8:96-104, 1966.
"Psychedelic therapy utilizing LSD in the treatment of the alcoholic patient. A preliminary report," by Kurland, A.A., et al. AMERICAN JOURNAL OF PSYCHIATRY. 123(10): 1202-1209, Nov., 1967.
"Psychodynamics of chronic lysergic acid diethylamide use," by Welpton, Douglas F. JOURNAL OF NERVOUS AND MENTAL DISEASE. 147(4):377-385, 1968.
"Psychological and drug variables in the LSD experiences of alcoholics," by Ditman, K.S., et al. PSYCHOTHERAPY AND PSYCHOSOMATICS. 15(1):15, 1967.

"Psychomycology: an interdisciplinary application of symbolism," by Boyd, Stuart, and Roberts, Alan H. AMERICAN PSYCHOLOGIST. 18(3):154-159, 1963.
"Psychopathology of LSD intoxication," by Kuramochi, Hiroshi, and Takahashi, Ryo. ARCHIVES OF GENERAL PSYCHIATRY. 11(2):151-161, 1964.
"The psychopharmacological revolution," by Jarvik, Murray E. PSYCHOLOGY TODAY. 1(1):51-59, 1967.
"Psychopharmacology and psychiatry - towards a classification of psychotropic drugs," by Delay, Jean. BULLETIN ON NARCOTICS. 19(1):1-5, Jan.-Mar., 1967.
"The psychopharmacology of hallucinogenic agents," by Freedman, D.X. ANNUAL REVIEW OF MEDICINE. 20:419-428, 1969.
"Psychophysiological effects of a large non-experimental dose of LSD-25," by Reynolds, H.H., and Peterson, G.K. PSYCHOLOGICAL REPORTS. 19(1):287-290, 1966.
"Psychotherapy under the influence of hallucinogens," by Leuner, H., and Holfeld, H. THE PHYSICIAN'S PANORAMA. 2:13, 1964.
"Psychotomimetic drugs and brain biogenic amines," by Freedman, D.X. AMERICAN JOURNAL OF PSYCHIATRY. 119:843, 1963.
"Reactions to psilocybin administered in a supportive environment," by Leary, T., et al. JOURNAL OF NERVOUS AND MENTAL DISEASE. 137(6):561-573, 1963.
"Regional localization of lysergic acid diethylamide in monkey brain," by Snyder, S.H., and Reivich, M. NATURE. 209:1093, 1966.
"The relation of expectation and mood to psilocybin reactions: a questionnaire study," by Metzner, Ralph, et al. PSYCHEDELIC REVIEW. no. 5:3-39, 1965.
"The relationship between serotonin antagonism and tranquilizing activity," by Gallant, D.M., et al. AMERICAN JOURNAL OF PSYCHIATRY. 119:882, 1963.
"Reports of wives of alcoholics of effects of LSD-25 treatment of their husbands," by Sarett, Mary, et al. ARCHIVES OF GENERAL PSYCHIATRY. 14(2):171-178, 1966.
"Research on the effects of isolation on cognitive functioning," by Holt, Robert R., and Goldberger, Leo. UNITED STATES AIR FORCE WRIGHT AIR DEVELOPMENT DIVISION TECHNICAL REPORT. no. 60-260, iii 22p., 1960.
"Retinal effects of high doses of LSD in the cat," by Schwartz, A.S. EXPERIMENTAL NEUROLOGY. 13(3):273-282, 1965.
"Retrospective alterations of the LSD-25 experience," by Linton, Harriet B., et al. JOURNAL OF NERVOUS AND MENTAL DISEASE. 138(5):409-423, 1964.
"Review of the evidence and qualifications regarding the effects of hallucinogenic drugs on chromosomes and embryos," by Houston, Kent. AMERICAN JOURNAL OF PSYCHIATRY. 126(2):251-254, Aug., 1969.
"The role of hallucinogens in depersonalization and allied syndromes," by De-Groot, M. PROCEEDINGS OF THE ROYAL MEDICOPSYCHOLOGICAL ASSOCIATION. pp. 97-100, 1963.
"The role of mescaline and d-lysergic acid in psychiatric

treatment," by Malitz, S. DISEASES OF THE NERVOUS SYS-
TEM. 27(7):39-42, 1966.
"The search for person-world isomorphism," by Murphy, Gard-
ner, and Cohen, Sidney. MAIN CURRENTS IN MODERN THOUGHT.
22(2):31-34, 1965.
"Self administration of minor tranquilizers as a function
of conditioning," by Harris, R.T., et al. PSYCHOPHARMA-
COLOGIA. 13(1):81-88, 1968.
"Serotonin binding to nerve ending particles of the rat
brain and its inhibition by LSD," by Marchbanks, R.M.,
et al. SCIENCE. 144:1135-1137, 1964.
"Serotonin release from brain slices by electrical stimulation: regional differences and effect of LSD," by
Chase, Thomas N., et al. SCIENCE. 157(3795):1461-4163,
1967.
"The significance of the temporal lobes and of hemispheric
dominance in the production of the LSD-25 symptomatology
in man: a study of epileptic patients before and after
temporal lobectomy," by Serafetinides, E.A. NEUROPSY-
CHOLOGIA. 3(1):69-79, 1965.
"Some comments concerning dosage levels of psychedelic com-
pounds for psychotherapeutic experiences," by Fisher,
Gary M. PSYCHEDELIC REVIEW. 1:209-218, Fall, 1963.
"Some effects of hallucinogenic drugs on electrical activity of the visual pathways of cats," by Apter, J.T., and
Pfeiffer, C.C. AMERICAN JOURNAL OF OPHTHALMOLOGY. 43:
206, 1960.
"Some effects of hallucinogenic morning-glory seeds on the
behavior of rats," by Gutherz, Keith, and Sperling, Sally
E. PSYCHOLOGICAL REPORTS. 19(3, pt.1):949-950, 1966.
"Some effects of LSD-25 on verbal communications," by Amar-
el, M., and Cheek, F.E. JOURNAL OF ABNORMAL PSYCHOLOGY.
70:453-456, 1965.
"Some effects of lysergic acid diethylamide on visual dis-
crimination in pigeons," by Becker, D.I., et al. PSY-
CHOPHARMACOLOGIA. 11(4):354-364, 1967.
"Some effects of the therapist's LSD experience on his work,"
by Kafka, J.S., and Gaarder, K.R. AMERICAN JOURNAL OF
PSYCHOTHERAPY. 18(20):236-243, 1964.
"Some narcotic antagonists in the benzomorphan series," by
Harris, L.C., and Pierson, A.K. JOURNAL OF PHARMACOLOGY
AND EXPERIMENTAL THERAPEUTICS. 143:141-148, 1964.
"Some observations on the resistance to the use of LSD in
psychotherapy," by Stern, Harold R. PSYCHEDELIC REVIEW.
no. 8:105-110, 1966.
"Some observations on the use of psychiatric drugs," by
Simons, J.E. ROCKY MOUNTAIN MEDICAL JOURNAL. 59:30-33,
1962.
"Some views of the formation of symptoms during alalytical
psychotherapy with the use of LSD," by Tautermann, P.
PSYCHOTHERAPY AND PSYCHOSOMATICS. 15(1):65, 1967.
"Stability of earliest memories under LSD-25 and placebo,"
by Langs, Robert J. JOURNAL OF NERVOUS AND MENTAL DI-
SEASE. 144(3):171-184, 1967.

"Standardization of scales which evaluate subjective effects of morphine, amphetamine, pentobarbital, alcohol, LSD-25, pyrahexl and chlorpromazine." PSYCHOPHARMACOLOGIA. 4(3):184-205, 1963.
"Structure-activity relationship studies on mescaline: II. Tolerance and cross-tolerance between mescaline and its analogues in the rat," by Smythies, J.R., et al. PSYCHO-PHARMACOLOGIA. 9(5):434-446, 1966.
"Structure-activity relationship studies on mescaline: III. The influence of the methoxy groups," by Smythies, J.R., et al. PSYCHOPHARMACOLOGIA. 10(5):379-387, 1967.
"Studies on alcoholism and LSD: I. The influence of therapist attitudes on treatment outcome," by Ludwig, Arnold M. AMERICAN JOURNAL OF ORTHOPSYCHIATRY. 37(2):212-213, 1967.
"Studies on mescaline: the effect of prior administration of various psychotropic drugs on different biochemical parameters. A preliminary report," by Dember, Herman C.B., et al. ANNALS OF THE NEW YORK ACADEMY OF SCIENCES. 96:14-36, 1962.
"Studies on the effects of drugs on performance of a delayed discrimination," by Roberts, M.H., and Bradley, P.B. PHYSIOLOGY AND BEHAVIOR. 2(4):389-397, 1967.
"Studies on the specificity of narcotic antagonists," by Foldes, F., et al. ANESTHESIOLOGY. 26:320-328, 1965.
"Study of lysergic acid diethylamide as an analgesic agent," by Kast, E.C., and Collins, V.J. ANAESTHESIA AND ANALGESIA; CURRENT RESEARCHES. 43(3):285-291, 1964.
"Temporal effects of LSD-25 and epinephrine on verbal behavior," by Honingfeld, Gilbert. NEWSLETTER FOR RESEARCH IN PSYCHOLOGY. 6(3):15-17, 1964; also in: JOURNAL OF ABNORMAL PSYCHOLOGY. 70(4):303-306, 1965.
"Ten months experience with LSD users admitted to county psychiatric receiving hospital," by Blumenfield, M., et al. NEW YORK STATE JOURNAL OF MEDICINE. 67:1849-1853, Jul. 1, 1967.
"Teratogenic property of LSD." BULLETIN ON NARCOTICS. 20 (2):8, Apr.-June, 1968.
"Theoretical aspects of LSD therapy," by Buchman, John. INTERNATIONAL JOURNAL OF SOCIAL PSYCHIATRY. 13(2):126-138, 1967.
"Therapeutic effect of LSD: a follow-up study," by Shagass, C., and Bittle, R.M. JOURNAL OF NERVOUS AND MENTAL DISEASE. 144(6):471-478, 1967.
"Time-series, frequency analysis, and electrogenesis of the EEG's of normals and psychotics before and after drugs," by Pfeiffer, Carl C., et al. AMERICAN JOURNAL OF PSYCHIATRY. 121(12):1147-1155, 1965.
"Tolerance and cross-tolerance among psychotomimetic drugs," by Appel, J.B., and Freedman, D.X. PSYCHOPHARMACOLOGIA. 13(3):267-274, 1968.
"Tolerance to LSD-25 in schizophrenic subjects," by Chessick, Richard D., et al. ARCHIVES OF GENERAL PSYCHIATRY. 10(6):653-658, 1964.

"Toxic effect of stramonium simulating LSD trip," by Di
Giacomo, Joseph N. JOURNAL OF THE AMERICAN MEDICAL
ASSOCIATION. 204(3):265-267, 1968.
"The treatment of alcoholics with psychedelic drugs," by
Metzner R., and editors of Psychedelic Review. PSYCHE-
DELIC REVIEW. no. 1:205-207, Fall, 1963.
"Treatment of alcoholism with lysergide," by Van Dusen, W.,
et al. QUARTERLY JOURNAL OF STUDIES ON ALCOHOL. 28(2):
295-304, 1967.
"The treatment of frigidity with LSD and ritalin," by Ling,
Thomas M., and Buckman, John. PSYCHEDELIC REVIEW. 1:
450-458, 1964.
"Two cases of altered consciousness with amnesia apparently
telepathically induced," by Paul, Margaret A. PSYCHEDEL-
IC REVIEW. no. 8:4-8, 1966.
"2,5-Dimethoxy-4-methylamphetamine (STP): a new hallucinogenic drug," by Snyder, S.H., et al. SCIENCE. 158:669-
670, Nov., 1967.
"Unpublicized hallucinogens - the dangerous Belladonna al-
kaloids (clinical note)," by Muller, D.J. JOURNAL OF
THE AMERICAN MEDICAL ASSOCIATION. 202(7):650-651, 1967.
"Untoward reactions to lysergic acid diethylamide (LSD) re-
sulting in hospitalization," by Frosch, W.A., et al.
NEW ENGLAND JOURNAL OF MEDICINE. 273:1235-1239, 1965.
"Urinary catecholamine excretion following lysergic acid
diethylamide in man," by Hollister, Leo E., and Moore,
Francis. PSYCHOPHARMACOLOGIA. 11(3):270-275, 1967.
"The use of LSD-25 in psychotherapy. An evaluation," by
Solursh, L.P. INTERNATIONAL JOURNAL OF NEUROPSYCHIATRY.
2(6):651-656, 1966.
"The use of LSD-25 in psychotherapy and some ideas on its
function in drug addiction," by Cutner, Margot. PSYCHO-
THERAPY AND PSYCHOSOMATICS. 15(1):14, 1967.
"The use of lysergic acid diethylamide in psychotherapy,"
by Baker, E.F.W. CANADIAN MEDICAL ASSOCIATION JOURNAL.
91:1200, 1964.
"The use of lysergic acid in individual psychotherapy," by
Ling, and Buckman. PROCEEDINGS OF THE ROYAL SOCIETY OF
MEDICINE. 53:927, 1960.
"A uterine stimulant effect of extracts of morning glory
seeds," by Der Marderosian, Ara H., et al. PSYCHEDELIC
REVIEW. no. 1:317-323, 1964.
"The witnesses: a schizophrenic patient's experience and
its relevance to psychiatry," by Osmond, Humphry. INTER-
NATIONAL JOURNAL OF PARAPSYCHOLOGY. 8(3):445-464, 1966.

MARIJUANA: Books and Essays

Aberle, D.F. THE PEYOTE RELIGION AMONG THE NAVAHO. Chicago: Aldine Press, 1966.

76

Abrams, S. "The Oxford scene and the law," THE BOOK OF GRASS, ed. G. Andrews, and S. Vinkenoog. New York: Grove Press, 1967, pp. 235-242.

Adams, R. "Marijuana," THE BOOK OF GRASS, ed. G. Andrews, and S. Vinkenoog. New York: Grove Press, 1967, pp. 150-152.

Aitken, D. GOING TO POT? (From 9th annual conference of the Student Humanist Federation, Jan., 1968). London: Student Humanist Federation, 1968.

Aldrich, M. DRUGS: A SEMINAR. Buffalo: Lemar-Sunyab, 1967.

American Medical Association. Committee on Alcoholism and Drug Dependence. Council on Mental Health. THE CRUTCH THAT CRIPPLES. Chicago: American Medical Association, 1968.

Andrews, G. "Steady roll," THE BOOK OF GRASS, ed G. Andrews, and S. Vinkenoog. New York: Grove Press, 1967, pp. 89-93.

Andrews, George, and Vinkenoog, S. THE BOOK OF GRASS: an anthology on Indian hemp. New York: Grove Press, 1967.

Anslinger, H., and Oursler F. THE MURDERERS. New York: Farrar,Straus, 1961.

Basham, A. "Soma," THE BOOK OF GRASS, ed. G. Andrews, and S. Vinkenoog. New York: Grove Press, 1967, pp. 1-3.

Battista, O. MENTAL DRUGS: chemistry's challenge to psychotherapy. Philadelphia: Chilton, 1960.

Baudelaire, C. "Concerning hasish," THE BOOK OF GRASS, ed. G. Andrews, and S. Vinkenoog. New York: Grove Press, 1967, pp. 38-44.

Baytop, T. MEDICINAL AND TOXIC PLANTS OF TURKEY. Istanbul: University of Istanbul, 1963.

Becker, H. "Becoming a marihuana user," NARCOTIC ADDICTION, ed. J. O'Donnell, and J. Ball. New York: Harper and Row, 1966, pp. 109-122.

Becker, H. THE OUTSIDERS: studies in the sociology of deviance. Glencoe: Free Press of Glencoe, 1963.

Benetowa, S. "Tracing one word through different languages: names of the plant," THE BOOK OF GRASS, ed. G. Andrews, and S. Vinkenoog. New York: Grove Press, 1967, pp. 15-18.

Bestic, A. TURN ME ON, MAN. London:Randem, 1966.

Bier, W. PROBLEMS IN ADDICTION: alcohol and drug addiction. New York: Fordham University Press, 1962.

Bischoff, William H. THE ECSTASY DRUGS. Delray Beach, Florida: University Circle Press, 1966.

Bloomquist, E.R. MARIJUANA. New York: Glencoe Press, 1968.

Blum, Richard H. "A history of cannabis," SOCIETY AND DRUGS. San Francisco: Jossey-Bass, 1969, pp. 61-84.

Blum, Richard, et al. UTOPIATES: the use and users of LSD-25. New York: Atherton Press, 1964.

Blumer, H., et al. THE WORLD OF YOUTHFUL DRUG USE. Berkeley: School of Criminology, University of California, 1967.

Boericke. "Materia Medica (a dictionary of hemeopathic substances)," THE BOOK OF GRASS, ed. G. Andrews, and S. Vinkenoog. New York: Grove Press, 1967, pp. 149-150.

Boughey, H. "Pot scenes east and west," MARIHUANA: myths

and realities, ed. J. Simmons. North Hollywood: Brandon House, 1967.

Bowles, P. A HUNDRED CAMELS IN THE COURTYARD. San Francisco: City Lights Books, 1962.

Bowles, P. "Kif: prologue and compendium of terms," THE BOOK OF GRASS, ed. G. Andrews, and S. Vinkenoog. New York: Grove Press, 1967, pp. 108-114.

Bowles, P. "The story of Lahcen and Idir," THE MARIHUANA PAPERS, ed. D. Solomon. Indianapolis: Bobbs-Merrill, 1966, pp. 163-170.

Bruin Humanist Forum. Issues Study Committee. DOCUMENTED FACTS ABOUT MARIJUANA: first preliminary draft. Los Angeles: Bruin Humanist Forum, Spring, 1966.

Bruin Humanist Forum. Issues Study Committee. DOCUMENTED FACTS ABOUT MARIJUANA: second preliminary draft. Los Angeles: Bruin Humanist Forum, Nov., 1966.

Bruin Humanist Forum. Issues Study Committee. MARIJUANA (CANNABIS) FACT SHEET. Los Angeles: Bruin Humanist Forum, 1967.

Budzikiewicz, H., et al. INTERPRETATION OF MASS SPECTRA OF ORGANIC COMPOUNDS. San Francisco: Holden-Day, 1964.

Burroughs, W. "Points of distinction between sedative and consciousness-expanding drugs," THE MARIHUANA PAPERS, ed. D. Solomon. Indianapolis: Bobbs-Merrill, 1966, pp. 388-393.

Carey, James T. THE COLLEGE DRUG SCENE. Englewood Cliffs, New Jersey: Prentice-Hall, 1968.

Cholst, S. "Notes on the use of hashish," THE MARIHUANA PAPERS, ed. D. Solomon. Indianapolis: Bobbs-Merrill, 1966, pp. 217-223.

Christozov, C. THE MAROCCAN ASPECT OF CANNABIS INTOXICATION BASED ON STUDIES OF CHRONIC MENTAL PATIENTS. Chicago: Special Libraries Association Translations Center, order no. 68-10338-06E, 1968.

Claus, E., and Tyler, V., Jr. PHARMACOGNOSY. Philadelphia: Lea and Febiger, 1965, pp. 243-246.

Clay, M. "Fragments from a search," THE BOOK OF GRASS, ed. G. Andrews, and S. Vinkenoog. New York: Grove Press, 1967, pp. 18-19.

Cortez, L., Jr., et al. ANALGESIC PROPERTIES OF CANNABIS PREPARATIONS AND TETRAHYDROCANNABINOL. Sao Paulo: International Pharmacological Conference (24-30 July, 1966) Abstracts, 1966.

Davies, A. "Nigeria whispers," THE BOOK OF GRASS, ed. G. Andrews, and S. Vinkenoog. New York: Grove Press, 1967, pp. 229-230.

Dosick, M. DRUG ABUSE IN TERMS OF THE FUNCTIONS OF SOCIAL DEVIANCE AND SOCIAL CONTROL. Carbondale: Southern Illinois University Delinquency Study Project, 26-30 June, 1967.

Ebin, D., ed. THE DRUG EXPERIENCE: first-person accounts of addicts, writers, scientists, and others. New York: Orion Press, 1961.

Eldridge, W. NARCOTICS AND THE LAW: A critique of the American experiments in narcotic drug control. New York:

New York University Press, 1962.
Eliade, M. "Ancient Scythia and Iran," THE BOOK OF GRASS, ed. G. Andrews, and S. Vinkenoog. New York: Grove Press, 1967, pp. 11-13.
Farmilo, C., and Davis, T. MARIHUANA IDENTIFICATION. London: Proceedings of the Third International Meeting (16-24 April, 1963) of Forensic Medicine, Immunology, Pathology, and Toxicology, 1963, pp. 1-19.
Farmilo, C. A REVIEW OF SOME RECENT RESULTS ON THE CHEMICAL ANALYSIS OF CANNABIS. United Nations: UN Document St-Soa-Ser. S-4, 1961.
Flynn, E. "Diego Rivera," THE BOOK OF GRASS, ed. G. Andrews, and S. Vinkenoog. New York: Grove Press, 1967, pp. 82-85.
Garattini, S. "Effects of a cannabis extract on gross behavior," HASHISH: its chemistry and pharmacology (Ciba Foundation Study Group 21, 21 October, 1964), ed. G. Wolstenholme, and J. Knight. London: J. and A. Churchill, 1965, pp. 70-82.
Gautier, T., tr. R. Gladstone. "The hashish club," THE MARIHUANA PAPERS, ed. D. Solomon. Indianapolis: Bobbs-Merrill, 1966, pp. 121-135.
Geller, Allen, and Boas, Maxwell. DRUG BEAT; a complete survey of the history, distribution, uses and abuses of marijuana, LSD, and amphetamines. New York: Cowles Book Company, 1969.
Gimlin, Joan S. LEGALIZATION OF MARIJUANA. Washington: Editorial Research Report, 1967 (v.2, no.6, Aug. 9).
Ginsberg, A. "First manifesto to end the bringdown," THE MARIHUANA PAPERS, ed. D. Solomon. Indianapolis: Bobbs-Merrill, 1966, pp. 183-200.
Ginsberg, A., ed. "Fact sheet: small anthology of footnotes on marijuana," BACKGROUND PAPERS ON STUDENT DRUG INVOLVEMENT, ed C. Hollander. Washington: United States National Student Association, 1967, pp. 9-14.
Ginsberg, A., and Fox, J. "Seminar on marijuana and LSD controls," BACKGROUND PAPERS ON STUDENT DRUG INVOLVEMENT, ed. C. Hollander. Washington: United States National Student Association, 1967, pp. 15-36.
Giordano, Henry L. THE DANGERS OF MARIHUANA...FACTS YOU SHOULD KNOW. Washington: United States Government Printing Office, 1968.
Goldstein, R. 1 IN 7: DRUGS ON CAMPUS. New York: Walker and Company, 1966.
Goldstein, R. "The college scene in the USA," THE BOOK OF GRASS, ed. G. Andrews, and S. Vinkenoog. New York: Grove Press, 1967, pp. 214-218.
Goode, Erich, comp. MARIJUANA. New York: Atherton Press, 1969.
Goodman, L., and Gilman, A. (ed.). THE PHARMACOLOGICAL BASIS OF THERAPEUTICS, 3rd edition. New York: Macmillan, 1965.
Great Britain. Stationery Office. REPORT ON CANNABIS PREPARED BY THE HALLUCINOGENS SUBCOMMITTEE OF THE HOME

OFFICE'S ADVISORY COMMITTEE ON DRUG DEPENDENCE. London: H.M. Stationery Office, 1968.

Grlic, L. A STUDY OF SOME CHEMICAL CHARACTERISTICS OF THE RESIN FROM EXPERIMENTALLY GROWN CANNABIS OF VARIOUS ORI- GINS. United Nations: UN Document St-Soa-Ser. S-10, 1964.

Groff, S. "Marijuana and the 'O' effect," THE BOOK OF GRASS, ed. G. Andrews, and S. Vinkenoog. New York: Grove Press, 1967, pp. 176-177.

Haertzen, C., et al. PREDICTION OF SUBJECTIVE RESPONSES TO DRUGS. San Juan: Presented to Study Group 11 at 5th Annual Meeting of the American College of Neuropsycho- pharmacology, 9 December, 1966.

Haislip, G. CURRENT ISSUES IN THE PREVENTION AND CONTROL OF MARIHUANA ABUSE. Washington: Presented to 1st Nation- al Conference on Student Drug Involvement (NSA sponsored), from United States Bureau of Narcotics, 16 August, 1967.

Harding, E. "The psychological significance of the Soma ritual," THE BOOK OF GRASS, ed. G. Andrews, and S. Vin- kenoog. New York: Grove Press, 1967, pp. 155-160.

Harney, Malachi L. DISCUSSION ON MARIJUANA: moderator's remarks. International Narcotic Enforcement Officer's Association, 8th Annual Conference Report. Louisville, Kentucky, Oct. 22-26, 1967.

Heaton, J. THE EYE: phenomenology and psychology of func- tion and disorder. London: Tavistock, 1968.

Hively, R. THE SYNTHESIS OF AN ISOMER OF TETRAHYDROCAN- NABINOL. Newark, Delaware: University of Delaware, 1962, (thesis).

Hively, R., and Hoffmann, F. UNITED STATES ARMY TECHNICAL REPORT EATR-4002 ON ISOMERS OF TETRAHYDROCANNABINOL. Edgewood, Maryland: United States Chemical/Biological war-weapons plant and arsenal, July, 1966.

Hollander, C., ed. BACKGROUND PAPERS ON STUDENT DRUG IN- VOLVEMENT. Washington: United States National Student Drug Association, 1967.

Huxley, A. "Culture and the individual," THE BOOK OF GRASS, ed. G. Andrews, and S. Vinkenoog. New York: Grove Press, 1967, pp. 192-201.

Huxley, A. ISLAND. New York: Harper and Row, 1962.

Huxley, J. "Psychometabolism," THE BOOK OF GRASS, ed. G. Andrews, and S. Vinkenoog. New York: Grove Press, 1967, pp. 184-192.

Hyde, Margaret O. MIND DRUGS. New York: McGraw-Hill, 1968.

International Narcotic Enforcement Officers Association. NON-NARCOTIC DRUG ABUSE. 5th Annual Conference, 1964, sponsored by Smith, Kline and French laboratories-- Philadelphia, 1965.

Joachimoglu, G. "Natural and smoked hashish," HASHISH: its chemistry and pharmacology (Ciba Foundation Study Group 21, 21 October, 1964), ed. G. Wolstenholme, and J. Knight. London: J. and A. Churchill, 1965, pp. 2-14.

Joyce, C. PSYCHOPHARMACOLOGY: DIMENSIONS AND PERSPECTIVES. London: Tavisock, 1968.

Kalant, Oriana J. AN INTERIM GUIDE TO THE CANNABIS (MARI-

HUANA). Bibliographic series no. 2 of the Addiction Research Foundation. Toronto: 1968.

Keniston, K. THE UNCOMMITTED: alienated youth in American society. New York: Harcourt, Brace and World, 1965.

Kluever, H. MESCAL AND MECHANISMS OF HALLUCINATIONS. Chicago: University of Chicago Press (Phoenix Science Series), 1966.

Korte, F., and Sieper, H. "Recent results of hashish analysis," HASHISH: its chemistry and pharmacology (Ciba Foundation Study Group 21, 21 October, 1964), ed. G. Wolstenholme, and J. Knight. London: J. and A. Churchill, 1965, pp. 15-36.

Kupferberg, T., ed. BIRTH (no. 3). New York: Birth Press, 1960.

La Barre, Weston. THE PEYOTE CULT. New enlarged edition. Hamden, Connecticut: Shoe String Press, 1964.

Laing, R., and Esterson, A. "Two letters," THE BOOK OF GRASS, ed. G. Andrews, and S. Vinkenoog. New York: Grove Press, 1967, pp. 179-181.

Land, Herman W. WHAT YOU CAN DO ABOUT DRUGS AND YOUR CHILD. New York: Hart Pub., 1969.

Lapa, A., and Abreu, L. THIN-LAYER CHROMATOGRAPHY OF CANNABIS AND BIOLOGICAL ASSAYS OF STRIP ELUATES. Sao Paulo: Abstracts of the International Pharmacological Conference, 24-30 July, 1966.

Laurie, Peter. DRUGS: MEDICAL PSYCHOLOGICAL, AND SOCIAL FACTS. Baltimore: Penguin Books, 1967.

Leary, T. "The politics, ethics, and meaning of marijuana," THE MARIHUANA PAPERS, ed. D. Solomon. Indianapolis: Bobbs-Merrill, 1966, pp. 82-99.

Leary, Timothy, and Alpert, R. "The politics of consciousness expansion," THE BOOK OF GRASS, ed. G. Andrews, and S. Vinkenoog. New York: Grove Press, 1967, PP. 208-210.

Leech, K., and Jordan B. DRUGS FOR YOUNG PEOPLE: THEIR USE AND MISUSE. Oxford: Religious Education Press, 1967.

Lemar-Detroit. THE CASE FOR THE RE-LEGALIZATION OF MARIJUANA. Detroit: Lemar-Detroit, 1966.

Lemar-SUNYAB. LEMAR-SUNYAB INFORMATION KIT. Buffalo: Lemar-SUNYAB, Box 71, Norton Hall, State University of New YORK at Buffalo.

Lerner, M., and Zeffert, J. "Determination of tetrahydrocannabinol isomers in marihuana and hashish." Baltimore: United States Customs Laboratory, 30 November, 1966.

Lewin, Lewis. "Indian hemp: cannabis indica," PHANTASTICA, by Lewis Lewin. New York: Dutton, 1964, pp. 107-123.

Lewis, B. THE ASSASSINS. New York: Basic Books, 1968.

Lindesmith, A. THE ADDICT AND THE LAW. Bloomington: Indiana University Press, 1965.

Lipton, L. "The holy barbarians," THE BOOK OF GRASS, ed. G. Andrews, and S. Vinkenoog. New York: Grove Press, 1967, p. 211.

Louria, D. NIGHTMARE DRUGS. New York: Pocket Books, 1966.

Lucena, J. "La symptomatologie du cannabisme," PROCEEDINGS OF THE 3RD WORLD CONGRESS OF PSYCHIATRY, v.1, ed.

R. Cleghorn, et al. Montreal-Toronto: University of Toronto Press and University of Montreal Press, 1962, pp. 401-406.

Ludlow, F. "Selections from 'The hasheesh eater'," THE MARIHUANA PAPERS, ed. D. Solomon. Indianapolis: Bobbs-Merrill, 1966, pp. 147-170.

MacDonald A. "Chairman's concluding remarks," HASHISH: its chemistry and pharmacology (Ciba Foundation Study Group 21, 21 October, 1964), ed. G. Wolstenholme, and G. Knight. London: J. and A. Churchill, 1965, p. 93.

Mc-Glothlin, W. "Cannabis: a reference," THE MARIHUANA PAPERS, ed. D. Solomon. Indianapolis: Bobbs-Merrill, 1966, pp. 401-416.

Mc-Glothlin, W. "Cannabis intoxication and its similarity to peyote and LSD," THE BOOK OF GRASS, ed. G. Andrews, and S. Vinkenoog. New York: Grove Press, 1967, pp. 165-176.

Mc-Glothlin, W. HALLUCINOGENIC DRUGS: a perspective with special reference to peyote and cannabis. Santa Monica: Rand Corporation Monograph, 1964, 81 pp.

Mc-Glothlin, W. "Toward a rational view of marijuana," MARIJUANA: MYTHS AND REALITIES. North Hollywood: Brandon House, 1967, pp. 163-214.

Mac-Kenzie, H. DREAMS AND DREAMING. London: Aldous Books, 1965.

Mandel, J. "Myths and realities of marihuana pushing," MARIJUANA: MYTHS AND REALITIES, ed. J. Simmons. North Hollywood: Brandon House, 1967, pp. 58-110.

Mandelkorn, Philip. "The drugs they use," THE HIPPIES, ed. J.D. Brown. New York: Time, 1967, pp. 171-184.

Masters, R., and Houston, J. PSYCHEDELIC ART. New York: Grove Press, 1968.

Masters, R., and Houston, J. THE VARIETIES OF PSYCHEDELIC EXPERIENCE. New York: Holt, Rinehart and Winston, 1966.

Michaux, Henri. LIGHT THROUGH DARKNESS. New York: Orion Press, 1963.

Milford, E. A STATISTICAL STUDY OF A MARIJUANA SUBCULTURE. Cambridge, Massachusetts: Social Relations Department, Harvard University, 1967.

Miller, D. "Narcotic drug and marijuana controls," BACKGROUND PAPERS ON STUDENT DRUG INVOLVEMENT, ed. C. Hollander. Washington: United States National Student Association, 1967, pp. 137-144.

Miras, C.J. "Some aspects of cannabis action," HASHISH: its chemistry and pharmacology (Ciba Foundation Study Group 21, 21 October, 1964), ed. G. Wolstenholme, and J. Knight. London: A. and J. Churchill, 1965, pp. 37-53.

Nowlis, Helen H. DRUGS ON THE COLLEGE CAMPUS. Garden City, New York: Doubleday, 1968.

Oursler, Will. MARIJUANA: THE FACTS, THE TRUTH. New York: Paul S. Eriksson, 1968.

Pauly, Adrienne. "The drug they use," THE HIPPIES, ed. J.D. Brown. Time, 1967, pp. 184-192.

Polsky, Ned. "The village beat scene: summer 1960," HUST-

LERS, BEATS AND OTHERS. Chicago: Aldine Publishing Company, 1967, pp. 150-185.
Regardie, I. ROLL AWAY THE STONE: an introduction to Aleister Crowley's essays on the psychology of hashish. St. Paul: Llewellyn Publishing, 1968.
Rose, P. THE HASHISH COOKBOOK. Los Angeles: Gnaoua Press, 1966.
—Rosevear, J. POT: A handbook of marijuana. New Hyde Park, New York: University Books, 1967.
Saltman, Jules. WHAT ABOUT MARIJUANA? New York: Public Affairs Committee, 1969, pamphlet no. 436.
Simmons, J.L., and Winograd, B. IT'S HAPPENING. Santa Barbara, California: Marc-Laird Publications, 1967.
Simmons, J.L. MARIHUANA: MYTHS AND REALITIES. North Hollywood: Brandon House, 1967.
Solomon, D., ed. THE MARIHUANA PAPERS. Indianapolis: Bobbs-Merrill, 1966.
Southern, T. RED-DIRT MARIJUANA AND OTHER TASTES. New York: New American Library (Signet), 1968.
Steinbeck, John. IN TOUCH. New York: Knopf, 1969.
—Surface, William. THE POISONED IVY. New York: Coward-McCann, 1968.
Taylor, Norman. "The pleasant assassin: the story of marihuana," NARCOTICS: NATURE'S DANGEROUS GIFTS. New York: Dell Publishing Company, 1966, pp. 7-28.
→United Nations. Economic and Social Council. THE QUESTION OF CANNABIS: CANNABIS BIBLIOGRAPHY. United Nations: Office of Public Information, 1965.
United States Congress. House. Committee on Government Operations. Intergovernmental Relations Subcommittee. PROBLEMS RELATING TO THE CONTROL OF MARIHUANA. Hearings before a subcommittee of the Committee on Government Operations, House of Representatives, 90th Congress, Second Session, Nov. 14 and 15, 1967. Washington: United States Government Printing Office, 1968.
—United States Department of Health, Education and Welfare. MARIHUANA; some questions and answers (Public Health Service Publication #1829). Washington: United States Government Printing Office, 1969.
United States National Student Association. MARIJUANA WHITE PAPER. Washington: United States National Student Association, 1968.
United States Senate. Committee on the Judiciary. JUVENILE DELINQUENCY: hearings pursuant to S. res. 240, pt. 19, March 4-6, 1968, LSD and marijuana among young people. 90th Congress. 2d session. Washington: United States Superintendent of Documents, Government Printing Office, 1968.
Vermes, Jean C. POT IS ROT. New York: Association Press, 1969.
Winick, C." "Marihuana use by young people," DRUG ADDICTION IN YOUTH, ed. E. Harms. New York: Pergamon Press, 1965, pp. 19-35.
Wolstenholme, G.E.W., and Knight, J., eds. HASHISH: its

chemistry and pharmacology. Boston: Little, Brown, and
Company, 1965.
Yablonsky, Lewis. THE HIPPIE TRIP. New York: Pegasus, 1968.
Yolles, Stanley F. RECENT RESEARCH ON LSD, MARIHUANA, AND
OTHER DANGEROUS DRUGS. Statement before the subcommittee
on juvenile delinquency of the Committee on the Judici-
ary, United States Senate, March 6, 1968. Washington:
Department of Health, Education and Welfare, 1968.

MARIJUANA: Periodical Literature

General Publications

"AMA lies about pot," by Fort, J. RAMPARTS MAGAZINE. 7:
12 passim, Aug. 24, 1968.
"Administrators forum: this month's problem; program on
drugs backfired when six students were picked up by ju-
venile authorities," SCHOOL MANAGEMENT. 11:25 passim,
Oct., 1967.
"Adverse reaction to marihuana," by Keeler, Martin H. AMER-
ICAN JOURNAL OF PSYCHIATRY. 124:674-677, Nov., 1967.
"America's social frontiers: why not smoke pot?" by Etzioni,
A. CURRENT. 95:38-41, May, 1968.
"The association of marijuana smoking with opiate addiction
in the United States," by Ball, J.C., et al. JOURNAL
OF CRIMINAL LAW, CRIMINOLOGY, AND POLICE SCIENCE. 59:
171-182, June, 1968.
"Authorities respond to growing drug use among high school
students." PHI DELTA KAPPAN. 50:213, Dec., 1968.
"Beyond the pleasure principle (review article)," by Coles,
R. PARTISAN REVIEW. 34:415-420, Summer, 1967.
"Boston pot party: research sponsored by the Boston Univer-
sity Medical Center." NEW REPUBLIC. 159:8, Dec. 21,
1968.
"A bust at gunpoint and an armed search at sunset." LIFE.
67:32-33, Oct. 31, 1969.
"But, mom, everibody smokes pot!" by Reice, S. MCCALLS.
95:68-69 passim, Sept., 1968; also READER'S DIGEST. 93:
81-85, Dec., 1968.
"Cannabis." DRUG AND THERAPEUTICS BULLETIN. 5:97-99, Dec.
8, 1967.
"Cannabis." MEDICAL JOURNAL OF AUSTRALIA. 1:99-101, 1968.
"Cannabis," by Hicks, J.T. HOSPITAL FORMULARY MANAGEMENT.
2:42-45, 1967.
"Cannabis, a toxic and dangerous substance: a study of
eighty takers," by Chapple, P.A.L. BRITISH JOURNAL OF
ADDICTION. 61:269-282, Aug., 1966.
"Cannabis and violence." UNITED NATIONS BULLETIN ON NAR-
COTICS. 20(2):44, 1968.
"Cannabis as a medicant," by Kabelik, J., et al. BULLETIN

ON NARCOTICS. 12(3):5-23, July/Sept., 1960.
"A cannabis concoction." BULLETIN ON NARCOTICS. 20(2):
55, Apr.-June, 1968.
"The cannabis habit: a review of recent psychiatric liter-
ature," by Murphy, H.D.M. BULLETIN ON NARCOTICS. 15(1):
15-23, Jan.-Mar., 1963.
"Cannabis hazard hotly disputed at congress." MEDICAL TRI-
BUNE. 9:1+, 1968.
"Cannabis in early pregnancy." BULLETIN ON NARCOTICS. 20
(2):8, Apr.-June, 1968.
"The cannabis problem: a note on the problem and the history
of international action." UNITED NATIONS BULLETIN ON
NARCOTICS. 14(4):27-31, 1962.
"The case against cannabis." PHARMACEUTICAL JOURNAL. 199:
399-400, 1967.
"Case against marijuana," by Brill, H. JOURNAL OF SCHOOL
HEALTH. 38:522-523, Oct., 1968.
"A case for cannabis?" BRITISH MEDICAL JOURNAL. 3:258-
259, Jul. 29, 1967.
"A case for cannabis?" by Stafford-Clark, D. BRITISH MED-
ICAL JOURNAL. 3:435, 1967.
"A case for cannabis?" by Tylden, E., et al. BRITISH MED-
ICAL JOURNAL. 3:556, Aug. 26, 1967.
"Case of the pot-smoking school principal; Mrs. G. Brennan
of Nicasio, California," by Alexander, S. LIFE. 63:25,
Nov. 17, 1967.
"Chat with an ad-man head." MARKETING COMMUNICATIONS.
296:63-65, Jan., 1968.
"Children of the drug age," by Simon, W., and Gagnon, J.H.
SATURDAY REVIEW. 51:60-63, 75-78, Sept. 21, 1968.
"Collapse after intravenous injection of hashish." BRITISH
MEDICAL JOURNAL. 3(5612):229-230, 1968.
"Concern over pot smoking," by Beavan, K.A. TIMES (London)
EDUCATIONAL SUPPLEMENT. 2809:916, Mar. 21, 1969.
"Confessions of a campus pot dealer." ESQUIRE. 68:100-101
passim, Sept., 1967.
"Confusion over effects." SCIENCE NEWS. 92:345-346,
Oct. 7, 1967.
"Constitutional objections to California's marijuana pos-
session statute," by Boyko, E., et al. UCLA LAW REVIEW.
14:773-795, 1967.
"Controversy over dangers of marijuana," by Gimlin, J.S.
EDITORIAL RESEARCH REPORT. 2:590-596, Aug. 9, 1967.
"Cool talk about hot drugs; misconceptions about heroin,
LSD, and marijuana," by Louria, D.B. NEW YORK TIMES
MAGAZINE. pp. 12-13 passim, Aug. 6, 1967; also READER'S
DIGEST. 91:111-117, Nov., 1967.
"Crime of marijuana." NEW REPUBLIC. 157:9-10, Oct. 7, 1967.
"Criminal justice notes: juveniles jailed for first mari-
juana offenses." NCCD News. 48(4):11, Sept./Oct., 1969.
"The criminogenic action of cannabis (marijuana) and narcot-
ics," by Andrade, O.M. BULLETIN ON NARCOTICS. 16:23-28,
Oct.-Dec., 1964.
"Dagga smoking in Rhodesia." CENTRAL AFRICA JOURNAL OF MED-
ICINE. 12:215-216, 1966.

"The dangerous drug problem," by Louria, D., et al. NEW
YORK MEDICINE. 22:3-8, 1966.
"Dependence on cannabis (marihuana)." JOURNAL OF THE AMER-
ICAN MEDICAL ASSOCIATION. 201:368-371, Aug. 7, 1967.
"Dissident youth," by Unwin, J.R. CANADA'S MENTAL HEALTH.
17:4-10, Mar./Apr., 1969.
"A doctor speaks of marijuana and other 'drugs'," by Dal-
rymple, W. JOURNAL OF THE AMERICAN COLLEGE HEALTH ASSOC-
IATION. 14:218-222, Feb., 1966.
"Does marijuana lead to heroin? New York City youthful
offenders studied." THE ATTACK ON NARCOTIC ADDICTION
AND DRUG ABUSE. 2(4):7, Nov., 1968.
"Dream farm; field of marijuana destroyed by narcotic
agents." TIME. 90:17-18, Sept. 8, 1967.
"Drinking and pot parties," by Rector, M.G. EDUCATION DI-
GEST. 33:45-47, Sept., 1967.
"Drop that pot!" NEWSWEEK. 72:61, July 1, 1968.
"Drowsed with the fume of poppies: opium and John Keats,"
by Ober, W. BULLETIN OF THE NEW YORK ACADEMY OF MED-
ICINE. 44:862-881, 1968.
"Drug dangers, the case gets stronger," by Snider, A.J.
SCIENCE DIGEST. 64:62-63, July, 1968.
"Drug dependence in Britain," by MacDonald, A. CURRENT
MEDICINE AND DRUGS. 6:23-30, 1966.
"Drug dependence of hashish type," by Watt, J.M. CIBA
FOUNDATION STUDY GROUP. 21:34-69, 1965.
"Drug effects and personality theory," by Lindmann, E,
and Von Felsinger, J. PSYCHOPHARMACOLOGIA. 2:69-92,
1961.
"The drug problem among young people. Use of both LSD and
marijuana entails significant risk," by Farnsworth, D.L.
RHODE ISLAND MEDICAL JOURNAL. 51:179-182 passim, Mar.,
1968.
"Drug use and experience in an urban college population,"
by Perlman, Samuel. AMERICAN JOURNAL OF ORTHOPSYCHIATRY.
37:297-299, Mar., 1967.
"Drug use: symptom, disease, or adolescent experimentation?
The task of therapy," by Liebert, R. JOURNAL OF THE
AMERICAN COLLEGE HEALTH ASSOCIATION. 16:25-29, 1967.
"Drugs and drug addiction: opinions on the taking of 'soft'
drugs." MEDICINE, SCIENCE AND THE LAW. 6:167-168, 1966.
"Drugs causing dependence," by Lendon, N. BRITISH JOURNAL
OF ADDICTION. 61:115-124, 1965.
"Drugs on the campus," by Shepherd, J. LOOK. 31:14-17,
Aug. 8, 1967.
"Drugs that move the mind," by Mandell, A. TRAUMA. 9:
73-115, 1968.
"Dust disease in hemp workers," by Barbero, A., and Flores,
R. ARCHIVES OF ENVIRONMENTAL HEALTH. 14:529-532, 1967.
"The effects of cannabis." BULLETIN ON NARCOTICS. 20(1):
38, Jan.-Mar., 1968.
"Effects of marijuana; findings of scientific tests." TIME.
92:52, Dec. 20, 1968.
"The effects of marijuana on human beings: a scientific re-

port," by Zinberg, Norman E., and Weil, Andrew T.
NEW YORK TIMES MAGAZINE. p. 28+, May 11, 1969.
"The essence of pot," by Collier, H. NEW SCIENTIST. 35:
436-438, 1967.
"Evaluation of marijuana for school physicians, nurses and
educators," by Alserver, W.D. JOURNAL OF SCHOOL HEALTH.
38:629-638, Dec., 1968.
"FCC wants in on pot party (WBBM-TV)." BROADCASTING. 74:
63-64, Mar. 25, 1968.
"Father's talk about marijuana," by Goldberg, M.J. GOOD
HOUSEKEEPING. 166:80-81 passim, Feb., 1968.
"Federal agents, alarmed at use, call colleges lax on mar-
ijuana ban," by Brunt, B. PHILADELPHIA BULLETIN. Nov.,
1965.
"Fiedler affair; Buffalo university group aims to legalize
marijuana." NEWSWEEK. 69:29, June 12, 1967.
"First double-blind findings on marijuana." MEDICAL WORLD
NEWS. 10:18-20, 1969.
"Flight from violence: hippies and the green rebellion,"
by Allen, James R., and West, Louise J. AMERICAN JOUR-
NAL OF PSYCHIATRY. 125(3):364-370, 1968.
"For the long distance runner who got caught a twenty-year
sentence," by Howard, Jane. LIFE. 67:30-31, Oct. 31,
1969.
"Free exercise: religion goes to pot," by Phillips, J.
CALIFORNIA LAW REVIEW. 56:100-115, 1968.
"From hard to soft drugs: temporal and substantive changes
in drug usage among gangs in a working-class community,"
by Klein, J., and Phillips, D. JOURNAL OF HEALTH AND
SOCIAL BEHAVIOR. 9:139-145, 1968.
"The furry with the syringe on top," by Schushnick, Irving.
EAST VILLAGE OTHER. pp. 5-20, Feb. 16-22, 1968.
"GH poll: should marijuana laws be changed?" GOOD HOUSE-
KEEPING. 167:10 passim, July, 1968.
"Getting tough with pot; marijuana smokers discovered at
New Jersey's Hun preparatory school." TIME. 90:110,
Dec. 8, 1967.
"The God in the flowerpot," by Barnard, M. AMERICAN SCHO-
LAR. 32:578-586, 1963; also PSYCHEDELIC REVIEW. no. 1:
244-251, 1963.
"Going to pot in Washington; a hippie party." U.S. NEWS
AND WORLD REPORT. 62:63, May 8, 1967.
"Graduate students as marijuana users." SCHOOL AND SOCIETY.
96:392, Nov. 9, 1968.
"Grand mal convulsions subsequent to marijuana use: case
report," by Keeler, M., and Reifler, C. DISEASES OF THE
NERVOUS SYSTEM. 28:474-475, 1967.
"Grass is good for business," by Firstenberg, M. MARIJUANA
REVIEW. 1(1), 1968.
"The great marijuana hoax: first manifesto to end the bring-
down," by Ginsberg, Allen. ATLANTIC. 218:104-112, Nov.,
1966.
"Great marijuana problem," by Gollan, A. NATIONAL REVIEW.
20:74-80, Jan. 30, 1968.

"Hallucinogenic drugs: a perspective with special reference to peyote and cannabis," by Mc-Glothlin, W. PSYCHEDELIC REVIEW. no. 6:16-57, 1965.

"The 'hang-loose' ethic and the spirit of drug use," by Suchman, Edward A. JOURNAL OF HEALTH AND SOCIAL BEHAVIOR. 9(2):146-155, 1968.

"The Hashbury is the capital of the hippies," by Thompson, H. NEW YORK TIMES MAGAZINE. p. 29 passim, May 14, 1967.

"Hashish." BRITISH MEDICAL JOURNAL. 5421:1348-1349, 1964.

"Hashish, assassins and the love of God," by Mandel, Jerry. ISSUES IN CRIMINOLOGY. 2:149-156, Fall, 1966.

"Hashish, avant gard and rearguard," by Krebs, Allen. STREETS. 1:17-22, May/June, 1965.

"Hashish consumption in Egypt, with special reference to psychosocial aspects," by Soueif, M.I. BULLETIN ON NARCOTICS. 19(2):1-12, Apr.-June, 1967.

"Hashish--contents, synthesis, and effects," by Runk, B., et al. MEDIZINISCHE MONATSSCHRIFT. 19:165-168, 1965.

"Have a high holiday; use of marijuana on campus." NEWSWEEK. 72:50-51, Dec. 30, 1968.

"The hemp plant." CIBA REVIEW. 1962-1965, pp. 2-32.

"High and low of marijuana and alcohol in the youth culture," by Hill, W.T. SOUNDINGS. 51:290-307, Fall, 1968.

"Hippies." TIME. 90:18-22, July 7, 1967; also READER'S DIGEST. 91:70-74, Oct., 1967.

"Hippies and early Christianity," by Mc-Glothlin, W. JOURNAL OF PSYCHEDELIC DRUGS. 1:24-35, 1967.

"History of the psychedelic drug experience," by Mahabir, W. CANADIAN PSYCHIATRIC ASSOCIATION JOURNAL. 13:189-190, 1968.

"How dangerous is marijuana? a top official sparks new debate; excerpts from statements," by Goddard, J.L. U.S. NEWS AND WORLD REPORT. 63:20, Oct. 30, 1967.

"How to handle a dope scandal: candor clears the air," by Goben, R.D. SCHOOL MANAGEMENT. 10:106-107, June, 1966.

"How to make a pot study legal." MEDICAL WORLD NEWS. 10:20, 1969.

"How to use pot; course description from the bulletin of the Midpeninsula free university, Stanford, California." SATURDAY REVIEW. 51:62, Sept. 21, 1968.

"I turned on 200 fellow students at the University of Michigan," by Ric. ESQUIRE. Sept., 1967, p. 101 passim.

"If is pot, don't panic." SCIENCE DIGEST. 64:62, Oct., 1968.

"In defence of pot: confessions of a Canadian marijuana smoker," by Ludlow, Peter. SATURDAY NIGHT. 80:28-29 passim, Oct., 1965.

"It's up to the young to solve the problem," by Wyzanski, C.E. NEW REPUBLIC. 157:15-16, Oct. 21, 1967.

"Keep off the grass?" NEW REPUBLIC. 156:5-6, June 17, 1967.

"Keeping on the grass," by Coleman, Kate. NEWSWEEK. 70:48-49, July 24, 1967.

"Kif cultivation in the Rif mountains," by Mikuriya, T.

ECONOMIC BOTANY. 21:3, July-Sept., 1967.
"LSD and marihuana: where are the answers?" by Davis, E.
SCIENCE. 160(3832):1063-1064, 1968.
"LSD and marihuana: where are the answers?" by Dohner, V.
SCIENCE. 169(3832):1061-1062, 1968.
"LSD and marihuana: where are the answers?" by Myers, W.A.
SCIENCE. 160(3832):1062, 1968.
"LSD and marihuana: where are the answers?" by Wertlake,
Paul T. SCIENCE. 160(3832):1064-1065, 1968.
"LSD and marijuana," by Abelson, P.H. SCIENCE. 159(3820):
1189, Mar. 15, 1968.
"LSD versus pot: effects compared." THE ATTACK ON NARCOTIC
ADDICTION AND DRUG ABUSE. 2(4):6, Nov., 1968.
"Later heroin use by marijuana-using and non-drug-using ad-
olescent offenders in New York City," by Glaser, D., et
al. THE INTERNATIONAL JOURNAL OF ADDICTION. 4(2):145-
155, June, 1969.
"Lemar International: the time is now," by Aldrich, M. MARI-
JUANA REVIEW. 1(2):2, 1968.
"Long road to Nirvana: dissertation on marijuana," by Pel-
ner, L. NEW YORK STATE JOURNAL OF MEDICINE. 67:952-
956, 1967.
"Madness to relax cannabis law." PHARMACEUTICAL JOURNAL.
199:122-123, 1967.
"Making of a hippie; with study-discussion guide," by Smal-
lenburg, C., and Smallenburg, H. PTA MAGAZINE. 63:6-9
passim, Jan., 1969; also EDUCATION DIGEST. 34:32-34,
Apr., 1969.
"Malignant anxiety in Africans," by Lambo T. JOURNAL OF
MENTAL SCIENCE. 108:256, 1962.
"Marihuana," by Harney, M. LANCET. 1:384-385, 1964.
"Marihuana," by Murphy, H.B. BULLETIN ON NARCOTICS. 2:
6, 1963.
"Marihuana," by Stungo, E. LANCET. 2:1124, 1963.
"Marihuana: a calling card to narcotic addiction," by Gior-
dano, Henry L. FBI LAW ENFORCEMENT BULLETIN. 37(11):
2-5, Nov., 1968.
"Marihuana: a product of controversy," by Johnson, G.
APPLED THERAPEUTICS. 10:458, 1968.
"Marihuana: ancient drug and modern social problem," by
Farnsworth, N.R. TILE AND TILL. 53(4):82-85, Dec.,
1967.
"Marihuana and alcohol," by Reuben, D. JOURNAL OF THE
AMERICAN MEDICAL ASSOCIATION. 204:407, 1968.
"Marihuana and crime," by Munch, James C. BULLETIN ON
NARCOTICS. 18(2):15-22, Apr.-June, 1966.
"Marihuana and its effects: statements by R.A. Schroth and
Addiction Research Foundation of Ontario." CATHOLIC
SCHOOL JOURNAL. 69:44-47, Sept., 1969.
"Marihuana and LSD usage among male college students:
prevalence rate, frequency, and self-estimates of future
use," by King, Francis W. PSYCHIATRY. 32:265-276, Aug.,
1969.
"Marihuana and society." JOURNAL OF THE AMERICAN MEDICAL

ASSOCIATION. 204(13):1181-1182, 1968.
"Marihuana and the law." CANADIAN MEDICAL ASSOCIATION JOUR-
NAL. 97:1359-1362, 1967.
"Marihuana and the new American hedonism," by Bleibtreu, J.
PSYCHEDELIC REVIEW. no. 9:72-79, 1967.
"Marihuana and young adults: a preliminary report," by Paul-
us, I., and Williams, H.R. ADDICTIONS. 13:26-33, 1966;
also BRITISH COLUMBIA MEDICAL JOURNAL. 8:240-244, 1966.
"Marihuana effects found to be mild." CANADA'S MENTAL
HEALTH. 17(3):45-46, May-Aug., 1969.
"The marihuana habit: some observations of a small group
of users," by Norton, W.A. CANADIAN PSYCHIATRIC ASSOC-
IATION JOURNAL. 13(2):163-173, Apr., 1968.
"Marihuana induced hallucinations," by Keeler, Martin H.
DISEASES OF THE NERVOUS SYSTEM. 29(5):314-315, 1968.
"The marihuana problem: an overview," by Mc-Glothlin, Wil-
liam H., and West, Louis J. AMERICAN JOURNAL OF PSYCHI-
ATRY. 125(3):370-378, 1968.
"Marihuana smoking and the onset of heroin use." BULLETIN
ON NARCOTICS. 20(3):29, July-Sept., 1968; also BRITISH
JOURNAL OF CRIMINOLOGY. 7(4):408-413, 1967.
"Marihuana smoking in the United States," by Pet, Donald D.,
and Ball, John C. FEDERAL PROBATION. 32:8-15, Sept.,
1968.
"Marihuana: social benefit or social detriment?" by Bloom-
quist, Edward R. CALIFORNIA MEDICINE. 106:346-353,
May, 1967.
"Marihuana thing." JOURNAL OF THE AMERICAN MEDICAL ASSOC-
IATION. 204(13):1187-1188, 1968.
"Marihuana: thirty-five years later," by Bromberg, W.
AMERICAN JOURNAL OF PSYCHIATRY. 125:391-393, Sept., 1968.
"Marijuana." THE ATTACK ON NARCOTIC ADDICTION AND DRUG
ABUSE. 3:3, Winter, 1969.
"Marijuana." MEDICAL LETTER ON DRUGS AND THERAPEUTICS.
9:73-74, 1967.
"Marijuana," by Austin, C.G. JOURNAL OF HIGHER EDUCATION.
40:477-479, June, 1969.
"Marijuana: an overview," by Burbridge, T.N. JOURNAL OF
SECONDARY EDUCATION. 43:197-199, May, 1968.
"Marijuana and drug addiction." UCLA DAILY BRUIN. 71(36,
1967 (entire no. 36).
"Marijuana and LSD: a survey of one college campus," by
Eells, K. JOURNAL OF COUNSELING PSYCHOLOGY. 15(5, pt.1):
459-467, 1968.
"Marijuana and mental disturbances," by Sonnenreich, C.,
and Goes, J. NEUROBIOLOGIA. 25:69-91, 1962.
"Marijuana and perceptual style: a theoretical note," by
Dinnerstein, A. PERCEPTUAL AND MOTOR SKILLS. 26:1016-
1018, 1968.
"Marijuana before the bench." TIME. 90:77 passim, Sept.
29, 1967.
"Marijuana causes psychic dependence, says physician."
TODAY'S HEALTH. 45:13, Sept., 1967.
"Marijuana control: a perspective," by Mc-Glothlin, W.H.

JOURNAL OF SECONDARY EDUCATION. 43:223-227, May, 1968.
"Marijuana: dangerous as alcohol." NEW REPUBLIC. 157:7-8,
Oct. 28, 1967.
"The marijuana famine," by Farrell, Barry. LIFE. 67:20B,
Aug. 22, 1969.
"Marijuana: how dangerous is it? Testimony of three doc-
tors with unique knowledge and experience," by Spencer,
S.M. READER'S DIGEST. 96(573):67-71, Jan., 1970.
"Marijuana impact on American youth," by Grimlin, J.S.
EDITORIAL RESEARCH REPORT. 2:579-586, Aug. 9, 1967.
"Marijuana in perspective," by Seevers, M.H. MICHIGAN
QUARTERLY REVIEW. 5:247-251, Oct., 1966.
"Marijuana is still illegal: Massachusetts ruling," by
Oteri, J. TIME. 90:38 passim, Dec. 29, 1967.
"Marijuana: just how harmless is it?" by Tunley, R. SEV-
ENTEEN. 27:138-139 passim, May, 1968.
"Marijuana, LSD, and other dangerous substances," by Quinn,
W. BULLETIN OF THE LOS ANGELES COUNTY MEDICAL ASSOCIA-
TION. 97:20-21, 1967.
"Marijuana law," by Shane, J. NEW REPUBLIC. 158:9-10,
Mar. 23, 1968.
"Marijuana madness," by DerMarderosian, A.H. JOURNAL OF
SECONDARY EDUCATION. 43:200-205, May, 1968.
"Marijuana mantras," by Aldrich M. INCENSE. 16:18-22, 1968.
"Marijuana: millions of turned-on users; with report," by
Rosenfeld, A. LIFE. 63:16-23, July 7, 1967.
"Marijuana or alcohol, which harms most?" U.S. NEWS AND
WORLD REPORT. 64:15, Feb. 5, 1968.
"The marijuana problem; pot is going middle class with pro-
found effects." NEWSWEEK. 70:46-52, July 24, 1967.
"Marijuana: real problems and the responsibilities of the
professions in solving them," by Fort, Joel. PSYCHI-
ATRIC OPINION. 5:9-15, Oct., 1968.
"Marijuana, sleeping pills and other drugs: peril for Amer-
ica," by Yolles, Stanley F. U.S. NEWS AND WORLD REPORT.
67:47-48, July 14, 1969.
"Marijuana: standardization, characterization and potential
therapeutic uses," by Feinglass, S.J. JOURNAL OF SECOND-
ARY EDUCATION. 43:206-210, May, 1968.
"Marijuana; the evidence begins to grow," by Toohey, J.V.
JOURNAL OF SCHOOL HEALTH. 38:302-303, May, 1968.
"Marijuana: the law vs. twelve million people." LIFE.
67:27-28, Oct. 31, 1969.
"Marijuana: the symbol and the ritual," by Ballante, A.
JOURNAL OF SECONDARY EDUCATION. 43:218-222, May, 1968.
"Marijuana warning." TIME. 91:61, June 28, 1968.
"Marijuana: what it is, and isn't." U.S. NEWS AND WORLD
REPORT. 67:48-50, Oct. 13, 1969.
"Marijuana witchhunt," by Brennan, Garnet E. EVERGREEN
REVIEW. 12:55-56 passim, June, 1968.
"Mary Jane in action: G I's arrested in Vietnam on charges
of smoking pot," by Donnelly, J. NEWSWEEK. 70:40,
Nov. 6, 1967.
"The medical view: not what the doctor ordered." NEWSWEEK.
70:46-47, July 24, 1967.

"Medico-social aspects of marijuana. Habituation to marijuana incompatible with productive college career," by Johnson, R.D. RHODE ISLAND MEDICAL JOURNAL. 51:171-178 passim, Mar., 1968.

"Mental illness and Indian hemp in Lagos," by Boroffka, A. EAST AFRICAN MEDICAL JOURNAL. 43:377-384, Sept., 1966.

"Morality of marijuana." TIME. 92:58, Aug. 16, 1968.

"Motivation for marihuana use: a correlate of adverse reaction," by Keeler, M. AMERICAN JOURNAL OF PSYCHIATRY. 125:386-390, 1968.

"Multiple drug use among marijuana smokers," by Goode, Erich. SOCIAL PROBLEMS. 17(1):48-64, Summer, 1969.

"The mystique of marijuana: why students smoke pot," by Shearer, L. PARADE. June 4, 1967, p. 8 passim.

"Narcotic analysis: a simple approach," by Lerner, M., et al. JOURNAL OF FORENSIC SCIENCES. 8:126-131, 1963.

"Narcotics and the law," by Sparks, W. COMMONWEAL. 74:467-469, Aug. 25, 1961.

"National Institute of Mental Health grows its own marihuana." CANADA'S MENTAL HEALTH. 17(3):34, May-Aug., 1969.

"Natural and smoked hashish," by Joachimoglu, G. CIBA FOUNDATION STUDY GROUP. 21:2-14, 1965.

"Never trust a man with a beard," by Schushnick, Irving. EAST VILLAGE OTHER. Jan. 12-Jan. 19, 1968, p. 4.

"New results on hashish-specific constituents," by Korte, Friedhelm, et al. BULLETIN ON NARCOTICS. 17(1):35-43, Jan.-Mar., 1965.

"Nixon's new plan to deal with the marijuana problem." U.S. NEWS AND WORLD REPORT. 67(17):14, Oct. 27, 1969.

"No martyr to marijuana: new Goddard line." NEW REPUBLIC. 157:6, Dec. 2, 1967.

"Oberlin's revised policy." SCHOOL AND SOCIETY. 96:167, Mar. 16, 1968.

"On marijuana," by Kissin, Benjamin. DOWNSTATE MEDICAL CENTER REPORTER, Brooklyn, New York. 2(7, pt.2), Apr., 1967.

"On the use of marihuana." NEDERLANDSCH MILITAIR GENEESKUNDE TIJDSCHRIFT. 13:108-112, 1960.

"One way or the other it all goes up in smoke." LIFE. 67:29, Oct. 31, 1969.

"Peyote and the definition of narcotic," by Barber, C.G. AMERICAN ANTHROPOLOGIST. 61:641-646, Aug., 1959.

"Physical, mental, and moral effects of marijuana: the Indian hemp drugs commission report," by Mikuriya, Tod H. THE INTERNATIONAL JOURNAL OF THE ADDICTIONS. 3:253-270, Spring, 1968.

"Politics of pot," by Sterba, J. ESQUIRE. 70:58-61 passim, Aug., 1968.

"Pop drugs: the high as a way of life." TIME. 94:68-78, Sept. 26, 1969.

"Pop'Pot'." LANCET. 2:989-990, 1963.

"Pot and Goddard." TIME. 90:54, Oct. 27, 1967.

"Pot and parents; high school students smoking marijuana."

TIME. 92:44-45, Aug. 30, 1968.
"'Pot' and politics: how they 'busted' Stony Brook," by
Greenberg, D. SCIENCE. 159:607-611, 1968.
"Pot boils," by McBroom, P. SCIENCE NEWS. 92:500-501,
Nov. 18, 1967.
"Pot bust at Cornell," by Sanford, D. NEW REPUBLIC. 156:
17-20, Apr. 15, 1967.
"Pot is good for business," by Harris, M. MARIJUANA RE-
VIEW. 1(1):12, 1968.
"Pot laws smashing our colleges!" by Harris, B. MARIJUANA
REVIEW. 1(1):8-9, 1968.
"Pot penalties too severe," by McBroom, P. SCIENCE NEWS.
90:270, Oct. 8, 1966.
"The pot plot," by Abrams, Stephen. [Oxford University News-
paper]CHERWELL. Feb., 1967, p.7.
"Pot: safer than alcohol?" TIME. 91:52-53, Apr. 19, 1968.
"Potheads in Missouri," by Shepherd, Jack. LOOK. Aug.8,
1967, pp. 14-17.
"Pot's luck; Massachusetts ban." NEWSWEEK. 71:14, Jan. 1,
1968.
"Potted ivy; alienated students smoking marijuana." TIME.
89:98 passim, May 19, 1967.
"Potty laws (in the U.S.)." ECONOMIST. 225:160, Oct. 14,
1967.
"Predictive value of marijuana use: a note to researchers
of student culture," by Messer, M. SOCIOLOGY OF EDUCA-
TION. 42:91-97, Winter, 1969.
"The problems of cannabis dependence," by Edwards, G. PRAC-
TITIONER. 200:226-233, Feb., 1968.
"The prodical powers of pot," by Wakefield, Dan. PLAYBOY.
Aug., 1962.
"Psychedelic drugs: cannabis and LSD." NURSING TIMES. 64:
326-327, Mar. 8, 1968.
"Psycho-pathological aspects of the cannabis situation in
Morocco," by Mikuriya, T. THE INTERNATIONAL JOURNAL OF
ADICTION. 3:397-398, 1968.
"The question of cannabis." (Note by the Secretary General).
United Nations: UN DOCUMENT E-CN.7-399, 5 Dec., 1960.
"The question of cannabis." (Note by the Secretary General).
United Nations: UN DOCUMENT E-CN.7-409, 1961.
"The question of pot," by Goldstein, R. MODERATOR. 4:9-10,
1965.
"Recent additions to a bibliography on cannabis," by Kwan,
V., and Rajeswaran, P. JOURNAL OF FORENSIC SCIENCES.
13:279-289, 1968.
"Risks of marijuana," by Sanford, D. NEW REPUBLIC. 156:
11-12, Apr. 22, 1967.
"Runaways, hippies, and marihuana," by Kaufman, J., et al.
AMERICAN JOURNAL OF PSYCHIATRY. 126(5):717-720, Nov.,
1969.
"Sack for pot?" TIMES (London) EDUCATIONAL SUPPLEMENT.
2813:1257, Apr. 18, 1969.
"Secret Chicago pot hearing held." BROADCASTING. 74:52-
53, Apr. 22, 1968.

"A screening technique for Indian hemp (cannabis sativa L.)," by Caddy, B., et al. JOURNAL OF CHROMATOGRAPHY. 31(2):584-587, 1967.

"Should it be legalized? Soon we will know," by Goddard, James L. LIFE. 67:34-35, Oct. 31, 1969; also READER'S DIGEST. 96(573):70, Jan., 1970.

"Similarities and differences between religious mysticism and drug-induced experiences," by Kurtz, P. JOURNAL OF HUMANISTIC PSYCHOLOGY. 3:146-154, 1963.

"Social control and marijuana use," by Curtis, J. CLINICAL TOXICOLOGY. 1:215-225, 1968.

"Socio-psychiatric problems of cannabis in Nigeria," by Asuni, T. BULLETIN ON NARCOTICS. 16(2):17-28, Apr.-June, 1964.

"Sociopsychological problems of cannabism," by dePinho, R., et al. NEUROBIOLOGIA. 25:9-19, 1962.

"Some aspects of cannabis action," by Miras, C.J. CIBA FOUNDATION STUDY GROUP. 21:37-53, 1965.

"Source of production of cannabis and other narcotic drugs entering the illicit traffic." United Nations: UN DOCUMENT GEN-NAR-65-CONF.2-5, 21 June, 1965.

"Spontaneous recurrence of marihuana effect," by Keeler, M.H., et al. AMERICAN JOURNAL OF PSYCHIATRY. 125:140-142, Sept., 1968.

"Staggers wants to harvest the grass first; WBBM-TV pot-party probe set for public Hill hearing." BROADCASTING. 74:68, May 6, 1968.

"Standard marijuana." SCIENCE NEWS. 91:461, May 13, 1967.

"Statement of cannabis." PHARMACEUTICAL JOURNAL. 199:142, 1967.

"Studies with the U.N. cannabis reference sample," by Joachimoglu, G., et al. BULLETIN ON NARCOTICS. 19(1):21-22, Jan.-Mar., 1967.

"Study of the Egyptian pot smoker." NEW SCIENTIST. 35:377, 1967.

"The teenager and drug abuse," by Johnson, F., and Westman, J. JOURNAL OF SCHOOL HEALTH. 38:646-654, 1968.

"Time and disease," by Nettleship, A., and Lair, C.V. JOURNAL OF CLINICAL AND EXPERIMENTAL PSYCHOPATHOLOGY AND QUARTERLY REVIEW OF PSYCHIATRY AND NEUROLOGY. 23:106-115, 1962.

"Toward a perspective on marijuana." WALL STREET JOURNAL. Mar. 25, 1968, p. 14.

"Truth about pot," by Gannon, R. POPULAR SCIENCE MONTHLY. 192:76-79 passim, May, 1968.

"Turning on: two views." TIME. 94:72-73, Sept. 26, 1969.

"Undesirable effects of marijuana," by Dally, P. BRITISH MEDICAL JOURNAL. Aug. 5, 1967, p. 367.

"Use of amphetamines, marihuana and LSD by students," by Blachly, P. NEW PHYSICIAN. 15:88-93, 1966.

"The use of marijuana and LSD on the college campus," by Kurtz, R.S. JOURNAL OF THE NATIONAL ASSOCIATION OF WOMEN'S DEANS AND COUSELORS. 30:124-128, Spring, 1967.

"Use of opium and cannabis in the traditional systems of

medicine in India," by Dwarakanath, Shri C. BULLETIN
ON NARCOTICS. 17(1):15-19, Jan.-Mar., 1965.
"Verdict on marijuana; findings of a team of Boston Univer-
sity investigators." NEWSWEEK. 72:48, Dec. 23, 1968.
"Violence and marijuana (Sixth Annual Conference Report of
the International Narcotic Enforcement Officers Assoc-
iation)." NEW YORK STATE DEPARTMENT OF HEALTH WEEKLY
BULLETIN. 20:26, 1967.
"What is marijuana?" TODAY'S EDUCATION. 58:39-41, Mar.,
1969.
"What price euphoria? The case against marijuana," by
McMorris, S.C. BRITISH JOURNAL OF ADDICTION. 62:203-
208, Mar., 1967; also MEDICO-LEGAL JOURNAL. 34:74-79,
1966.
"What's wrong with pot?" NEWSWEEK. 70:30, Oct. 2, 1967.
"Wheeling and dealing with tragedy," by Shepherd, J. LOOK.
32:56-59, Mar. 5, 1968.
"Who says marijuana use leads to heroin addiction?" by Man-
del, J. JOURNAL OF SECONDARY EDUCATION. 43:211-217,
May, 1968.
"Why marijuana?" by Wolk, D.W. THE UNIVERSITY OF BRIDGE-
PORT QUARTERLY. 2:8-11, Spring, 1968.
"Why they do it," by Garvin, Andrew. NEWSWEEK. 70:52,
July 24, 1967.
"Wild grass chase," by Mount, F. NATIONAL REVIEW. 20:
81-84, Jan. 30, 1968.
"William Burroughs speaks!" by Burroughs, W. MARIJUANA
NEWSLETTER. 1, 1966.

MARIJUANA: Periodical Literature

Scientific Publications

"Antibiotic activity of various types of cannabis resin,"
by Radosevic, A., et al. NATURE. 195:1007-1009, 1962;
also UN DOCUMENT ST-SOA-SER.S-6, 1962.
"Behavioral effects in monkeys of racemates of two biologically active marijuana constituents," by Scheckel, C.,
et al. SCIENCE. 160(3835):1467-1469, 1968.
"Bioassay of cannabis preparations based on abolition of
the rabbit blink test," by Valle, J., et al. FARMACO
EDIZIONE SCIENTIFICA. 22:27-36, 1967.
"Byosinosis in hemp workers," by Bouhuys, A., et al. AR-
CHIVES OF ENVIRONMENTAL HEALTH. 14:533-544, 1967.
"Blocking action of tetrahydrocannabinol upon transmission
in the trigeminal system of the cat," by Lapa, A., et
al. JOURNAL OF PHARMACY AND PHARMACOLOGY. 20:373-376,
1968.
"Cannabichromene, a new active principle in hashish," by
Gaoni, Y., and Mechoulam, R. CHEMICAL COMMUNICATIONS.
1:20-21, 1966.

"Cannabis. A toxic and dangerous substance. A study of
eighty takers," by Chapple, P.A. BRITISH JOURNAL OF
ADICTION. 61:269-282, Aug., 1966.
"Cannabis as a medicament," by Kebelik, J., et al. BUL-
LETIN ON NARCOTICS. 12(3):5-23, 1960.
"Cannabis as a medicament: a brief survey of the methods
of isolation and the physical and chemical properties
and structures of the isolated antibacterial substances,"
by Santavi, F., and Krejci, Z. BULLETIN ON NARCOTICS.
12(3):8-12, 1960.
"Cannabis as a medicament: treatment with cannabis in ancient, folk and official medicine up to the beginning
of the twentieth century," by Kabelik, J. BULLETIN ON
NARCOTICS. 12(3):508, 1960.
"Cannabis as a medicament: methods and results of the bacteriological experiments: I. Preliminary bacteriological experiments with extracts from cannabis sativa var.
indica. II. Bacteriological experiments carried out
with isolated and purified resin from cannabis," by Krejci, Z BULLETIN ON NARCOTICS. 12(3):12-19, 1960.
"Cannabis as a medicament: survey of clinical experiences,"
by Krejci, Z. BULLETIN ON NARCOTICS. 12(3):19-22, 1960.
"Cannabis in early pregnancy," by Persaud, T., and Ellington, A. LANCET. 2:1306, 1967.
"Chemical and pharmacological investigations on cannabis
sativa (linn): I," by Bose, B., et al. ARCHIVES INTER-
NATIONALES DE PHARMACODYNAMIE ET DE THERAPIE. 146:99-
105, 1963.
"Chemical studies on hashish: a synthesis of dl-cannabidiol
dimethylether," by Kochi, H., and Matsui, M. AGRICUL-
TURAL AND BIOLOGICAL CHEMISTRY (Tokyo). 31:625-627, 1967.
"Chromatographic identification of cannabis," by Betts,
T.J., et al. JOURNAL OF PHARMACY AND PHARMACOLOGY. 19
(Supplement):97S-102S, 1967.
"Chromatographic separation of the phenolic compounds of
cannabis sativa," by deRopp, R. JOURNAL OF THE AMERICAN
PHARMACEUTICAL ASSOCIATION (Sci. ed.). 49:756-758, 1960.
"Chromatography of edestin (from cannabis sativa) at 50
degrees," by Stockwell, D., et al. BIOCHIMICA ET BIO-
PHYSICA ACTA. 82:221-230, 1964.
"Clinical and psychological effects of marihuana in man,"
by Weil, A., et al. SCIENCE. 162:1234-1242, Dec.13,
1968.
"Collapse after intravenous injection of hashish," by Henderson, A., et al. BRITISH MEDICAL JOURNAL. 3:229-230,
1968.
"A combined spectrophotometric differentiation of samples
of cannabis," by Grlić, Ljubiša. BULLETIN ON NARCOTICS.
20(3):25-29, July-Sept., 1968.
"Comparative assay of the constituents from the sublimate
of smoked cannabis with that from ordinary cannabis,"
by Miras, C.J., et al. BULLETIN ON NARCOTICS. 16:13-
15, Jan., 1964.
"A comparative study of some chemical and biological char-

acteristics of various samples of cannabis resin," by
Grlic, L. BULLETIN ON NARCOTICS. 14(3):37-46, 1962.
"A comparison of LSD-25 with (----)-Δ^9-transtetrahydrocan-
nabinol (THC) and attempted cross tolerance between LSD
and THC," by Isbell, H., and Iasinski, D.R. PSYCHO-
PHARMACOLOGIA. 14(2):115-123, 1969.
"Concerning the isomerization of Δ^1- to $\Delta^{1\ 6}$-tetrahydrocan-
nabinol," by Gaoni, Y., and Mechoulam, R. JOURNAL OF
THE AMERICAN CHEMICAL SOCIETY. 88:5673-5675, 1966.
"Conjugate deviation of the eyes after cannabis indica in-
toxication," by Mohan, H., et al. BRITISH JOURNAL OF
OPHTHAMOLOGY. 48:160-161, 1964.
"The content of acid fraction in cannabis resin of various
age and provenance," by Grlic, L., and Andrec, A. EX-
PERIENTIA. 17:325-326, 1961.
"Degradation products of gambogic acid (preparation of can-
nabinolactonic acid)," by Hunt, B., and Rigby, W. CHEM-
ISTRY AND INDUSTRY. 42:1790-1791, 1967.
"Determination of tetrahydrocannabinol isomers in marijuana
and hashish," by Lerner, Melvin, and Zeffert, Judith T.
BULLETIN ON NARCOTICS. 20(2):53-54, Apr.-June, 1968.
"Drug use: symptom, disease, of adolescent experimentation,
the task of therapy," by Liebert, R.S. JOURNAL OF THE
AMERICAN COLLEGE HEALTH ASSOCIATION. 16:25-29, 1967.
"The effect of cannabis indica on carbohydrate metabolism
in rabbits," by El-Sourogy, M., et al. JOURNAL OF THE
EGYPTIAN MEDICAL ASSOCIATION. 49:626-628, 1966.
"Effect of cannabis indica on hexobarbital sleeping time
and tissue respiration of rat brain," by Bose, B., et
al. ARCHIVES INTERNATIONALES DE PHARMACODYNAMIE ET DE
THERAPIE. 146:520-524, 1963.
"Effect of hemp dust on certain functions of the organism,"
by Milenkov, Kh. R., et al. GIGIENA I SANITARIYA. 26:
25-32, 1961.
"Effect of 2-thiouracil on cell differentiation and leaf
morphogenesis in cannabis sativa," by Heslop-Harrison,
J. ANNALS OF BOTANY (London). 1962, pp. 375-387.
"Effects of (-) delta^9 trans-tetrahydrocannabinol in man,"
by Isbell, Harris. PSYCHOPHARMACOLOGIA. 11:184-188,
1967.
"Effects of a cannabis extract on gross behavior," by Gar-
attini, S. CIBA FOUNDATION STUDY GROUP. 21:70-82, 1965.
"Effects of a tetrahydrocannabinol derivative on some motor
systems in the cat," by Boyd, E., and Meritt, D. AR-
CHIVES INTERNATIONALES DE PHARMACODYNAMIE ET DE THERAPIE.
153:1-12, 1965.
"Effects of barbiturates and a tetrahydrocannabinol derivative on recovery cycles of medial lemniscul, thalamus
and reticular formation in the cat," by Boyd, E.S., and
Meritt, D.A. JOURNAL OF PHARMACOLOGY AND EXPERIMENTAL
THERAPEUTICS. 151:376-384, 1966.
"Effects of cannabis sativa and chlorpromazine on mice, as
measured by two methods used for evaluation of tranquilizing agents," by Salustiano, J., et al. MEDICINA ET
PHARMACOLOGIA EXPERIMENTALS. 15:153-162, 1966.

"Effects of cannabis sativa (marihuana) on maze performance of the rat," by Carlini, E., and Kramer, C. PSYCHOPHAR-MACOLOGIA. 7:175-181, 1965.

"Effects of cannabis sativa (marihuana) on the fighting behavior of mice," by Santos, M., et al. PSYCHOPHARMACOL-OGIA. 8:437-444, 1966.

"Effects of pharmacological agents on male sexual functions," by Mann, T. JOURNAL OF REPRODUCTION AND FERTILITY. suppl. 4:101-114, 1968.

"Effects of some tetrahydrocannabinols on hexobarbital sleeping time and amphetamine-induced hyperactivity in mice," by Garriott, J.C., et al. LIFE SCIENCE. 6(19):2119-2128, 1967.

"Effects of strychnine and cannabis sativa(marihuana) on the nucleic acid content in brain of the rat," by Carlini, G., and Carlini, E. MEDICINA ET PHARMACOLOGIA EXPERIMENTALS. 12:21-26, 1965.

"Effects of tetrahydrocannabinols and other drugs on operant behavior in rats," by Boyd, E., et al. ARCHIVES INTERNATIONALES DE PHARMACODYNAMIE ET DE THERAPIE. 144:533-554, 1963.

"Effects of the organic layer of hashish smoke extract and preliminary results of its chemical analysis," by Amaral Vieira, F.J., et al. PSYCHOPHARMACOLOGIA. 10(4):361-362, 1967.

"Effects of thiopental and a tetrahydrocannabinol derivative on arousal and recruiting in the cat," by Boyd, E.S., et al. JOURNAL OF PHARMACOLOGY AND EXPERIMENTAL THERAPEUTICS. 149:138-145, 1965.

"Essential oil from fresh cannabis sativa and its use in identification," by Martin, L., et al. NATURE. 191:774-776, 1961.

"Examination of cannabis resin by means of ferric chloride test," by Grlic, L., and Tomic, N. EXPERIENTIA. 19:267-268, 1963; also UN DOCUMENT St-Soa-Ser. S-8, 1963.

"Experimental studies of marihuana," by Clark, L.D., and Nakashima, E.N. AMERICAN JOURNAL OF PSYCHIATRY. 125(3):379-384, 1968.

"Extraction of the phenolic compounds of cannabis sativa and preparation of a synthetic intermediate," by Davis, D., et al. PHARMACOLOGIST. 4:161, 1962.

"Further neuropsychiatric observations in Nigeria, with comments on the need for epidemiological study in Africa," by Lambo, T. BRITISH MEDICAL JOURNAL. 2:1696, 1960.

"Ganja (cannabis sativa 1.), a review," by Stuart, K.L. WEST INDIAN MEDICAL JOURNAL. 12:156-160, 1963.

"Gas chromatography of Indian hemp (cannabis sativa)," by Caddy, B., et al. JOURNAL OF PHARMACY AND PHARMACOLOGY. 19(12):851-852, 1967

"General toxicodermatitis following acute poisoning caused by smoking Indian hemp," by Beliaev, N.V. VESTNIK DER-MATOLOGII I VENEROLOGII. 38:77-78, 1964.

"Grand mal convulsions subsequent to marijuana use," by Keeler, M.H., and Reifler, C.B. DISEASES OF THE NERVOUS

SYSTEM. 28(7):474-475, 1967.
"Hashish: a total synthesis of dl-Δ^1-tetrahydrocannabinol, the active constituent of hashish," by Machoulam, R. JOURNAL OF THE AMERICAN CHEMICAL SOCIETY. 87:3273-3275, 1965.
"Hashish: the isolation and constitution of a new component, cannabigerol," by Gaoni, Y., and Machoulam, R. PROCEEDINGS OF THE 33RD MEETING OF THE ISRAELI CHEMICAL SOCIETY. 1:229-230, 1963.
"Hashish: isolation, structure and partial synthesis of an active constituent of hashish," by Gaoni, Y., and Machoulam, R. JOURNAL OF THE AMERICAN CHEMICAL SOCIETY. 86:1646-1647, 1964.
"Hashish: the isolation and structure of cannabinolic, cannabidiolic and cannabizerolic acids," by Mechoulam, R. TETRAHEDRON. 21:1223-1229, 1965.
"Hashish: the structure of cannabidiol," by Mechoulam, R. TETRAHEDRON. 19:2073-2078, 1963.
"Histological reactions of hemp plant cannabis sativa to gibberellic acid," by Herich, R. PHYTON ANNALES REI BOTANICAE. 9:126-134, 1960.
"Hybridization of Southern dioecious varieties with monoecious varieties of hemp (cannabis sativa)," by Nevinnykh, V.A. AGROBIOLOGIYA. 2:205-212, 1962.
"Identification and origin determinations of cannabis by gas and paper chromatography," by Davis, T.W.M., et al. ANALYTICAL CHEMISTRY. 35(6):1751-1755, 1963.
"An improved and rapid test for detection of marihuana with diazotized p-nitroaniline," by Irudayasamy, A., and Natarajan, A. INDIAN JOURNAL OF CHEMISTRY. 3:327-328, 1965.
"Increased fibre content in hemp (cannabis sativa) and sunn (crotalaria juncea) by application of gibberelline," by Atal, C., and Sethi, J. CURRENT SCIENCE. 30:177-179, 1961.
"Influence of cannabis, tetrahydrocannabinol and pyrahexyl on the linguomandibular reflex of the dog," by Sampaio, C., et al. JOURNAL OF PHARMACY AND PHARMACOLOGY. 19:552-554, 1967.
"Influence of the age of pollen and stigmas on sex determination in hemp," by Laskowska, R. NATURE. 192:147-148, 1961.
"Isolation of edestin from aleurone grains of cannabis sativa," by St.Angelo, A., et al. ARCHIVES OF BIOCHEMISTRY AND BIOPHYSICS. 124:199-205, 1968.
"Isolation of trans-Δ^6-tetrahydrocannabinol from marijuana," by Hively, R., et al. JOURNAL OF THE AMERICAN CHEMICAL SOCIETY. 88:1832-1833, 1966.
"Isolation, structure, and partial synthesis of an active constituent of hashish," by Gaoni, Y., and Mechoulam,R.R. JOURNAL OF THE AMERICAN CHEMICAL SOCIETY. 86(8):1646-1647, 1964.
"Lack of cross-tolerance in rats among (-)Δ^9-trans-tetrahydrocannabinol (Δ^9-THC), cannabis extract, mescaline

and lysergic acid diethylamide (LSD-25)," by Silva, M.T.,
et al. PSYCHOPHARMACOLOGIA. 13(4):332-340, 1968.
"Long road to nirvana. Dissertation on marijuana," by Pel-
ner, L. NEW YORK STATE JOURNAL OF MEDICINE. 67:952-
956, 1967.
"Marihuana: tetrahydrocannabinol and related compounds,"
by Lerner, M. SCIENCE. 140(3563):175-176, 1963.
"Methods for the identification of cannabis: a study of
methods for the identification of cannabis by means of
ultraviolet absorption spectrophotometry." United Nations: UN DOCUMENT ST-SOA-SER. S-2, 1960.
"Methods for the identification of cannabis: a study of
the behavior of certain plant constituents when tested
with chemical reaction for the identification of cannabis." United Nations: UN DOCUMENT ST-SOA-SER.S-5, 1961.
"Methods for the identification of cannabis: a study of
the specificity of some chemical reactions for the identification of cannabis." United Nations: UN DOCUMENT
ST-SOA-SER. S-1, 1960.
"Methods of distinguishing biologically active cannabis
and fibre cannabis," by Toffoli, F., et al. BULLETIN
ON NARCOTICS. 20(1):55-59, Jan.-Mar., 1968.
"The methods used for the identification of cannabis by the
authorities in the United States of America." United
Nations: UN DOCUMENT ST-SOA-SER.S-3, 1960.
"The morphology and embryology of cannabis sativa," by Ram,
H., and Nath, R. PHYTOMORPHOLOGY. 14:414-429, 1964.
"Notes on the structure of cannabidiol compounds," by San-
tavi, F.. ACTA UNIVERSITATIS PALACKIANAE OLOMUCENSIS
FACULTATIS MEDICAE. 35:5-8, 1964.
"Observations on the pharmacological actions of cannabis
indica: 2," by Bose, B., et al. ARCHIVES INTERNATION-
ALES DE PHARMACODYNAMIE ET DE THERAPIE. 147:285-290,
1964.
"Occurrence of endosperm haustorium in cannabis sativa 1.,"
by Ram, H. ANNALS OF BOTANY. 24:79-82, 1960.
—"On the effect of hashish on the psyche," by Aal 'Tsman,
G.I., and Lenskii, G.P. ZDRAVOOKHRANENIE KAZAKHSTANA.
22:30-35, 1962.
"On the pharmacology of the hemp seed oil," by Vieira, J.,
et al. MEDICINA ET PHARMACOLOGIA EXPERIMENTALS. 16:
219-224, 1967.
"Paper and gas chromatogrphic analysis of cannabis," by
Farmilo, C., and Davis, T. JOURNAL OF PHARMACY AND
PHARMACOLOGY. 13:767-768, 1961.
—"Peripheral effects of a tetrahydrocannabinol," by Dagir-
manjian, R., and Boyd, E. FEDERATION PROCEEDINGS. 19:
267, 1960.
"Peroxide-sulphuric acid tests as an indication of the ripe-
ness and physiological activity of cannabis resin," by
Grlic, L. JOURNAL OF PHARMACY AND PHARMACOLOGY. 13:
637-638, 1961.
"Pharmacologic properties of some cannabis-related com-
pounds," by Garriott, J., et al. ARCHIVES INTERNATION-

ales de pharmacodynamie et de therapie. 171:425-434, 1968.

"Pharmacological activity of cannabis according to the sex of the plant," by Valle, J., et al. JOURNAL OF PHARMACY AND PHARMACOLOGY. 20:798-799, 1968.

"Pharmacological effects of two active constituents of marijuana," by Bicher, H., and Mechoulam, R. ARCHIVES INTERNATIONALES DE PHARMACODYNAMIE ET DE THERAPIE. 172: 24-31, 1968.

"Physiologically active nitrogen analogs of tetrahydrocannabinols: tetrahydrobenzopyzano(3,4-D) pyridines," by Pars, H., et al. JOURNAL OF THE AMERICAN CHEMICAL SOCIETY. 88:3664-3665, 1966.

"The precise determination of tetrahydrocannabinol in marihuana and hashish," by Lerner, Pauline. BULLETIN ON NARCOTICS. 21(3):39-42, July-Sept., 1969.

"Preliminary report on the separation and quantitative determination of cannabis constituents present in plant material, and when added to urine, by thin-layer and gas chromatography," by Parker, K., et al. BULLETIN ON NARCOTICS. 20(4):9-14, Oct.-Dec., 1968.

"Rabbit reactivity to cannabis preparations, pyrahexyl and tetrahydrocannabinol," by Valle, J., et al. JOURNAL OF PHARMACY AND PHARMACOLOGY. 18:476-478, 1966.

"Recent advances in the chemical research on cannabis," by Grlic, L. BULLETIN ON NARCOTICS. 16(4):29-38, 1964.

"Recent advances in the chemistry of hashish," by Mechoulam, R. FORTSCHRITTE DER CHEMIE ORGANISCKER NATURSTOFFE. 25:175-213, 1967.

"Recent results of hashish analysis," by Korte, F., and Sieper, H. CIBA FOUNDATION STUDY GROUP. 21:15-36, 1965.

"Research on cannabis (and addendum 1)." United Nations: UN DOCUMENT E-CN.7-442 ; also E-CN.7-442-ADD.1, Jan. 28, 1963.

"Rf values of some hashish constituents." JOURNAL OF CHROMATOGRAPHY. 6:D8, 1961.

"Scientific research on cannabis (note by the secretary general). United Nations: UN DOCUMENT E-CN.7-418, Jan. 25, 1962.

"Scientific research on cannabis (note by the secretary general): addendum 1." United Nations: UN DOCUMENT E-CN.7-418-ADD.1, Apr. 6, 1962.

"A screening technique for Indian hemp (cannabis sativa 1.)," by Caddy, B., and Fish, F. JOURNAL OF CHROMATOGRAPHY. 31:584-587, 1967.

"Separation of components of marijuana by gas-liquid chromatography," by Kingston, C., and Kirk, P. ANALYTICAL CHEMISTRY. 33:1794-1795, 1961.

"Some pharmacological effects of two tetrahydrocannabinols," by Dagirmanjian, R., and Boyd, E. JOURNAL OF PHARMACOLOGY AND EXPERIMENTAL THERAPEUTICS. 135:25-33, 1962.

"Spectrophotometric identification of marihuana," by Scaringelli, F. JOURNAL OF THE ASSOCIATION OF OFFICIAL AGRICULTURAL CHEMISTS. 44:296-303, 1961.

"Stereoelectronic factor in the chloranil dehydrogenation of cannabinoids: total synthesis of dl-cannabichromene," by Mechoulam, R., et al. JOURNAL OF THE AMERICAN CHEMICAL SOCIETY. 90:2418-2420, 1968.

"A stereospecific synthesis of $(-)$-Δ^1- and $(-)$-$\Delta^{1 \cdot 6}$-tetrahydrocannabinols," by Mechoulam, R., et al. JOURNAL OF THE AMERICAN CHEMICAL SOCIETY. 89:4552-4554, 1967.

"Stereospecifically labeled Δ^1-6-tetrahydrocannabinol," by Burstein, S., and Mechoulam, R. JOURNAL OF THE AMERICAN CHEMICAL SOCIETY. 90:2420-2421, 1968.

"The structure and synthesis of cannabigerol, a new hashish constituent," by Gaoni, Y., and Mechoulam, R. PROCEEDINGS OF THE AMERICAN CHEMICAL SOCIETY. p. 92, Mar., 1964.

"Studies on pharmacological actions of cannabis indica (linn): 3," by Bose, B., et al. ARCHIVES INTERNATIONALES PHARMACODYNAMIE ET DE THERAPIE. 147:291-297, 1964.

"Studies on the chemical analysis of marihuana," by Farmilo, C., et al. PROCEEDINGS OF THE CANADIAN SOCIETY OF FORENSIC SCIENTISTS. 1:1-50, 1962; also UN DOCUMENT ST-SOA-SER.S-7, 1962.

"Studies on the constituents of the hemp plant (cannabis sativa l.): isolation and identification of piperidine and several amino acids in the hemp plant," by Obata, Y., et al. BULLETIN OF THE AGRICULTURAL CHEMICAL SOCIETY OF JAPAN. 24:670-672, 1960.

"Studies on the constituents of the hemp plant)cannabis sativa l.): isolation of a Gibbs-positive compound from Japanese hemp," by Obata, Y. AGRICULTURAL AND BIOLOGICAL CHEMISTRY. 30:619-620, 1966.

"Studies on the constituents of the hemp plant (cannabis sativa l.): volatile phenol fraction," by Obata, Y., and Ishikawa, Y. BULLETIN OF THE AGRICULTURAL CHEMICAL SOCIETY OF JAPAN. 24:667-669, 1960.

"Studies of the dependence-producing potential of the narcotic antagonist 2-cyclopropylmethyl-2'-hydroxy-5, 9-dimethyl-6, 7-benzomorphan (cyclazocine, win-20, 740, arc II-C-3)," by Martin, W., et al. JOURNAL OF PHARMACOLOGY AND EXPERIMENTAL THERAPEUTICS. 150:426-436, 1965.

"Studies with the UN cannabis reference sample," by Joachimoglu, G., et al. BULLETIN ON NARCOTICS. 19(1):21-22, 1967.

"A study of infra-red spectra of cannabis resin," by Grlic, L. PLANTA MEDICA. 13:1281-1295, 1965; also UN DOCUMENT ST-SOA-SER.S-14, 1965.

"Study of the pharmacology of hashish," by Joachimoglu, G., and Miras, C. BULLETIN ON NARCOTICS. 15(3-4):7-8, July-Dec., 1963.

"Suppressive effects of 2-thiouracil on differentiation and flowering in cannabis sativa," by Heslop-Harrison, J. SCIENCE. 132:1943-1966, 1960.

"Synthesis gives active marihuana component: tetrahydrocannabinol isomer is identical to physiologically active compound isolated from hashish." CHEMICAL AND ENGINEERING NEWS. 44(4):38-39, 1966.

"Synthesis of d,1-cannabichromene, franklinone and other natural chromenes," by Cardillo, G., et al. TETRAHEDRON. 24:4825-4831, 1968.

"The synthesis of some model compounds related to tetrahydrocannabinol," by Taylor, E., and Strojny, E. JOURNAL OF THE AMERICAN CHEMICAL SOCIETY. 82:5198-5202, 1960.

"Synthesis of the eight stereoisomers of a tetrahydrocannabinol congener," by Aaron, H., and Ferguson, C. JOURNAL OF ORGANIC CHEMISTRY. 33:684-689, 1968.

"Tentative and rigorous proof in the identification of organic compounds and application of these concepts to the detection of the active principles of marihuana," by Cheronis, N. MICROCHEMICAL JOURNAL. 4:555-567, 1960.

"Teratogenic activity of cannabis resin," by Persaud, T., and Ellington, A. LANCET. 2(7564):406-407, 1968.

"Tetrahydrocannabinol analogs: synthesis of 2-(3-Methyl-2-Octyl)-3-Hydroxy-6,6,9-Trimethyl-7,8,9,10-Tetrahydrodibenzo(B,D)Pyran," by Taylor, E., et al. TETRAHEDRON. 23:77-85, 1967.

"Tetrahydrocannabinolcarboxylic acid. a component of hashish: part I," by Korte, F., et al. ANGEWANDTE CHEMIE INTERNATIONAL EDITION IN ENGLISH. 4:872, 1965.

"Tetrahydrocannabinols and analgesia." BULLETIN ON NARCOTICS. 21(1):29, Jan.-Mar., 1969.

"Tolerance to chronic administration of cannabis sativa (marihuana) in rats," by Carlini, E. PHARMACOLOGY (Basel). 1:135-142, 1968.

"Total synthesis of Δ^8-($\Delta^{1<6>}$)-tetrahydrocannabinol, a biologically active constituent of hashish (marijuana)," by Jen, T., et al. JOURNAL OF THE AMERICAN CHEMICAL SOCIETY. 89:4551-4552, 1967.

"The total synthesis of dl-Δ^9-tetrahydrocannabinol and four of its isomers," by Fahrenholtz, K., et al. JOURNAL OF THE AMERICAN CHEMICAL SOCIETY. 89:5934-5941, 1967.

"Total synthesis of dl-Δ^9-tetrahydrocannabinol and of dl-8-tetrahydrocannabinol, racemates of active constituents of marihuana," by Fahrenholtz, K., et al. JOURNAL OF THE AMERICAN CHEMICAL SOCIETY. 88:2079-2080, 1966.

"Toxicologic note on the varieties of hemp cultivated in Anjou," by Herisset, A. ANNALES PHARMACEUTIQUES FRANCAISES. 23:631-635, 1965.

"Vegetative hybridization of hemp as a method of obtaining starting material for selection," by Sustrina, V. AGROBIOLOGIIA. 3:386-391, 1960.

NARCOTIC ADDICTION: Books and Essays

Adams, S., and Zietz, D. PATTERNS OF NARCOTIC INVOLVEMENT: the autobiographies of five juvenile offenders. Sacramento, California: Department of Youth Authority, Division of Research, 1962.

Addiction Research Foundation, Toronto, Canada. PRELIMINARY REPORT ON ATTITUDES AND BEHAVIOUR OF TORONTO STUDENTS IN RELATION TO DRUGS. Toronto, 1967.

American Bar Association and The American Medical Association Joint Committee on Narcotic Drugs. DRUG ADDICTION: CRIME OR DISEASE? Bloomington, Indiana: Indiana University Press, 1961.

American Medical Association. Committee on Alcoholism and Drug Dependence and Council on Mental Health. THE CRUTCH THAT CRIPPLES: DRUG DEPENDENCE. Chicago, 1967.

American Medical Association. Council on Mental Health. DRUG DEPENDENCE: a guide for physicians. Chicago, 1969.

American Medical Association. Department of Mental Health. NARCOTIC ADDICTION. Chicago, 1963.

Andry, R.C. PSYCHOLOGICAL ASPECTS OF DRUG-TAKING; proceedings of a one day conference held at University College, London, Sept. 25, 1964. New York: Pergamon Press, 1965.

Anslinger, Harry Jacob, and Oursler, W. THE MURDERERS; the story of the narcotic gangs. New York: Farrar, Strauss and Cudahy, 1961.

Ausubel, David P. DRUG ADDICTION; physiological, psychological and sociological aspects. New York: Random House, 1968.

Barish, Herbert, and Brown, E. BEHAVIOR TRAITS OF THE MOTHER OF THE MALE ADDICT. New York: Lower Eastside Information Center for Narcotic Addiction, Inc., 1964.

Becker, Howard S., ed. THE OTHER SIDE; perspectives and deviance. New York: Free Press, 1964.

Becker, Howard Saul. OUTSIDERS; studies in the sociology of deviance. London: Free Press of Glencoe, 1963.

Bestic, Alan. TURN ME ON, MAN. New York: Award Books, 1968.

Bier, W.C. PROBLEMS IN ADDICTION: alcohol and drug addiction. New York: Fordham University Press, 1962.

Bill, Keith. SHOT TO HELL. Westwood, New Jersey: Revell Company, 1967.

Biological Council Symposium. DRUG DEPENDENCE. Boston: Little, Brown, 1969.

Bloch, H.A., and Geis, Gilbert. "Narcotic addicts," MAN, CRIME AND SOCIETY. New York: Random House, 1962, pp. 355-361.

Blum, Eva. "Horatio Alger's children: case studies," STUDENT AND DRUGS, by Blum, R.H. San Francisco: Jossey-Bass, 1969, pp. 243-273.

Blum, Richard H. "Bad outcomes on campus," STUDENT AND DRUGS. San Francisco: Jossey-Bass, 1969, pp. 147-167.

--"Correlations and factor analysis," STUDENT AND DRUGS. San Francisco: Jossey-Bass, 1969, pp. 101-109.

--"A cross-cultural study," SOCIETY AND DRUGS. San Francisco: Jossey-Bass, 1969, pp. 135-186.

--"Drugs on five campuses," STUDENT AND DRUGS. San Fran-

cisco: Jossey-Bass, 1969, pp. 31-47.
--"Life style interviews," STUDENT AND DRUGS. San
Francisco: Jossey-Bass, 1969, pp. 209-231.
--"Normal drug use," SOCIETY AND DRUGS. San Fran-
cisco: Jossey-Bass, 1969, pp. 245-275.
--"On the presence of demons," SOCIETY AND DRUGS.
San Francisco: Jossey-Bass, 1969, pp. 323-341.
--"Psychological tests," STUDENT AND DRUGS. San
Francisco: Jossey-Bass, 1969, pp. 233-241.
--"Student characteristics and major drugs," STUDENT
AND DRUGS. San Francisco: Jossey-Bass, 1969, pp.
63-81.
--"Student characteristics, minor drugs, and motiva-
tion," STUDENT AND DRUGS. San Francisco: Jossey-
Bass, 1969, pp. 83-98.
--"Student ideologies compared," STUDENT AND DRUGS.
San Francisco: Jossey-Bass, 1969, pp. 195-207.
--"Students' drug diaries," STUDENT AND DRUGS. San
Francisco: Jossey-Bass, 1969, pp. 169-182.
--"Those who do, those who do not," STUDENT AND
DRUGS. San Francisco: Jossey-Bass, 1969, pp.
49-61.
--"Users of approved drugs," STUDENT AND DRUGS. San
Francisco: Jossey-Bass, 1969, pp. 111-131.
--"Users of illicit drugs," STUDENT AND DRUGS. San
Francisco: Jossey-Bass, 1969, pp. 133-144.
Blum, Richard H., and Ferguson, Bruce. "Predicting who
will turn on," STUDENT AND DRUGS. San Francisco:
Jossey-Bass, 1969, pp. 275-288.
Blum, Richard H., and Garfield, Emily. "A follow-up
study," STUDENT AND DRUGS. San Francisco: Jossey-
Bass, 1969, pp. 185-193.
Blum, Richard H., et al. "Drugs and high school students,"
STUDENT AND DRUGS. San Francisco: Jossey-Bass, 1969,
pp. 321-348.
Blum, Richard H., et al. SOCIETY AND DRUGS. social and
cultural observations. San Francisco: Jossey-Bass,
1969.
Blum, Richard H., et al. STUDENT AND DRUGS; college and
high school observations. San Francisco: Jossey-Bass,
1969.
Blumer, Herbert, et al. THE WORLD OF YOUTHFUL DRUG USE.
Berkeley: University of California, 1967.
Borgatta, Edgar F. SOME PROBLEMS IN THE STUDY OF DRUG
USE AMONG COLLEGE STUDENTS. Based on presentation
at the NASPA Drug Education Conference. Washington,
1966.
Bredemeier, H., and Toby, J. SOCIAL PROBLEMS IN AMERICA.
New York: Wiley, 1963.
Brill, Leon, et al. AUTHORITY AND ADDICTION. Boston:
Little, Brown, 1969.
Brotman, Richard, et al. A COMMUNITY MENTAL HEALTH AP-
PROACH TO DRUG ADDICTION. Washington: United States
Department of Health, Education and Welfare, 1968.
Brown, C. MANCHILD IN THE PROMISED LAND. New York:

American Library, 1966.

Brown, T. THE ENIGMA OF DRUG ADDICTION... Springfield, Illinois: C.C. Thomas, 1963.

Burroughs, William. JUNKIE (Originally published as 'Junk' under the pen-name of William Lee). New York: Ace Books, 1964.

Cain, Arthur H. YOUNG PEOPLE AND DRUGS. New York: John Day Company, 1969.

California. Department of Justice. REPORTS ON: comparative studies on the detection of narcotic users with chemical tests and effect of narcotic antagonists on the pupil diameter of nonaddicts. Sacramento: S. Mosk, 1961.

California. Narcotic Enforcement Bureau. THE NARCOTIC PROBLEM: a brief study. Sacramento, 1965.

Carey, James T. THE COLLEGE DRUG SCENE. Englewood Cliffs, New Jersey: Prentice-Hall, 1968.

Casper, E. NARCOTICS ADDICTION: a response to structured strain. Philadelphia: Pennsylvania Parole Board, 1965.

Casriel, D. SO FAIR A HOUSE: the story of Synanon. Englewood Cliffs, New Jersey: Prentice-Hall, 1963.

Chein, I., et al. THE ROAD TO H; narcotics, delinquency and social policy. New York: Basic Books, 1964.

Chopra, R.N., and Chopra, I.C. DRUG ADDICTION. New Delhi: Delhi Press, 1965.

Clark, Janet, pseud. THE FANTASTIC LODGE; the autobiography of a girl drug addict, ed. Helen MacGill Hughes. Boston: Houghton Mifflin, 1961.

Cloward, Richard A., and Oblin, L. DELINQUENCY AND OPPORTUNITY: a theory of delinquent gangs. Glencoe, Illinois: Free Press, 1960.

Cohen, Sidney. DRUG DILEMMA. New York: McGraw-Hill, 1969.

Cole, Jonathan O., and Wittenborn, J.R. DRUG ABUSE: social and psychopharmacological aspects. Springfield, Illinois: C.C. Thomas, 1969.

Curtis, Jack H. "Drugs and Catholic students," STUDENT AND DRUGS, by Blum, R.H. San Francisco: Jossey-Bass, 1969, pp. 305-319.

Dawtry, F., ed. SOCIAL PROBLEMS OF DRUG ABUSE. London: Butterworth and Company, 1968.

De Quincey, Thomas. CONFESSIONS OF AN ENGLISH OPIUM EATER, ed. A. Ward. New York: New American Library, 1966.

De Ropp, Robert S. DRUGS AND THE MIND. New York: Grove Press, 1960.

Duncan, Tommie L. UNDERSTANDING AND HELPING THE NARCOTIC HABIT. Philadelphia: Fortress Press, 1968.

Ebin, David, ed. THE DRUG EXPERIENCE; first-person accounts of addicts, writers, scientists and others. New York: Orion Press, 1961.

Eddy, N.B. "Chemopharmacologic approach to the addiction problem," NARCOTICS, ed. D.M. Wilner, and G.G.Kassebaum. New York: McGraw-Hill, 1965, pp. 67-84.

Ely, Virginia. SOME OF MY BEST FRIENDS WERE ADDICTS. Westwood, New Jersey: Revell Company, 1968.

Endore, Guy. SYNANON: controversial drug addiction cure.

New York: Doubleday, 1968.

Farber, S.M., and Wilson, R.H.L., eds. CONFLICT AND CRE-
ATIVITY: control of the mind. New York: McGraw-Hill,
1963.

Fiddle, Seymour. PORTRAITS FROM A SHOOTING GALLERY: life
styles from the drug addict world. New York: Harper,
1967.

Fort, J. "Social values, American youth, and drug use,"
BACKGROUND PAPERS ON STUDENT DRUG INVOLVEMENT, ed. C.
Hollander. Washington: United States National Student
Association, 1967, pp. 131-146.

Fort, Joel M. THE PLEASURE SEEKERS; the drug crisis, youth
and society. Indianapolis: Bobbs-Merrill, 1969.

Freyhan, F. DRUG ADDICTION. New York: Grune and Stratton,
1963.

Geller, Allen, and Boas, Maxwell. THE DRUG BEAT. New York:
Cowles, 1969.

Gimenez, John, and Meredith, C. UP TIGHT. Waco, Texas:
Word Books, 1967.

Gioscia, Victor. "Adolescence, addiction and achrony,"
PERSONALITY AND SOCIAL LIFE, by Endleman, R. New York:
Random House, 1967.

Glaser, Daniel, et al. LATER HEROIN USE BY ADOLESCENT MAR-
IJUANA AND HEROIN USERS, AND BY NON-DRUG USING ADOLESCENT
OFFENDERS. Albany: New York State Narcotic Addiction
Control Commission, 1968.

Glazer, N., and Moynihan, D.P. BEYOND THE MELTING POT.
Cambridge: The M.I.T. Press and Harvard University Press,
1963.

Great Britain. Interdepartmental Committee on Drug Addiction. DRUG ADDICTION. London: H.M. Stationery Office,
1961.

Great Britain. Stationery Office. REPORT OF THE INTERDE-
PARTMENTAL COMMITTEE, MINISTRY OF HEALTH, SCOTTISH HOME
AND HEALTH DEPARTMENT. London: H.M. Stationery Office,
1961.

Great Britain. Stationery Office. SECOND REPORT OF THE
INTERDEPARTMENTAL COMMITTEE, MINISTRY OF HEALTH, SCOT-
TISH HOME AND HEALTH DEPARTMENT. London: H.M.Station-
ery Office, 1965.

Harms, E. DRUG ADDICTION IN YOUTH. New York: Pergamon
Press, 1965.

Harney, Maleachi L. THE NARCOTIC OFFICER'S NOTEBOOK.
Springfield, Illinois: C.C. Thomas, 1961.

Harris, J.D. THE JUNKIE PRIEST - FATHER DANIEL EGAN, S.A.
New York: Coward-McCann, 1964; Pocket Books, 1965.

Hentoff, N. A DOCTOR AMONG THE ADDICTS. Chicago: Rand
McNally, 1968.

Hess, A.G. CHASING THE DRAGON: a report on drug addiction
in Hong Kong. New York: Free Press, 1965.

THE HIPPIES, by the correspondents of Time, ed. Joe David
Brown. New York: Time, Inc., 1967.

Hofling, C. "Personality disorders: narcotic addiction,"
TEXTBOOK OF PSYCHIATRY FOR MEDICAL PRACTICE, by Hofling,
C. Philadelphia: Lippincott, 1963, pp. 414-416.

107

Hollander, Charles, ed. STUDENT DRUG INVOLVEMENT. Washington: United States National Student Association, 1967.

Hong Kong Government. THE PROBLEM OF NARCOTIC USE IN HONG KONG: a white paper laid before legislative council Nov. 11, 1959. Hong Kong: Government Printer, 1959.

Hong Kong Government. A PROBLEM OF PEOPLE. Hong Kong: Government Printer, 1960.

Howe, Hubert S. NARCOTICS AND YOUTH; a doctor discusses the problem of teen-age addiction and its effects. West Orange, New Jersey: The Brook Foundation, 1964.

Hyde, Margaret O., ed. MIND DRUGS. New York: McGraw-Hill, 1968.

Illinois. Department of Public Instruction. PROGRAM DEVELOPMENT FOR FOUNDATIONS IN ALCOHOL AND NARCOTIC EDUCATION. Springfield, 1963.

Jaffe, Jerome H. "Drug addiction and drug abuse," THE PHARMACOLOGICAL BASIS OF THERAPEUTICS, ed. Goodman and Gillman, 3rd edition. New York: Macmillan, 1965, pp. 300-301.

Jeffe, S. NARCOTICS: an American plan. New York: Paul S. Eriksson, Inc., 1966.

Kalant, Harold, et al. EXPERIMENTAL APPROACHES TO THE STUDY OF DRUG DEPENDENCE. Toronto: University of Toronto Press, 1969.

Kane, J.J. SOCIAL PROBLEMS: a situational-value approach. Englewood Cliffs, New Jersey: Prentice-Hall, 1962.

Keniston, Kenneth. "Drug use and student values," BACKGROUND PAPERS ON STUDENT INVOLVEMENT, ed. C. Hollander. Washington: United States National Student Association, 1967, pp. 121-130.

Keniston, Kenneth. THE UNCOMMITTED: alienated youth in American society. New York: Dell Publishing Company, 1967.

Kitzinger, A., and Hill, P.J. DRUG ABUSE: a source book and guide for teachers. Sacramento: California State Department of Education, 1967.

Kolb, L. DRUG ADDICTION: a medical problem. Springfield, Illinois: C.C. Thomas, 1962.

Kron, Yves J., and Brown, E.M. MAINLINE TO NOWHERE; the making of a heroin addict. New York: Pantheon Books, 1965.

Laing, R.D. THE DIVIDED SELF; a study of sanity and madness. Chicago: Quadrangle Books, 1960.

Land, Herman W. WHAT YOU CAN DO ABOUT DRUGS AND YOUR CHILD. New York: Hart Pub., 1969.

Larimore, Granville, and Brill, Henry. CONTROLLING THE ADDICT. New York: Random House, 1961.

Larner, J. THE ADDICT IN THE STREET, tape recordings collected by Ralph Tefferteller. New York: Grove Press, 1964.

Laurie, Peter. DRUGS: medical, psychological and social facts. Baltimore: Penguin Books, 1967.

Lawrence, D.R., and Bacharuch, A.L. EVALUATION OF DRUG ACTIVITIES. London: Academic Press, 1964.

Lee, William, pseud., see Burroughs, William.
Leeds, David Paul. PERSONALITY PATTERNS AND MODES OF BE-
HAVIOR OF MALE ADOLESCENT NARCOTIC ADDICTS AND THEIR MO-
THERS. New York: Yeshiva University, 1965.
Lindesmith, A.R. THE ADDICT AND THE LAW. Bloomington,
Indiana: Indiana University Press, 1965.
Lindesmith, Alfred R. ADDICTION AND OPIATES, revised ed-
ition. Chicago: Aldine Publishing Company, 1968.
Lindesmith, Alfred R. "Basic problems in the social psy-
chology of addiction and a theory," CHATHAM CONFERENCE
ON PERSPECTIVES ON NARCOTIC ADDICTION. Chatham, Massa-
chusetts, Sept. 9-11, pp. 1-16.
Lindesmith, Alfred R. DRUG ADDICTION: crime or disease.
Bloomington: Indiana University Press, 1961.
Lindesmith, Alfred R. "Problems in the social psychology
of addiction," NARCOTICS, ed. Wilner and Kassebaum.
New York: McGraw-Hill, 1965.
Listen (Washington, D.C.). NOW YOU'RE LIVING! Basic information for scientific education for the prevention of
alcoholism and drug addiction, revised edition. Washington: Narcotics Education Inc., 1964.
Listen (Washington, D.C.). REALLY LIVING; basic information for scientific education for the prevention of alcoholism and drug addiction, revised edition. Washington: Narcotics Education Inc., 1960.
Livingston, Robert B., ed. NARCOTIC DRUG ADDICTION PROBLEM.
United States Department of Health, Education and Wel-
fare, Public Health Service publication no. 1050. Wash-
ington: Government Printing Office, 1963.
Louria, Donald B. DRUG SCENE. New York: McGraw-Hill, 1968.
Los Angeles County Narcotics and Dangerous Drug Commission,
et al. DARKNESS ON YOUR DOORSTEP. Los Angeles: The Los
Angeles County Board of Supervisors, 1964.
Maddux, J.F. "Hospital management of the narcotic addict,"
NARCOTICS, ed. D.M. Wilner, and G.G.Kassebaum. New York:
McGraw-Hill, 1965, pp. 159-176.
Marks, John. THE SCIENTIFIC BASIS OF DRUG THERAPY IN PSY-
CHIATRY. Oxford: Pergamon Press, 1965.
Mathison, R. FAITHS, CULTS, AND SECTS OF AMERICA. Indian-
apolis: Bobbs-Merrill, 1960.
Maurer, David W. WHIZ MOB: a correlation of the argot of
pickpockets with their behavior pattern. New Haven:
College and University Press Services, 1964.
Maurer, David W., and Vogel, Victor H. NARCOTICS AND NAR-
COTIC ADDICTION, 3rd. edition. Springfield, Illinois:
C.C. Thomas, 1967.
Meiselas, H. A REPORT OF SOME EARLY CLINICAL EXPERIENCES
FROM THE NEW YORK STATE DEPARTMENT OF MENTAL HYGIENE'S
NARCOTIC RESEARCH UNIT, presented before the 24th Meet-
ing of the Committee on Drug Addiction and Narcotics,
National Academy of Science and National Research Coun-
cil, Jan. 29, 1962.
Menconi, L. NARCOTIC PROBLEM, a brief study. Sacramento,
California: Bureau of Narcotic Enforcement, 1962.

Michaux, Henry. LIGHT THROUGH DARKNESS. New York: Orion Press, 1963.

Mills, J., et al. THE DRUG TAKERS. New York: Time-Life Books, 1965.

Mills, James. THE PANIC IN THE NEEDLE PARK. New York: Farrar, Straus and Giroux, 1966.

Mulcahy, J.R., and Mulcahy, John F. PERSPECTIVES ON NARCOTIC ADDICTION. The Chatham Conference, Cape Cod, Massachusetts, Sept. 9-11, 1963, April 9, 1964.

Myrdal, Gunnar. AN AMERICAN DILEMMA. New York: Harper and Row, 1962.

Mitchell, Alexander Ross Kerr. DRUGS; the parents dilemma, ed. C. Morris. Royston, England: Priory, 1969.

NARCOTIC DRUG ADDICTION PROBLEMS. Symposium on the history of narcotic drug addiction, Bethesda, Maryland, 1958. Washington: Government Printing Office, 1963.

NARCOTICS ADDICTION; official actions of the American Medical Association. Washington: Department of Health, 1963.

National Academy of Sciences. National Research Council. Addiction and Narcotics Committee. MINUTES OF THE TWENTY-SEVENTH MEETING, 1965. Washington, 1965.

New Jersey. Legislature. Narcotic Drug Study Commission. AN INTERIM REPORT: a study of the administration of narcotic control relating to the causes, prevention and control of drug addiction, constituted pursuant to Senate joint resolution no. 16, Laws of 1963. Trenton, New Jersey, 1964.

New Jersey. State Education Department. DRUG ABUSE; a reference for teachers. 1967.

New York. Regional Mental Health Planning Committee. Subcommittee on Addiction. REPORT. New York: Community Mental Health Board, 1965.

New York (State) Division of Parole. AN EXPERIMENT IN THE SUPERVISION OF PAROLE OFFENDERS ADDICTED TO NARCOTIC DRUGS. Final report of the special narcotic project. Albany, 1960.

New York (State) Division of Parole. RECENT DEVELOPMENTS IN THE TREATMENTS OF PAROLE OFFENDERS ADDICTED TO NARCOTIC DRUGS, by Diskind, Meyer H., and Klonsky, George. Albany, 1964.

New York (State) Education Department. Curriculum Development Center. DRUG ABUSE: supplementary information for teachers on the use, misuse and abuse of drugs. Albany, 1967.

New York (State) Narcotic Addiction Control Commission. ANNUAL REPORT FOR 1968. Albany, 1969.

New York (State) Narcotic Addiction Control Commission. THE STATE OF NEW YORK AND THE DRUG ADDICT. Albany, 1968.

New York (State) University. DRUGS ON CAMPUS: an assessment. Proceedings of the joint conference sponsored by State University of New York and Narcotic Addiction Control Commission, Nov. 20-22. Albany, 1968.

The New York Times. THE DRUG SCENE; a series on the use

and abuse of drugs in the United States. New York, 1968.
Nowlis, Helen H. DRUGS ON THE COLLEGE CAMPUS. Garden City, New York: Doubleday, 1968.
Nowlis, Helen H. "Overview for administrators," STUDENT AND DRUGS, by Blum, R.H. San Francisco: Jossey-Bass, 1969, pp. 351-358.
O'Donnell, J.A., and Ball, J.C. NARCOTIC ADDICTION. New York: Harper and Row, 1966.
O'Donnell, John A. A FOLLOW-UP OF NARCOTIC ADDICTS: mortality, relapse and abstinence. Washington: National Academy of Science, 1964.
O'Donnell, John A. THE RELAPSE RATE IN NARCOTIC ADDICTION; a critique of follow-up studies. Albany: Narcotic Addiction Control Commission, 1968.
Oklahoma. State Department of Health. NARCOTIC ADDICTION AND DRUG ABUSE. Oklahoma City, 1964.
Parks, D.C. NARCOTICS AND NARCOTICS ADDICTION. New York: Carlton Press, 1969.
Patrick, S.W., and Krug, D.C. LET'S TALK ABOUT NARCOTIC ADDICTION. New York City: Department of Health, Research Unit on Narcotics Addiction, 1962.
Paulsen, James. "Psychiatric problems," STUDENT AND DRUGS, by Blum, R.H. San Francisco: Jossey-Bass, 1969, pp. 291-303.
Pearl, A. "An addict tells his story," MENTAL HEALTH OF THE POOR, ed. F. Riesman, J. Cohen, and A. Pearl. New York: Free Press, 1964.
PSYCHOSOCIAL ASPECTS OF DRUG-TAKING. Foreward by R.G. Andry, summarized by Derrick Sington. Long Island City, New York: Pergamon Press Inc., 1965.
Purtell, Thelma C. TONIGHT IS TOO LATE. New York: Paul S. Ericksson, 1965.
Rado, Sandor. "Narcotic bondage: a general theory of the dependence on narcotic drugs," PSYCHOANALYSIS OF BEHAVIOR, by Rado, Sandor. New York: Grune and Stratton, 1962, vol 2, pp. 21-29.
Redlich, Frederick C., and Friedman, Daniel X. THE THEORY AND PRACTICE OF PSYCHIATRY. New York: Basic Books, 1966.
Relin, Louis. A DOCTOR DISCUSSES NARCOTICS AND DRUG ADDICTION. Chicago: Budlong Press, 1968.
Retterstol, N., and Sund, A. DRUG ADDICTION AND HABITUATION. Oslo, Norway: The Norwegian Research Council for Science and the Humanities, 1965.
Robertson, J.P.S., and Walton, D. ADDICTION TO ANALGESIC DRUGS: resumé of research. Document no. 5, prepared for the British Psychological Society Working Party on Drug Addiction, 1960.
St. Charles, Alwyn J. NARCOTICS MENACE. Alhambra, California: Borden, 1968.
Saltman, Jules. WHAT WE CAN DO ABOUT DRUG ABUSE. New York: Public Affairs Committee, Inc., 1966.
Samuels, Gertrude. THE PEOPLE VS. BABY. Garden City, New York: Doubleday, 1967.
Schaap, Richard. TURNED ON: the Friede-Crenshaw case. New

York: New American Library, 1967.

Schmidt, Jacob E. NARCOTICS, LINGO AND LORE. Springfield, Illinois, C.C. Thomas, 1960.

Schoenfeld, E. DEAR DOCTOR HIP POCRATES. New York: Grove Press, 1968.

Schur, E.M. CRIMES WITHOUT VICTIMS: deviate behavior and public policy, abortion, homosexuality, drug addiction. Englewood Cliffs, New Jersey: Prentice-Hall, 1965.

Schur, E.M. NARCOTIC ADDICTION IN BRITAIN AND AMERICA: the impact of public policy. Bloomington, Indiana: Indiana University Press, 1962.

Shaffer, H.B. NARCOTICS ADDICTION: punishment or treatment. Washington: Editorial Research Reports, 1962.

Sharoff, Robert L., et al. DOCTOR DISCUSSES NARCOTICS AND DRUG ADDICTION. Chicago: Budlong Press, 1969.

Shoham, Shlomo. SURVEY OF PROSTITUTION IN ISRAEL. Treatment of offenders. Ministry of Welfare, 1962.

Simmons, J., and Winograd, B. IT'S HAPPENING. Santa Barbara: Marc-Laird Publications, 1966.

Sington, Derrick, and Klare, H.S. PSYCHOLOGICAL ASPECTS OF DRUG-TAKING. New York: Pergamon Press, 1966.

Slim, Iceberg. PIMP; the story of my life. Los Angeles, California: Holloway House Publishing Company, 1967.

Smith, Kline and French Laboratories. DRUG ABUSE; a manual for law enforcement officers. Philadelphia, 1965.

Smith, Kline and French Laboratories. DRUG ABUSE: ESCAPE TO NOWHERE; a guide for educators. Philadelphia: Smith, Kline and French Laboratories in cooperation with the American Association for Health, Physical Education, and Recreation; distributed by National Education Association, Washington. 1967.

Smith, M., et al. THE RAS TAFARI MOVEMENT IN KINGSTON, JAMAICA. Kingston: University College of the West Indies, 1960.

Society for the Study of Addiction to Alcohol and other drugs. PHARMACOLOGICAL AND EPIDEMIOLOGICAL ASPECTS OF ADOLESCENT DRUG DEPENDENCE, ed. Cedric W.M. Wilson. New York: Pergamon Press, 1968.

Sprigge, Elizabeth, and Kihm, J.J. JEAN COCTEAU; the man and the mirror. New York: Coward-McCann, 1968.

Stearn, Jess. THE SEEKERS. New York: Doubleday, 1969.

Stringfellow, W. MY PEOPLE IS THE ENEMY. New York: Holt, 1964.

Symposium on the History of Narcotic Drug Addiction Problems. Bethesda, Maryland, 1958. NARCOTIC DRUG ADDICTION PROBLEMS; proceedings, ed. B. Livingston. Washington: United States Department of Health, Education and Welfare, Public Health Service. Government Printing Office, 1963.

Texas. Alcohol and Narcotic Education. THE ALCOHOL-NARCOTIC PROBLEM; a handbook for teachers, revised edition. Dallas: Tane Press, 1964.

Time, Inc. THE DRUG TAKERS. New York: Time-Life Books, 1965.

Time, Inc. HOW TO IDENTIFY WHAT DRUGS A TEEN MAY BE TAKING. New York: Time-Life Books, 1966.
Trocchi, Alexander. CAIN'S BOOK. New York: Grove Press, 1960.
Turkel, Peter. THE CHEMICAL RELIGION; facts about drugs and teens. Glen Rock, New Jersey: Paulist Press, 1969.
Uhr, L . and Miller, J.G., eds. DRUGS AND BEHAVIOR. New York: Wiley, 1967.
United Kingdom. Ministry of Health. Department of Health for Scotland. DRUG ADDICTION: report of the Interdepartmental Committee. London: H.M. Stationery Office, 1961.
United States. Bureau of Narcotics. CONTROL AND REHABILITATION OF THE NARCOTIC ADDICT. Washington, 1961.
United States. Bureau of Narcotics. LIVING DEATH: the truth about drug addiction. Washington: United States Superintendent of Documents, Government Printing Office, 1965.
United States. Department of Defense. Armed Forces Information Service. DRUG ABUSE: game without winners, a basic handbook for commanders. Washington: United States Superintendent of Documents, Government Printing Office, 1968.
United States Interdepartmental Committee on Narcotics. REPORT TO THE PRESIDENT OF THE UNITED STATES. Washington: Government Printing Office, 1961.
United States. National Institute of Mental Health. NARCOTIC DRUG ADDICTION. Mental Health Monograph no. 2. Washington: United States Superintendent of Documents, Government Printing Office, 1963.
United States. National Institute of Mental Health. Demonstration Center, New York. REHABILITATION IN DRUG ADDICTION; a report on a five-year community experiment of the New York Demonstration Center. Washington: Government Printing Office, 1963.
United States. Advisory Committee on Narcotic and Drug Addiction. FINAL REPORT. Washington: Government Printing Office, 1963.
United States. Treasury Department. Bureau of Narcotics. ACTIVE NARCOTIC ADDICTS AS OF DEC. 31, 1963. Annual tabulation. Washington: Government Printing Office, 1964.
Wakefield, Dan. THE ADDICT. Greenwich, Connecticut: Fawcett Publications, 1963.
Walker, K. THE CONSCIOUS MIND. London: Rider and Company, 1962.
Watts, Alan W. THE JOYOUS COSMOLOGY; adventures in the chemistry of consciousness. New York: Pantheon Books, 1962.
Weakland, John H. "Hippies: what the scene means," SOCIETY AND DRUGS, by Blum, R.H. San Francisco: Jossey-Bass, 1969, pp. 343-372.
White House Ad Hoc Panel on Drug Abuse. PROGRESS REPORT. Washington, 1962.
Wikler, Abraham. THE ADDICTIVE STATES. Baltimore: Williams and Wilkins, 1968.

Wilkerson, David. THE CROSS AND THE SWITCHBLADE. New York:
Pyramid Books, 1963.
Williams, John B., ed. NARCOTICS AND HALLUCINOGENICS: a
handbook. Beverly Hills: Glencoe Press, 1967.
Wilner, Daniel, and Kassebaum, G.G. NARCOTICS. New York:
McGraw-Hill, 1965.
Winick, C. "Epidemiology of narcotics use," NARCOTICS, ed.
D.M. Wilner, and G.G.Kassebaum. New York: McGraw-Hill,
1965, pp. 3-18.
Winick, C. THE NARCOTIC ADDICTION PROBLEM. New York: Amer-
ican Social Health Association, 1962.
Wisconsin. Division for Children and Youth. NARCOTICS
AND YOUTH, revised edition by Harvey W. Rowe. Madison,
1961.
Wittenborn, J.R., et al, eds. DRUGS AND YOUTH: proceedings
of the Rutgers Symposium on drug abuse. Springfield,
Illinois: C.C. Thomas, 1969.
World Health Organization. Scientific Group on the Eval-
uation of Dependence-Producing Drugs. EVALUATION OF
DEPENDENCE-PRODUCING DRUGS: a report of a WHO scientif-
ic group. Geneva: World Health Organization, 1964.
Yablonsky, Lewis. THE HIPPIE TRIP. New York: Pegasus, 1968.
Yablonsky, Lewis. THE TUNNEL BACK: SYNANON. New York:
Macmillian, 1965.

NARCOTIC ADDICTION: Doctoral Dissertations

Ahmed, Samir N. "Patterns of juvenile drug use" (Thesis,
unpublished, University of California at Berkeley).
DISSERTATION ABSTRACTS. 28(11-A):4703, 1968.
Birner, L. "Level of self-esteem of imprisoned addicted
users of narcotic drugs" (Thesis, unpublished, Yeshiva
University), 1961.
Bret, S.R. "Group interaction techniques and their influ-
ence on 'addict identification'." DISSERTATION ABSTRACTS.
26:2309-2310, 1965.
Cutler, Rhoda. "An assessment of the meaning of work to
the male narcotic addict in a voluntary treatment center" (Thesis, unpublished, New York University). DIS-
SERTATION ABSTRACTS. 28(10-A):3881, 1968.
Einstein, Stanley. "The influence of the self-system, eth-
nicity and drug addiction upon future time perspective"
(Thesis, unpublished, Yeshiva University). DISSERTATION
ABSTRACTS. 26(6):3674, 1964.
Garrett, June J. "Personality variables associated with
sociometric status among institutionalized narcotic drug
addicts" (Thesis, unpublished, North Texas State University). DISSERTATION ABSTRACTS. 28(6-B):2661-2662, 1967.
Gold, L. "Reaction of male adolescent addicts to frustra-
tion as compared to two adolescent non-addicted groups"

(Thesis, unpublished, New York University). DISSERTA-
TION ABSTRACTS. 20:4716, 1960.
Grupp, Stanley E. "The nalline test and addict attitudes"
(Thesis, unpublished, Indiana University). DISSERTATION
ABSTRACTS. 28(5-A):1910-1911, 1967.
Hughes, James W. "The American medical profession and the
narcotics policy controversy" (Thesis, unpublished, In-
diana University). DISSERTATION ABSTRACTS. 28(11-A):
4718, 1968.
Leeds, David P. "Personality patterns and modes of behav-
ior of male adolescent narcotic addicts and their mothers"
(Thesis, unpublished, Yeshiva University). DISSERTATION
ABSTRACTS. 26(5):2861-2862, 1965.
Leibowitz, Marvin. "Effects of psychological support on
test performance of four types of narcotic addicts" (The-
sis, unpublished, New York University). DISSERTATION
ABSTRACTS. 27(8-B):2873, 1967.
Levine, Esther E. "An experimental investigation of the
role of disruptive stress reactions in narcotic addicts"
(Thesis, unpublished, New York University). DISSERTATION
ABSTRACTS. 25(1):630, 1964.
Sand, Walter T. "Psychosocial factors and the types of
sociopathy" (Thesis, unpublished, University of Maryland)
DISSERTATION ABSTRACTS. 27(4-A):1112-1113, 1966.
Schiff, Stanley. "A self-theory investigation of drug ad-
diction in relation to age of onset" (Thesis, unpublish-
ed, New York University). DISSERTATION ABSTRACTS. 27
(5-A):1449-1450, 1966.
Weinrebe, Claire K. THE MALE ADOLESCENT DRUG ADDICT AND
HIS MOTHER: their concepts of themselves, each other,
and the addict's father. New York: Columbia University,
1967. DISSERTATION ABSTRACTS. 28(9-A):3792, 1968.

NARCOTIC ADDICTION: Periodical Literature

General Publications

"Abuse of belladonna alkaloids." BULLETIN ON NARCOTICS.
20(2):55, Apr.-June, 1968.
"The abuse of drugs," by Hessler, W. PRAXIS. 50:1091-
1093, 1961.
"Abuse of drugs, a growing menace; symposium. UNESCO
COURIER. 21:4-29, May, 1968.
"The abuse of paregoric in Detroit, Michigan (1956-1965),"
by Lerner, A. Martin. BULLETIN ON NARCOTICS. 18(3):
13-19, July-Sept., 1966.
"Accidental therapeutic drug addiction," by Friend, D.G.
CLINICAL PHARMACOLOGY AND THERAPEUTICS. 7:832-834,
Nov.-Dec., 1966.
"Action research in a treatment center," by Freedman,

Alfred M. AMERICAN JOURNAL OF NURSING. 63:57-60, July, 1963.
"The addict, a drama by eight ex-dope addicts," by Young-blom, B. CHRISTIAN YOUTH CRUSADE. 1(1), 1965.
"The addict and his drugs," by Gelber, Ida. AMERICAN JOUR-NAL OF NURSING. 7:52-56, July, 1963.
"The addict and the physician," by Berger, H. MEDICAL TIMES. 94:710-720, 1966.
"The addict and treatment," by Raskin, H.A. ILLINOIS MED-ICAL JOURNAL. 130:465-473, 1966.
"The addict as a rehab client," by Richman, S. REHABILI-TATION RECORD. 7:24-26, 1966.
"The addict as an inpatient," by Rohde, Ildaura M. AMER-ICAN JOURNAL OF NURSING. 63:61-66, July, 1963.
"Addict at your door," by Friedman, J. NEW YORK STATE DENTAL JOURNAL. 31:256-257, 1965.
"Addict builds habit." NEWSWEEK. 78:179, Sept. 17, 1960.
"The addict culture and movement into and out of hospitals," by Fiddle, S. NEW YORK COUNCIL ON NARCOTICS ADDICTION, 1962.
"Addict, heal thyself," by Champlin, C.D. ISLAND LANTERN. pp. 20-25, June, 1965.
"Addict helps build habit." SCIENCE NEWS LETTER. 78:179, Sept. 17, 1960.
"Addict program launched," by McBroom, P. SCIENCE NEWS. 90:410, Nov. 12, 1966.
"Addicted! addiction to diet pills." GOOD HOUSEKEEPING. 164:12 passim, May, 1967.
"Addiction among physicians," by Overstreet, S.A. JOURNAL OF THE KENTUCKY MEDICAL ASSOCIATION. 65:683-684, July, 1967.
"Addiction among the hill tribes of Thailand." BULLETIN ON NARCOTICS. 20(4):8, Oct.-Dec., 1968.
"Addiction an illness, not a sin or crime." SCIENCE NEWS LETTER. 81:8, Jan. 6, 1962.
"Addiction and criminal responsibility," by Caplan, L. MEDICO-LEGAL JOURNAL. 30:85-97, 1962.
"Addiction and criminal responsibility. A joint meeting with the Medico-Legal Society, March 8, 1962." THE BRITISH JOURNAL OF ADDICTION. 58(2):65-85, 1962.
"Addiction and existence," by Von Kaam, Adrian. REVIEW OF EXISTENTIAL PSYCHOLOGY AND PSYCHIATRY. 8(1):54-64, 1968.
"Addiction and habituation," by Gabriel, E. MUENCHENER MEDIZINISCHE WOCHENSCHRIFT. 102:2074-2078, 1960.
"Addiction and the campus," by Lippincott, W.T. JOURNAL OF CHEMICAL EDUCATION. 45:687, Nov., 1968.
"Addiction as a public health problem," by Edwards, G. MEDICAL OFFICER. 113(13):177-179, 1965.
"Addiction: beginning of wisdom," by Lindesmith, A.R. NATION. 196:49-52, Jan. 19, 1965.
"Addiction by overuse." SCIENCE NEWS LETTER. 87:69, Jan. 30, 1965.
"Addiction. Cases treated on a psychiatric service," by Koutsky, C.D., et al. MINNESOTA MEDICINE. 50:189-194, Feb., 1967.

"Addiction: current issues," by Cameron, D.C. AMERICAN
JOURNAL OF PSYCHIATRY. 120(4):313-319, 1963.
"Addict on dope." AMERICA. 108:251-252, Feb. 23, 1963.
"Addiction drugs: narcotics and non-narcotics," by Mason,
O. JOURNAL OF THE MOUNT SINAI HOSPITAL, NEW YORK.
33(1):28-31, 1966.
"The addiction epidemic (annotations)." LANCET. 2(7404:
169, 1965.
"The addiction epidemic (letter to the editor)," by Chap-
ple, P.A.L., and Marks, V. LANCET. 2:288-289, 1965.
"The addiction epidemic (London Letter)." CANADIAN MED-
ICAL ASSOCIATION JOURNAL. 93:723-724, 1965.
"Addiction; everybody's business." ELECTRONIC NEWS. 11:
1 passim, Dec. 5, 1966.
"Addiction liability of albino rats: breeding for quanti-
tative differences in morphine drinking," by Nichols,
J.R., and Hsiao, S. SCIENCE. 157:561-563, Aug. 4, 1967.
"Addiction new style." LANCET. 1:852-853, Apr. 20, 1968.
"Addiction new style," by Norman-Taylor, W. LANCET. 1:
925, Apr. 27, 1968.
"Addiction of petrol vapour." LANCET. 1:707, 1964.
"Addiction or drug-dependence?" by Terry, E.N. PSYCHO-
SOMATICS. 6:241-242, 1965.
"'Addiction' reactions in cultured human cells," by Cors-
sen, G., and Skora, I.A. JOURNAL OF THE AMERICAN MED-
ICAL ASSOCIATION. 187(5):328-332, 1964.
"Addiction research center inventory: development of a
general drug estimation scale," by Haertzen, C. JOUR-
NAL OF NERVOUS AND MENTAL DISEASE. 141:300-307, 1965.
"The addiction research center inventory: Appendix I.
Items comprising empirical scales for seven drugs.
II. Items which do not differentiate placebo from any
drug condition," by Hill, H. PSYCHOPHARMACOLOGIA.
4:184-205, 1963.
"Addiction to chlorodyne." BRITISH MEDICAL JOURNAL.
5368:1284-1285, 1963.
"Addiction to chlorodyne." BRITISH MEDICAL JOURNAL.
5370:1472, 1963.
"Addiction to chlorodyne," by Conlon, M.F. BRITISH MEDICAL
JOURNAL. 5366:1177-1178, 1963.
"Addiction to daprisal," by Sours, J.A. JOURNAL OF THE
AMERICAN MEDICAL ASSOCIATION. 205:940, Sept. 23, 1968.
"Addiction to drugs by medical and paramedical personnel,"
by Lundy, J.S. JOURNAL OF THE AMERICAN OSTEOPATHIC
ASSOCIATION. 64:591-595, 1965.
"Addiction to ethchlorvynol. A report of two cases," by
Garza-Perez, J., et al. MEDICAL SERVICES JOURNAL CAN-
ADA. 23:775-778, May, 1967.
"Addiction to innocuous drugs," by Kelman, Harvey. MED-
ICAL TIMES. 93:155-158, Feb., 1965.
"Addiction to intravenous darvon, case report," by Collins,
M.S., et al. JOURNAL OF THE OKLAHOMA STATE MEDICAL
ASSOCIATION. 60:609-610, Nov., 1967.
"Addiction to methadone among patients at Lexington and

Fort Worth," by Sapira, J.D., et al. PUBLIC HEALTH REPORTS. 83:691-694, Aug., 1968.

"Addiction to nonbarbiturate sedative and tranquilizing drugs," by Essig, C.F. CLINICAL PHARMACOLOGY AND THERAPEUTICS. 5:334-343, 1964.

"Addiction to poppy-heads in England," by Glatt, M.M., and Hossain, M.M. BRITISH MEDICAL JOURNAL. 5349:102, 1963.

"Addiction to poppy heads (unbalanced capsules of papaver somniferum 'post')." BRITISH JOURNAL OF ADDICTION. 59(2):149-155, 1963.

"Addiction to stimulants," by Bell, D.C. MEDICAL JOURNAL OF AUSTRALIA. 1:41-45, Jan. 14, 1967.

"Addictions and their effects on community health," by Born, G.V. ROYAL SOCIETY OF HEALTH JOURNAL. 84:264-267, 1964.

"Addictive society: habitual users of narcotics." CHRISTIAN CENTURY. 84:331-334, Mar. 15, 1967.

"Addicts among your patients?" MEDICAL ECONOMICS. Feb. 27, 1961.

"Addicts as patients," by Taylor, S.D. NURSING OUTLOOK. 13:41-44, 1965.

"Addicts run a station; and double its volume. With hard work and guidance a synanon team is winning friends in San Francisco." NATIONAL PETROLEUM NEWS. 58:99, Oct., 1966.

"Administrators forum: this month's problem; program on drugs backfired when six students were picked up by juvenile authorities." SCHOOL MANAGEMENT. 11:25 passim, Oct., 1967.

"Admissions of narcotic drug addicts to public health service hospitals, 1935-1963," by Ball, J., and Cottrell, E. PUBLIC HEALTH REPORTS. 80:471-475, June, 1965.

"Adolescence: a subculture in United States society," by Milman, Doris H. BULLETIN OF THE NEW YORK ACADEMY OF MEDICINE. 45:347-352, Apr., 1965.

"The adolescent drug addict: an Adlerian view," by Laskowitz, D. JOURNAL OF INDIVIDUAL PSYCHOLOGY. 17:68-79, May, 1961.

"Advice on addiction." LANCET. 2:1131-1132, Nov. 25, 1967.

"Affective differentiation: comparison of emotion profiles gained from clinical and patient self report," by Sheppard, C., et al. PSYCHOLOGICAL REPORTS. 22(3, pt.1): 809-814, 1968.

"Aftercare of drug addicts: the missing link in rehabilitation," by Egan, D. ILLINOIS MEDICAL JOURNAL. 130: 500-512, Oct., 1966.

"The agony of Dr. Wells (Wells H)," by Brown, C.T. MILITARY MEDICINE. 132:101-102, Feb., 1967.

"Alarming rise in dope traffic." U.S. NEWS AND WORLD REPORT. 65:43-45, Sept. 2, 1968.

"Alcohol and drug addiction in physicians," by Lamere, F. NORTHWEST MEDICINE. 64:196-198, 1965.

"Alcohol and other drug dependencies," by Birchard, Carl. CANADA'S MENTAL HEALTH. 15(5-6):31-33, 1967.

"Alcohol, drugs, and the adolescent," by Glatt, M.M.
  PUBLIC HEALTH. 80:284-294, 1966.
"Alcohol - narcotics - poison," by Dattoli, J.A. PENN-
  SYLVANIA MEDICAL JOURNAL. 68:41-43, 1965.
"The alcohol-narcotic addict," by Chessick, R.D., et al.
  QUARTERLY JOURNAL OF STUDIES ON ALCOHOL. 22:261-268,
  1961.
"Alcoholism, addiction, depression: a nurse's story."
  NURSING OUTLOOK. 13:48-49, 1965.
"Alcoholism and addiction in general practice," by Cooney,
  J.G. JOURNAL OF THE IRISH MEDICAL ASSOCIATION. 53:
  54-56, 1963.
"Alcoholism and drug addiction in Israel," by Wislicki, L.
  BRITISH JOURNAL OF ADDICTION. 62:367-373, Dec., 1967.
"Alcoholism and addiction in urbanized Sioux Indians," by
  Kuttner, R.E., et al. MENTAL HYGIENE. 51:530-542,
  Oct., 1967.
"Alcoholism and drug dependence in doctors and nurses,"
  by Glatt, M.M. BRITISH MEDICAL JOURNAL. 1:380-381,
  Feb. 10, 1968.
"Alcoholism in a geriatric setting. IV. Incidence of drug
  addiction and disease," by Harrington, L.G., and Price,
  A.C. JOURNAL OF THE AMERICAN GERIATRIC SOCIETY. 10:
  207-208, 1962.
"All-time high; drug situation in Britain," by Wenham, B.
  NEW REPUBLIC. 157:13, Aug. 19, 1967.
"An alternative proposal for dealing with drug addiction,"
  by Celler, E. FEDERAL PROBATION. 27(2):2-26, 1963.
"Ambulatory withdrawal treatment of heroin addicts," by
  Berle, B.B., and Nyswander, M. NEW YORK JOURNAL OF
  MEDICINE. 64:1846-1848, 1964.
"Analgesic habits of 500 veterans: incidence and compli-
  cations of abuse," by Gault, M.H., et al. CANADIAN
  MEDICAL ASSOCIATION JOURNAL. 98(13):619-626, Mar. 30,
  1968.
"Answer to youthful drug addiction," by Luce, C.B. MCCALLS.
  93:70 passim, Mar., 1966.
"Anti-narcotic testing: a physician's point of view."
  FEDERAL PROBATION. 27(2):32-38, 1963.
"Apropos of the abuse of certain drugs," by Dreyfuss, R.
  PRAXIS. 50:1093-1094, 1961.
"Aspects of drug addiction (symposium)." CATHOLIC PSYCHO-
  LOGICAL RECORD. 6:134-168, Fall, 1968.
"Attack on dope." AMERICA. 108:251-252, Feb. 23, 1963.
"Attitude of families in the treatment of the drug addicts,"
  by Imada, Y. JOURNAL OF MENTAL HEALTH. 14:85-94, 1965.
"Attitudes toward addicts: some general observations and
  comparative findings," by Schur, E.M. AMERICAN JOURNAL
  OF ORTHOPSYCHIATRY. 34(1):80-90, 1964.
"Authorities respond to growing drug use among high school
  students." PHI DELTA KAPPAN. 50:213, Dec., 1968.
"Background paper on narcotic addiction," by Goff, D.H.
  JOURNAL OF PASTORAL CARE. 18(20):71-76, 1964.
"Bad habits and social deviation; a proposed revision in

conflict theory," by Astin, A.W. JOURNAL OF CLINICAL
PSYCHOLOGY. 18:227-231, 1962.
"A bag full of laughs," by Danto, B.L. AMERICAN JOURNAL
OF PSYCHIATRY. 121:612-613, 1964.
"Baleful influence of gambling from the two-dollar bet to
narcotics," by Kennedy, R.F. ATLANTIC MONTHLY. 209:
76-79, 1962.
"Beat wanderers," by Gennrich, C. ATLAS. 11:146-151,
Mar., 1966.
"Beautiful affair." TIME. 84:44, Oct. 30, 1964.
"Bemoaning the lost dream--Coleridge's Kubla Khan and ad-
diction," by Marcovitz, E. INTERNATIONAL JOURNAL OF
PSYCHO-ANALYSIS. 45:411-425, 1964.
"Benevolent coercion: New York's dope nostrum; Nelson
Rockefeller's program," by Prisendorf, A. NATION. 204:
486-489, Apr. 17, 1967.
"The big fix," by Joseph, J. NEW YORK JOURNAL AMERICAN.
pp. 4-5 passim, May 19, 1963.
"Bizarre addictions in children," by Allison, G.E. MANI-
TOBA MEDICAL REVIEW. 47:288-290, June-July, 1967.
"Boy and girl; case of C. Crenshaw and R. Friede." NEWS-
WEEK. 67:31B, Feb. 21, 1966.
"Bridge for addicts." AMERICA. 110:213, Feb. 15, 1964.
"Bridging the gap between institution and community in
the treatment of narcotic addicts," by Berliner, A.K.
MENTAL HYGIENE. 52:263-271, Apr., 1968.
"A brief survey of a drug dependency unit in a psychiatric
hospital," by George, H., and Glatt, M. BRITISH JOURNAL
OF ADDICTION. 62:147-153, 1967.
"Britain's Px for our drug addicts," by Kobler, J. SATUR-
DAY EVENING POST. 239:74-78, Aug. 13, 1966.
"Britain's secret junkies," by Hardiment, M. TWENTIETH
CENTURY. 171:59-66, Winter 1962/1963.
"British way with the junkie," by Samuels, G. NEW YORK
TIMES MAGAZINE. p. 37+, Oct. 18, 1964.
"The Bureau of Narcotics and American pharmacy," by Gior-
dano, H.L. MILITARY MEDICINE. 130:763-767, 1965.
"A bureaucratic mess - narcotics addiction in the U.S.A.
AMERICAN JOURNAL OF PSYCHOTHERAPY. 17:169-173, 1963.
"California's nalline program: its use in detecting and
combating narcotics addiction," by Mosk, S. STATE GOV-
ERNMENT. 34:112-117, Spring, 1961.
"Campus dope addiction up," by Anderson, J. BUFFALO COUR-
IER EXPRESS. Nov. 21, 1965.
"Campus drug abuse gets second look." THE ATTACK ON NAR-
COTIC ADDICTION AND DRUG ABUSE. 2(4):1, Nov., 1968.
"The campus drug problem," by Philip, A.F. JOURNAL OF THE
AMERICAN COLLEGE HEALTH ASSOCIATION. 16:150-160, Dec.,
1967.
"Canada: who's got it?" NEWSWEEK. 55:61, May 9, 1960.
"A Canadian programme of voluntary treatment of drug de-
pendence: the work of the narcotic addiction foundation
of British Columbia," by Hoskin, H. BULLETIN ON NARCOT-
ICS. 20(2):45-48, 1968.

120

"Cancer, cocaine and courage," by Bechard, A.J., and Crane, W.D. LISTEN. 15:4, July-Aug., 1962.
"The case against narcointerrogation," by Gall, J.C., Jr. JOURNAL OF FORENSIC SCIENCES. 7(1):29-55, 1962.
"The case against the drug culture," by Anderson, H. ADDICTIONS. 14(1):42-48, 1967.
"Case history of an addict patient." LOOK. 29:25-27, Nov. 30, 1965.
"Case... Narcotics addiction (editorial)." PUBLIC HEALTH REPORTS. 79:698, 1964.
"A case of chloral hydrate addiction," by Robinson, J.T. INTERNATIONAL JOURNAL OF SOCIAL PSYCHIATRY. 12:66-71, Winter, 1966.
"A case of morphine addiction," by Baker, A.A. LANCET. 2:946-947, 1963.
"Case of the hypnotic hippie." NEWSWEEK. 74(24):30-37, Dec. 15, 1969.
"Causes and types of narcotic addiction: a psycho-social view," by Ausabel, D.P. PSYCHIATRIC QUARTERLY. 35: 523-531, 1961.
"Census of drug addicts in Brazil - the incidence and nature of drug addiction," by Parreiras, D. BULLETIN ON NARCOTICS. 17(1):21-23, Jan.-Mar., 1965.
"Centres for treatment of drug addiction. Importance of research," by Connell, P.H. BRITISH MEDICAL JOURNAL. 2:499-500, May 20, 1967.
"Certain aspects of toxicomanias," by Petran V. CASOPIS LEKARU CESKYCH. 99:1079-1082, 1960.
"Cessation patterns among neophyte heroin users," by Schasre, R. INTERNATIONAL JOURNAL OF THE ADDICTIONS. 1(2): 23-32, 1966.
"Changes in public attitudes on narcotic addiction," by Pattison, E.M., et al. AMERICAN JOURNAL OF PSYCHIATRY. 125(2):160-167, Aug., 1968.
"Changing friendship patterns in addict groups," by Stein, R. PENNSYLVANIA PSYCHIATRIC QUARTERLY. 6(2):3-10, 1966.
"Characteristics of hospitalized narcotic addicts," by Ball, J.C., et al. HEALTH, EDUCATION AND WELFARE INDICATORS. pp. 17-26, Mar., 1966.
"The characteristics of opium users studied at the treatment centres in Lekhapani and North Lakhimpur, India," by Ahmed, R.Z. BULLETIN ON NARCOTICS. 19(2):45-49, Apr.-June, 1967.
"Chat with an ad-man head." MARKETING COMMUNICATIONS. 296:63-65, Jan., 1968.
"Chatorpan: a culturally defined form of addiction in North India," by Vatuk, V.P., and Vatuk, S.J. INTERNATIONAL JOURNAL OF THE ADDICTIONS. 2(1):103-113, 1967.
"Chet Baker's tale of woe," by Gitler, I. DOWN BEAT. 31: 22-24, 1964.
"A child on drugs," by Wyden, B.W. NEW YORK TIMES MAGAZINE. pp. 63 passim, Aug. 20, 1967.
"Childhood and adolescent addictive disorders," by Freedman, A.M. PEDIATRICS. 34:283-292, 1964.

"Childhood and adolescent addictive disorders," by Freedman, A.M., and Wilson, E.A. PEDIATRICS. 34:425-439, 1964.
"Children of the drug age; high school students," by Simon, W., and Gagnon, J.H. SATURDAY REVIEW. 51:60-63 passim, Sept. 21, 1968.
"Chinese narcotic addicts in the United States," by Ball, J.C., and Lau, M.P. SOCIAL FORCES. 45:68-72, Sept., 1966.
"The chronic addict--and why he turned to drugs," by Chein, I. REHABILITATION RECORD. 7:16-18, May-June, 1966.
"The chronic hopers are still at it in Corona, California," by Dean, R.L. WESTERN MEDICINE. 7:60-63, 1966.
"Civil commitment for narcotic addicts," by Kuh, R.H. FEDERAL PROBATION. 27(2):21-23, 1963.
"Civil commitment for addicts: the California program," by Kramer J.C., et al. AMERICAN JOURNAL OF PSYCHIATRY. 125(6):816-824, 1968.
"Clamping down." ECONOMIST. 223:118+, Apr. 8, 1967.
"A clergyman looks at drug abuse," by Starkey, L.M. THE JOURNAL OF SCHOOL HEALTH. 39:478-486, Sept., 1969.
"Codeine addiction with death possibly due to abrupt withdrawal," by Margolis, J. JOURNAL OF THE AMERICAN GERIATRICS SOCIETY. 15:951-953, 1967.
"Cold turkey inhumane," by Marley, F. SCIENCE NEWS LETTER. 85:102, Feb. 15, 1964.
"College drug scene," by Larner, J. ATLANTIC MONTHLY. 216:127-130, Nov., 1965.
"The college drug scene," by Pearlman, S. CHOICE. 6:181-187, Apr., 1969.
"College guidance on drugs; Columbia University." SCHOOL AND SOCIETY. 95:139, Mar. 4, 1967.
"Commentary on the above paper: why compulsory closed-ward treatment of narcotic addicts?" by Schlich, R. ILLINOIS MEDICAL JOURNAL. 130:485-487, Oct., 1966.
"Comments on narcotic addiction," by Hoch, P.H. COMPREHENSIVE PSYCHIATRY. 4:140-144, June, 1963.
"The community's response to substance misuse," by Cavior, N., et al. INTERNATIONAL JOURNAL OF THE ADDICTIONS. 2(1):139-142, 1967.
"Commuting to the border (story by a narcotic addict)." CALIFORNIA YOUTH AUTHORITY QUARTERLY. 15(1):3-9, 1962.
"Compulsive, addictive personality problems," by Bennett, A.E. MEDICAL TIMES. 92:433-442, 1964.
"Conference on narcotic addiction mental health logistics," by Visotsky, H.M. ILLINOIS MEDICAL JOURNAL. 130:520-522, Oct., 1966.
"Conference on narcotic studies liaison of medicine, law." JOURNAL OF THE MEDICAL ASSOCIATION OF THE STATE OF ALABAMA. 36:1156-1157, 1967.
"Confession of a goof ball addict," by Davidson, H.A. AMERICAN JOURNAL OF PSYCHIATRY. 120(8):750-759, 1964.
"Congenital neonatal narcotics addiction: a natural history," by Rosenthal, T., et al. AMERICAN JOURNAL OF

PUBLIC HEALTH AND THE NATION'S HEALTH. 54(8):1252-1262, 1964.
"Connecting with addicts." ECONOMIST. 204:1030, Sept. 15, 1962.
"Contradictions in addiction." PUBLIC HEALTH REPORTS. 78:669-672, 1963.
"Control of dangerous drugs on university campuses," by Bruyn, H.B. JOURNAL OF THE AMERICAN COLLEGE HEALTH ASSOCIATION. 16:13-19, 1967.
"Controlling the addict: British system." NEWSWEEK. 55:80, Jan. 11, 1960.
"Controversial issues in the management of drug addiction: legalization, ambulatory treatment and the British system," by Ausabel, D.P. MENTAL HYGIENE. 44:535-544, Oct., 1960
"Cops in the world of junk: narcotic squad, New York City," by Lipsyte, R.M. NEW YORK TIMES MAGAZINE. p. 63+, Oct. 14, 1962.
"Cornered crook with $3 million worth of heroin." LIFE. 52:40, Jan. 26, 1962.
"A correctional dilemma: the narcotics addict," by Nahrendorf, R.O. SOCIOLOGY AND SOCIAL RESEARCH. 53:21-33, Oct., 1968.
"A counseling center for drug addicts," by Osnos, R., and Laskowitz, D. BULLETIN ON NARCOTICS. 18(4):31-46, 1966.
"Counseling the adolescent addict," by Telson, S. JOURNAL OF REHABILITATION. 30(5):10-12, 1964.
"Counter culture," by Roszak, T. NATION. 206:466-471, Apr. 8, 1968.
"Crash program on drug abuse," by Pinkerton, P.B. JOURNAL OF SECONDARY EDUCATION. 43:228-232, May, 1968.
"Crime or disease." MODERN MEDICINE. p. 4, May 15, 1961.
"Crime, the untouchables." TIME. 80:21, July 20, 1962.
"Criminal justice notes: drug abuse up 1,500 per cent." NCCD NEWS. 48(4):10, Sept.-Oct., 1969.
"Criminal justice notes: juvenile drug data; Arizona. NCCD NEWS. 48(4):7, Sept.-Oct., 1969.
"The critical dilemma of the school drop out," by Taber, R.C. AMERICAN JOURNAL OF ORTHOPSYCHIATRY. 33(3):501-508, 1963.
"Crutch that cripples: drug dependence; excerpts." TODAY'S HEALTH. 46:11-12 passim, Sept., 1968, 46:12-15 passim, Oct., 1968.
"Cure not permanent." SCIENCE NEWS LETTER. 81:75, Feb. 3, 1962.
"Current trends in the rehabilitation of narcotics addicts," by Lieberman, L. SOCIAL WORK. 12(2):53-59, 1967.
"The curse of addiction." SPRING 3100. 36(5):11-27, 1965.
"The cycle of abstinence and relapse among heroin addicts," by Raz, M.B. SOCIAL PROBLEMS. 9:132-140, 1961.
"Dagga in South Africa," by Watt, J. BULLETIN ON NARCOTICS. 13(3):9-14, 1961.
"Damage caused by drugs," by Saenger, S. DAPIM REFUIIM. 24:10-24, 1965.

"Dangerous Drugs Act 1967. Restrictions on the prescribing of heroin or cocaine to addicts. NURSING TIMES. 64: 486, Apr. 12, 1968.

"The dangerous drug problem. Report of subcommittee on narcotics addiction (New York County Medical Society)." NEW YORK MEDICINE. 22(9):3-8, 1966.

"Dangers of drug abuse," by Clark, M. EDUCATION DIGEST. 34:15-18, Oct., 1968.

"Dangers of drug reform," by Sayle, M., and Page, B. NEW STATESMAN. 72:246-247, Aug. 19, 1966.

"Death and disability in drug addiction and abuse," by Brill, H. ANNALS OF INTERNAL MEDICINE. 67:205-207, July, 1967.

"Death of a hooked heiress; case of C. Crenshaw and R. Friede," by Schaap, D. LOOK. 30:19-25, July 26, 1966.

"Death of opium Jones (apomorphine treatment)," by Burroughs, W. NEW STATESMAN. 71:304-305, Mar. 4, 1966.

"Death of Tommy." SATURDAY EVENING POST. Sept. 20, 1962.

"Deaths from narcotism in New York City. Incidence, circumstances, and postmortem findings," by Helpern, M., and Rho, Y.M. NEW YORK JOURNAL OF MEDICINE. 66:2391-2408, 1966.

"The descriminalization of narcotics addiction," by McMorris, S.C. AMERICAN CRIMINAL LAW QUARTERLY. 3(2):84-88, 1965.

"Defiance and deviates," by Becker, H.S. NATION. 201: 120-124, Sept. 20, 1965.

"Deliberate aspirin intoxication," by Madden, J.S., et al BRITISH MEDICAL JOURNAL. 5495:1090, Apr. 30, 1966.

"'Delirium tremens' following withdrawal of ethchlorvinol," by Wood, H.P., and Flippin, H.F. AMERICAN JOURNAL OF PSYCHIATRY. 121:1127-1129, 1965.

"Demographic factors associated with negro opiate addiction," by Chambers, C.D., et al. INTERNATIONAL JOURNAL OF THE ADDICTIONS. 3:329-343, Spring, 1968.

"Dental care for narcotic addicts at the northern dispensary," by Ferber, I., et al. NEW YORK STATE DENTAL JOURNAL. 34:485, Oct., 1968.

"Dependence on alcohol and other drugs." WHO CHRONICLE. 21:219-226, June, 1967.

"Dependency on methaqualone hydrochloride (melsedin)," by Martin, G.J. BRITISH MEDICAL JOURNAL. 5505:114, July 9, 1966.

"Derelictions of the medical profession concerning narcotic addiction," by Stokes, R.C. TEXAS JOURNAL OF MEDICINE. 59:839-842, 1963.

"Determinants for the classification of drug addicts," by Pinney, E.L., Jr. DISEASES OF THE NERVOUS SYSTEM. 27 (suppl.):55-59, July, 1966.

"The development and validation of a heroin addiction scale with the MMPI," by Cavior, N., et al. INTERNATIONAL JOURNAL OF THE ADDICTIONS. 2(1):129-137, 1967.

"Development of a 'psychopathic' scale for the Addiction Research Center Inventory (ARCI)," by Haertzen, C.A.,

and Panton, J.H. INTERNATIONAL JOURNAL OF THE ADDIC-
TIONS. 2(1):115-127, 1967.
"Development of scales based on patterns of drug effects,
using the Addiction Research Center Inventory," by
Haertzen, C. PSYCHOLOGICAL REPORTS. 18:163-194, 1966.
"Dextro propoxyphene addiction, observations of a case,"
by Elson, A., and Domino, E.F. JOURNAL OF THE AMERICAN
MEDICAL ASSOCIATION. 183:482-485, 1963.
"Diagnosis and management of depressant drug dependence,"
by Ewing, J.A., and Bakewell, W.E. AMERICAN JOURNAL OF
PSYCHIATRY. 123(8):909-917, 1967.
"Diagnosis and therapy in drug addiction," by Kielhotz, P.
PRAXIS DER PSYCHOTHERAPIE. 10:257-267, 1965.
"Diagnosis of autonomic disorders in the neonate (Drug ad-
diction--Riley's disease)," by Behrendt, H. PROCEEDINGS
OF THE RUDOLPH VIRCHOW MEDICAL SOCIETY IN THE CITY OF
NEW YORK. 23:94-96, 1964.
"The diagnosis of death from intravenous narcotism, with
emphasis on the pathologic aspect," by Siegel, H. JOUR-
NAL OF FORENSIC SCIENCES. 11:1-16, 1966.
"Diethylpropion dependence," by Jones, H.S. MEDICAL JOUR-
NAL OF AUSTRALIA. 1:267, Feb. 17, 1968.
"Differential association and the rehabilitation of drug
addicts," by Volkman, R., and Cressey, D.R. AMERICAN
JOURNAL OF SOCIOLOGY. 69(2):129-142, 1963; also BRIT-
ISH JOURNAL OF ADDICTION. 61:91-100, Nov., 1965.
"Diffusion of the intravenous technique among narcotic
addicts in U.S.," by O'Donnell, John, and Jones, J.P.
JOURNAL OF HEALTH AND SOCIAL BEHAVIOR. 9(2):120-130,
1968.
"Dilemma for drug addicts," by Murtagh, J.M. AMERICA.
108(21):740-742, May 25, 1963.
"The dimensions of narcotism: a study of medical and social
policy," by Howell, J.B. JOURNAL OF THE MISSISSIPPI
STATE MEDICAL ASSOCIATION. 6:1-5, 1965.
"Discharge of narcotic drug addicts against medical advice,"
by Levine, J., and Monroe, J.J. PUBLIC HEALTH REPORTS.
79(1):13-18, 1964.
"Disciplining drug users; drugs on campus." SCHOOL AND
SOCIETY. 95:381, Oct. 28, 1967.
"Discussion on drug addiction." PRACTITIONER. 198:842-
844, June, 1967.
"Diseases caused by drugs," by Harlem, O.K. TIDSSKRIFT
FOR DEN NORSKE LAEGEFORENING. 83:1672-1674, 1963.
"Dissident youth," by Unwin, J.R. CANADA'S MENTAL HEALTH.
17:4-10, Mar.-Apr., 1969.
"Don't be fooled by drug addicts," by Morrison, L.W. MED-
ICAL ANNALS OF THE DISTRICT OF COLUMBIA. 29:234-235,
1960.
"Dope has nothing to do with addicts," by Casselman, B.W.
JOURNAL OF ORAL THERAPEUTICS AND PHARMACOLOGY. 1:533,
1965.
"Dope invades the suburbs," by Goldman, R.P. SATURDAY
EVENING POST. 237:19-25, Apr. 4, 1964.

"Dope problem in Detroit." LISTEN. 13:6, Nov./Dec., 1960.
"Doping of athletes (editorial)." BRITISH MEDICAL JOURNAL.
5408:525-526, 1964.
"Drowsed with the fume of poppies: opium and John Keats,"
by Ober, W.B. BULLETIN OF THE NEW YORK ACADEMY OF MED-
ICINE. 44:862-881, Jul., 1968.
"Drug abuse," by Larimore, G.W. NATIONAL ASSOCIATION OF
SECONDARY SCHOOL PRINCIPALS BULLETIN. 52:30-38, Mar.,
1968.
"Drug abuse," by Talmey, A. VOGUE. 152:138-139, Sept. 15,
1968.
"Drug abuse and abusers," by Osbourn, R.A. MEDICAL ANNALS
OF THE DISTRICT OF COLUMBIA. 37:98-99 passim, Feb., 1968.
"Drug abuse and addiction. Reporting in a general hospital,"
by Schremly, J.A., and Solomon, F. JOURNAL OF THE AMER-
ICAN MEDICAL ASSOCIATION. 189(6):512-514, 1964.
"Drug abuse abd control," by Smythe, H.A. CANADIAN HOSPI-
TAL. 45:41-42, Apr., 1968.
"Drug abuse and social policy." CANADA'S MENTAL HEALTH.
17:26-32, Jan.-Feb., 1969.
"Drug abuse and the new generation," by Demos, G.D. PHI
DELTA KAPPAN. 50:214-217, Dec., 1968.
"Drug abuse and the value crisis," by Richards, L.G.
SENIOR SCHOLASTIC. 91(suppl.):13-14, Nov. 16, 1967.
"Drug abuse and the young," by Ledger, L. THE TEXAS OUT-
LOOK. 51:33-35, Dec., 1967.
"Drug abuse as a social problem," by Brill, L. INTERNA-
TIONAL JOURNAL OF THE ADDICTIONS. 1(2):7-21, 1966.
"Drug abuse, dependence, and drug addiction," by Wang, R.I.
WISCONSIN MEDICAL JOURNAL. 65:122-125, 1966.
"Drug - drug dependence." TILE AND TILL. 55(1):16-19,
Mar., 1969.
"Drug abuse education," by Weinswig, M.H., et al. PHI
DELTA KAPPAN. 50:222, Dec., 1968.
"Drug abuse education program," by Barr, M. SCHOOL AND
SOCIETY. 97:273, Summer, 1969.
"Drug abuse in Czechoslovakia." BULLETIN ON NARCOTICS.
21(1):30, Jan.-Mar., 1969.
"Drug abuse in our society," by Rogers, P.G. JOURNAL OF
THE AMERICAN PHARMACEUTICAL ASSOCIATION. 8:122-124,
Mar., 1968.
"Drug abuse in Sweden, part 1: 1. Development of drug abuse.
2. The present situation," by Goldberg, L. BULLETIN ON
NARCOTICS. 20(1):1-31, 1968.
"Drug abuse in Sweden, part 2: 3. Medical complications.
4. Drug identification, metabolism and effects. 5. Ther-
apeutic approaches. 6. Turnover of drugs and syringes.
7. Law enforcement. 8. Factors of importance for the
emergence of drug dependence. 9. New elements in the
pattern of drug abuse," by Goldberg, L. BULLETIN ON
NARCOTICS. 20(2):9-36, 1968.
"Drug abuse in the eyes of the law," by Ledger, L. THE
TEXAS OUTLOOK. 51:37-39, Nov., 1967.
"Drug abuse in the nursing profession," by Bloomquist, E.R.,

et al. GP. 34:133-139, Nov., 1966.
"Drug abuse is hitting younger children," by Leach, G.
THE INSTRUCTOR. 79:60-61, Aug., 1969.
"Drug abuse - now a community problem," by Publey, H.C.
CALIFORNIA MEDICINE. 108:340-341, Apr., 1968.
"Drug abuse of the modern man," by Bay, R. DEUTSCHE MED-
IZINISCHE WOCHENSCHRIFT. 85:1676-1680, 1960.
"Drug abuse: our new challenge," by Davoli, E. CLINICAL
PROCEEDINGS OF THE CHILDREN'S HOSPITAL OF THE DISTRICT
OF COLUMBIA. 24:151-152, May, 1968.
"Drug abuse potential: a developing program," by Joffe,
M.H. JOURNAL OF CLINICAL PHARMACOLOGY. 8:20-24, Jan.-
Feb., 1968.
"Drug abuse problems of identification," by Lehman, D.J.
JOURNAL OF THE AMERICAN PHARMACEUTICAL ASSOCIATION.
8:35, Jan., 1968.
"Drug abuse programs on campus," by Doerr, D.W., et al.
JOURNAL OF THE AMERICAN PHARMACEUTICAL ASSOCIATION.
7:478-481 passim, Sept., 1967.
"Drug abuse project, Coronado, California," by Jordan, C.W.
JOURNAL OF SCHOOL HEALTH. 38:692-695, Dec., 1968.
"Drug abusers include 500,000 middle-classers." AMERICAN
DRUGGIST. 157:16, Jan. 29, 1968.
"Drug addiction." BULLETIN OF THE NEW YORK ACADEMY OF
MEDICINE. 41:825-829, 1965.
"Drug addiction." JOURNAL OF THE IRISH MEDICAL ASSOCIATION.
61:105-106, Mar., 1968.
"Drug addiction." LANCET. 2(7422):1113-1114, 1965.
"Drug addiction." NURSING TIMES. 63:1646, Dec. 8, 1967.
"Drug addiction." NURSING TIMES. 64:386, Mar. 22, 1968.
"Drug addiction." ROYAL SOCIETY OF HEALTH JOURNAL. 86:
1-2, 1966.
"Drug addiction," by Bewley, T.H. BRITISH MEDICAL JOURNAL.
3:603-605, Sept. 2, 1967.
"Drug addiction," by Brain, Lord. PHARMACEUTICAL JOURNAL.
195(5327):560-562, 1965.
"Drug addiction," by Chapple, P.A. LANCET. 1:365, 1966.
"Drug addiction," by Gibson, J. CANADIAN NURSE. 56:156-
158, 1960.
"Drug addiction," by Kolb, L.C. BULLETIN OF THE NEW YORK
ACADEMY OF MEDICINE. 41:306-309, 1965.
"Drug addiction," by Macdonald, A.D. JOURNAL OF PHARMACY
AND PHARMACOLOGY. 14(suppl.):9T-16T, 1962.
"Drug addiction," by Mullin, P., et al. LANCET. 2:1294,
Dec. 18, 1965.
"Drug addiction," by Murray, J.B. JOURNAL OF GENERAL PSY-
CHOLOGY. 77(1):41-68, 1967.
"Drug addiction," by Parry, W.H. NURSING TIMES. 62:37-
39, 1966.
"Drug addiction," by Rees, W.L. ROYAL SOCIETY OF HEALTH
JOURNAL. 84:276-281, 1964.
"Drug addiction," by Simon, W. MINNESOTA MEDICINE. 47:
541-542, 1964.
"Drug addiction," by Tylden, E. LANCET. 2:284, 1966.

"Drug addiction. A medical hazard," by Krantz, J.C., Jr.
MARYLAND STATE MEDICAL JOURNAL. 15:43-45, 1966.
"Drug addiction; a pharmacist's viewpoint," by Kesling, J.H.
JOURNAL OF SCHOOL HEALTH. 39:174-179, Mar., 1969.
"Drug addiction: a review," by Meyerstein, A.N. JOURNAL
OF SCHOOL HEALTH. 34:77-87, Feb., 1964.
"Drug addiction: a social problem. United Nations: UN DOC-
UMENT NAR-AFRI-SEM-DOC.2, 9 Sept., 1963.
"Drug addiction: a way back," by McCarrick, H. NURSING
TIMES. 63:569-570, 1967.
"Drug addiction. Action research in a treatment center,"
by Freedman, A.M. AMERICAN JOURNAL OF NURSING. 63:57-
60, 1963.
"Drug addiction among pimps and prostitutes, Israel 1967,"
by Friedman, I., and Peer, I. INTERNATIONAL JOURNAL OF
THE ADDICTIONS. 3:271-300, Spring, 1968.
"Drug addiction: an eclectic view," by Freedman, A.M. JOUR-
NAL OF THE AMERICAN MEDICAL ASSOCIATION. 197(11):878-
883, 1966.
"Drug addiction and abuse." POSTGRADUATE MEDICINE. 43:196,
Jun., 1968.
"Drug addiction and crime," by Winick, C. CURRENT HISTORY.
52:349-353 passim, June, 1967.
"Drug addiction and habit formation: an attempted integra-
tion," by Walton, D. JOURNAL OF MENTAL SCIENCE. 106:
1195-1229, 1960.
"Drug addiction and 'hyper-sexuality': related modes of
mastery," by Hoffman, M. COMPREHENSIVE PSYCHIATRY.
5(4):262-270, 1964.
"Drug addiction as a deviant career," by Rubington, E.
INTERNATIONAL JOURNAL OF THE ADDICTIONS. 2(1):3-20, 1967.
"Drug addiction. Assessment of the function of the gen-
eral practitioner," by Ollendorff, R.H. PROCEEDINGS OF
THE ROYAL SOCIETY OF MEDICINE. 61:181-184, Feb., 1968.
"Drug addiction; clamping down." ECONOMIST. 223:118 pas-
sim, Apr. 8, 1967.
"Drug addiction: criminal or medical problem," by Morgan,
J.P., Jr. POLICE. 9(6):6-9, 1965.
"Drug addiction debate." MD. 7(5):77-78, 1963.
"Drug addiction; epidemic." STATIST. 190:1407, Dec. 9,
1966.
"Drug addiction - five views on a vexing problem." MEDICAL
TRIBUNE. 6(121):8-26, 1965.
"Drug addiction in adolescence," by Bender, L. COMPREHEN-
SIVE PSYCHIATRY. 4:181-194, June, 1963.
"Drug addiction in America and England," by Schur, E.M.
COMMENTARY. 30:241-248, Sept., 1960.
"Drug addiction in Britain now," by Laurence, D.R. NATURE.
210(5042):1203-1204, 1966.
"Drug addiction in East Africa," by Tanner, R.E.S. INTER-
NATIONAL JOURNAL OF THE ADDICTIONS. 1(1):9-29, 1966.
"Drug addiction in Egypt, and its sociological aspects," by
Abdelnabi, A., and El-nagbi, A. MEDICO-LEGAL JOURNAL.
28:200-202, 1960.

"Drug addiction in Great Britain," by Partridge, M. COM-
PREHENSIVE PSYCHIATRY. 4:208-213, June, 1963.
"Drug addiction in Great Britain today with special refer-
ence to prognosis," by Clark, J.A. COMPREHENSIVE PSY-
CHIATRY. 4:214-224, June, 1963.
"Drug addiction in Hong Kong." EASTERN WORLD. 18:10, Jan.,
1964.
"Drug addiction in Israel," by Wislicki, L. BRITISH JOUR-
NAL OF ADDICTION. 59(2):37-45, 1963.
"Drug addiction in pregnant women." BULLETIN ON NARCOTICS.
20(3):17, July-Sept., 1968.
"Drug addiction in pregnant women," by Perlmutter, J.F.
AMERICAN JOURNAL OF OBSTETRICS AND GYNECOLOGY. 99:569-
572, Oct. 15, 1967.
"Drug addiction in the United Kingdom: the second report
of the Interdepartmental Committee (1965). BULLETIN ON
NARCOTICS. 18(2):23-28, Apr.-June, 1966.
"Drug addiction in youth," ed. E. Harms. INTERNATIONAL
SERIES OF MONOGRAPHS IN CHILD PSYCHIATRY. 3:1-224, 1965.
"Drug addiction; just beginning," by Newell, P. STATIST.
191:147, Feb. 3, 1967.
"Drug addiction: new approaches to an old problem," by Skom,
J.H., et al. POSTGRADUATE MEDICINE. 43:74-81, June,
1968.
"Drug addiction out of control?" by Wansell, G. TIMES (Lon-
don) EDUCATIONAL SUPPLEMENT. 2765:1664, May 17, 1968.
"Drug addiction: problem of law or morality?" by Miller,
H.M. RELIGION IN LIFE. 36:590-604, Winter, 1967.
"Drug addiction, special issue." COMPREHENSIVE PSYCHIATRY.
4:135-235, 1963.
"Drug addiction studied." SCIENCE NEWS LETTER. 88:87,
Aug. 7, 1965.
"Drug addiction. The addict and his drugs," by Gelber, I.
AMERICAN JOURNAL OF NURSING. 63:52-56, July, 1963.
"Drug addiction. The addict as an inpatient," by Rohde,
I.M. AMERICAN JOURNAL OF NURSING. 63:61-66, 1963.
"Drug addiction. The medico-legal conflict," by Ostrow, S.
AMERICAN JOURNAL OF NURSING. 63:67-71, 1963.
"Drug addiction under British policy," by Schur, E.M.
SOCIAL PROBLEMS. 9:156-166, Fall, 1961.
"Drug addiction up; findings of survey in Britain. SCIENCE
NEWS. 92:495, Nov. 18, 1967.
"Drug addiction wave among adolescents," by Harms, E. NEW
YORK JOURNAL OF MEDICINE. 62:3996-3997, 1962.
"Drug addiction: young mainliners." ECONOMIST. 216:700-
701, Aug. 21, 1965.
"Drug addicts, part 1," by Mills, J., and Eppridge, B.
LIFE. 58:92B passim, 1965.
"Drug addicts: are we creating them?" by Kennedy, J.D.
MANITOBA MEDICAL REVIEW. 47:207-212, Apr., 1967.
"Drug addicts as folk devils; dangers of intolerance," by
Sanders, K. TIMES (London) EDUCATIONAL SUPPLEMENT.
2750:353, Feb. 2, 1968.
"Drug addicts in a casualty department," by Elliott, H.

NURSING TIMES. 63:478-480, Apr. 14, 1967.
"Drug addicts in a therapeutic community: outline on California Rehabilitation Center Program," by Fischmann, V.S. PSYCHOTHERAPY AND PSYCHOSOMATICS. 15(1):21, 1967; also INTERNATIONAL JOURNAL OF THE ADDICTIONS. 3:351-359, Spring, 1968.
"Drug addicts; in search of a prescription." ECONOMIST. 226:15-16, Feb. 3, 1968.
"Drug addicts need medicine not punishment." SCIENCE NEWS LETTER. 84:4, July 6, 1963.
"Drug addicts's lang of jargon," by 'Consultant psychiatrist of a boys' approved school'. APPROVED SCHOOLS GAZETTE. 61(5):234-236, 1967.
"Drug addicts who cure each other," by Robinson, L. EBONY. 18:116-118, Feb., 1963.
"Drug centre that cures," by McKerron, J. NEW STATESMAN. 74:248, Sept. 1, 1967.
"Drug dependence." BRITISH MEDICAL JOURNAL. 5407:461, 1964.
"Drug dependence." NATURE (London). 208:825-827, Nov. 27, 1965.
"Drug dependence," by Marjot, D.H. JOURNAL OF THE ROYAL NAVAL MEDICAL SERVICE. 52:150-156, Winter, 1966.
"Drug dependence: a symptom." LANCET. 1:853. Apr. 20, 1968.
"Drug dependence and abuse in England," by Gillespie, D., et al. BRITISH JOURNAL OF ADDICTION. 62:155-170, Mar., 1967.
"Drug dependence and alcohol problems." AMERICAN JOURNAL OF PSYCHIATRY. 122(7):721-840, 1966.
"Drug dependence in admission centre patients," by Sainsbury, M.J. MEDICAL JOURNAL OF AUSTRALIA. 2:18-20, July 1, 1967.
"Drug dependence in Britain," by Macdonald, A.D. CURRENT MEDICINE AND DRUGS. 6:23-30, Jan., 1966.
"Drug-dependence in psychiatric patients," by Whitlock, F.A., et al. MEDICAL JOURNAL OF AUSTRALIA. 1:1157-1166, June 10, 1967.
"Drug dependence in the U.S.A.," by Bewley, T.H. BULLETIN ON NARCOTICS. 21(2):13-30, Apr.-June, 1969.
"The drug dependence problem among young people," by Farnsworth, D.L. THE WEST VIRGINIA MEDICAL JOURNAL. 63:433-437, Dec., 1967.
"Drug dependence: threat to society," CANADA'S MENTAL HEALTH. 17:39, Mar.-Apr., 1969.
"Drug dependency," by Willis, J.H. NURSING TIMES. 63:474-476, Apr. 14, 1967.
"Drug experience and attitudes among seniors in a liberal arts college," by Pearlman, Samuel. NASPA, JOURNAL OF THE ASSOCIATION OF DEANS AND ADMINISTRATORS OF STUDENT AFFAIRS. 4:121-126, Jan., 1967.
"Drug for addicts," by Hentoff, N. TIME. 77:74-76, May 12, 1961.
"Drug habit." NEW REPUBLIC. 142:6, Feb. 8, 1960.
"Drug habits and immaturity," by Minckler, L.S. SCIENCE. 161:419, Aug. 2, 1968.

"Drug intoxication (Symposium on emergencies in dental practice)," by Steiner, R.B. DENTAL CLINICS OF NORTH AMERICA. pp. 727-754, 1965.

"Drug offenders in Israel: a survey," by Drapkin, I., and Landau, S. BRITISH JOURNAL OF CRIMINOLOGY. 6(4): 376-391, Oct., 1966.

"Drug problems in Haight-Ashbury," by Sankot, M., and Smith, D.E. AMERICAN JOURNAL OF NURSING. 68(8):1686-1689, 1968.

"Drug-taking among teachers; misrepresented." TIMES (London) EDUCATIONAL SUPPLEMENT. 2778:290, Aug. 16, 1968.

"Drug-taking by the young." BRITISH MEDICAL JOURNAL. 2: 67-68, Apr. 8, 1967.

"Drug usage and the law: the adolescent and an archaic concept," by Barton, W. CLINICAL PROCEEDINGS OF THE CHILDRENS HOSPITAL OF THE DISTRICT OF COLUMBIA. 24:180-184, 1968.

"Drug use among adolescents," by Stanton, A.H. AMERICAN JOURNAL OF PSYCHIATRY. 122:1282-1283, May, 1966.

"Drug use: an emotional storm signal," by Hollister, W.G. PTA MAGAZINE. 62:25-26, Mar., 1968.

"Drug use and abuse among youth," by Strack, A.E. JOURNAL OF HEALTH, PHYSICAL EDUCATION AND RECREATION. 39:26-28 passim, Jan., 1968.

"Drug use and experience in an urban college population," by Pearlman, S. AMERICAN JOURNAL OF ORTHOPSYCHIATRY. 38(3):503-514, 1968.

"Drug use in a normal population of young negro men," by Robins, L., and Murphy, G. AMERICAN JOURNAL OF PUBLIC HEALTH. 57:1580-1596, Sept., 1967.

"Drug use in an urban college population." BULLETIN ON NARCOTICS. 20(4):2, Oct.-Dec., 1968.

"Drug use on high school and college campuses," by Cwalina, G. JOURNAL OF SCHOOL HEALTH. 38:638-646, Dec., 1968.

"Drug users seek the 'happiness pill'," by Dunn, M.L. MENTAL HYGIENE NEWS. 40:4, Oct. 31, 1969.

"Drug Warren-- the refugee slums that have spawned 300,000 addicts," by Markham, G. (with photographs by Alexander Low). DAILY TELEGRAPH (London). No. 49: 13-17 passim, Aug., 1965.

"Drugs: a student report," by Lake, A. SEVENTEEN. 25: 170-171 passim, Sept., 1966.

"Drugs and confusion." PUBLIC HEALTH. 81:265-266, 1967.

"Drugs and driving," by Perry, C.J.G., and Morgenstern, A.L. JOURNAL OF THE AMERICAN MEDICAL ASSOCIATION. 195(5):376-379, 1966.

"Drugs and drug addiction," by Sands, S.L. JOURNAL OF THE IOWA MEDICAL SOCIETY. 53:785-789, 1963.

"Drugs and drug addiction: opinions on the taking of 'soft' drugs." MEDICINE, SCIENCE AND THE LAW. 6:167-168, 1966.

"Drugs and drug addiction: unjust operation of the dangerous drugs act." MEDICINE, SCIENCE AND THE LAW. 6:168, 1966

"Drugs and teenagers," by Jones, A. JOURNAL OF FORENSIC SCIENCES. 7:12-16, Jan., 1967.

"Drugs and the generation gap," by Woodring, P. (an editor-
ial). SATURDAY REVIEW. 52:86-88, Oct. 18, 1969.
"Drugs and the young law-breaker," by Gibbens, T.C. MENTAL
HEALTH. 25(3):36-37, 1966.
"Drugs and tobacco; films," by Falconer, V. SENIOR SCHOL-
ASTIC. 91(suppl.):15-16, Nov. 16, 1967.
"Drugs and youth." SENIOR SCHOLASTIC. 88:4-7, Apr. 29,
1966.
"Drugs, behavior, and crime," by Blum, R.H. ANNALS OF THE
AMERICAN ACADEMY OF POLITICAL AND SOCIAL SCIENCE. 374:
135-146, Nov., 1967.
"Drugs causing dependence," by Lendon, N.C. BRITISH JOUR-
NAL OF ADDICTION. 61:115-124, 1965.
"Drugs hook eleven percent of narcotics victims," by Frazer,
H.F. OIL, PAINT AND DRUG REPORT. 186:4, July 6, 1964.
"Drugs in jazz and rock music," by Curry, A. CLINICAL TOX-
ICOLOGY. 1:235-244, 1968.
"Drugs in the great society," by Turkel, P. CATHOLIC WORLD.
203:265-269, Aug., 1966.
"Drugs: mounting menace of abuse; symposium." LOOK. 31:
11-28, Aug. 8, 1967.
"Drugs, narcotics and the flight from reality; with inter-
view and press comments." SENIOR SCHOLASTIC. 90:4-12,
Feb. 10, 1967.
"Drugs of abuse on stamps." JOURNAL OF THE AMERICAN PHARM-
ACEUTICAL ASSOCIATION. 8:15, Jan., 1968.
"Drugs on campus." COLLEGE MANAGEMENT. Aug., 1966, pp. 20-
25.
"Drugs on campus," by Goldstein, R. SATURDAY EVENING POST.
239:40-44 passim, May 21, 1966; also 239:34-38 passim,
June 4, 1966.
"Drugs on campus: turned on and tuned out," by Freedman,
M.B., and Powelaon, H. THE NATION. 202:125-127, Jan.
31, 1966.
"Drugs; problems of addiction." STATIST. 190:83-84, July
8, 1966.
"Drugs settle in." ECONOMIST. 225:628, Nov. 11, 1967.
"Drugs that even scare hippies," by Rosenfeld, A. LIFE.
63:81-82, Oct. 27, 1967.
"Drugs; the middle line." ECONOMIST. 222:402, Feb. 4, 1967.
"Drugs: the synthetic crisis," by Page, B. NEW STATESMAN.
74:109-110, July 28, 1967.
"Drugs, uses and abuses: young doctor's crusade," by Luce,
J. LOOK. 31:24-28, Aug. 8, 1967.
"The dysleptics: note on a No Man's Land," by Elkes, J.
COMPREHENSIVE PSYCHIATRY. 4:195-198, 1963.
"Economic impact of drug addiction," by Wilson, O.W. ILLI-
NOIS MEDICAL JOURNAL. 130:522-523, Oct., 1966.
"Education is the answer to drug abuse by our young people,"
by Goddard, J.L. JUNIOR COLLEGE JOURNAL. 38:8-9, Sept.,
1967.
"Efficiency in inhalation as a mode of administering heroin,"
by Mo, P.B.N., et al. FEDERATION PROCEEDINGS. 24(2,
part I):300, 1965.

"Emergency cases at Hesperia Hospital, Helsinki, during 1962," by Achté, K.A., and Seppala, K.R. PSYCHIATRIC QUARTERLY (Supplement). 38:537-543, 1964.

"Employment status of narcotic addicts one year after hospital discharge," by Baganz, P.C., and Maddux, J.F. PUBLIC HEALTH REPORTS. 80:615-621, 1965.

"Ending campus drug incidents," by Becker, H.S. TRANS-ACTION. 5(5):4-5, Apr., 1968.

"Ending campus drug incidents," by Friedson, E. TRANS-ACTION. 5(8):75-81, July-Aug., 1968.

"The epidemiology of drug addiction and reflections on the problem and policy in the U.S.," by Mattick, H.W. ILLINOIS MEDICAL JOURNAL. 130:436-447, Oct., 1966.

"Establishment of a new drug addiction program," by McIsaac, W.M. PSYCHOPHARMACOLOGY BULLETIN; NATIONAL CLEARING HOUSE FOR MENTAL HEALTH INFORMATION. 3(4):40-44, 1966.

"Ethchlorvynol addiction," by Magness, J.L. APPLIED THERAPEUTICS. 7:649-653, 1965.

"Excessive drug consumption and the pharmacist," by Meyer, H. SVENSKA FARMACEUTISK TIDSKRIFT. 68:694-703, 1964.

"Exiles from the American dream: the junkie and the cop," by Jackson, B. ATLANTIC MONTHLY. 219:44-51, Jan., 1967.

"Exodus House - for Harlem addicts." REHABILITATION RECORD. 7:18, 1966.

"Experiment for addicts," by Winslow, W. NATION. 192:371-373, Apr. 29, 1961.

"Facilities for treatment and rehabilitation of narcotic drug users and addicts," by Winick, C., and Bynder, H. AMERICAN JOURNAL OF PUBLIC HEALTH AND THE NATION'S HEALTH. 57:1025-1035, 1967.

"Factors in addiction: overwork, fatigue, illness." JOURNAL OF THE AMERICAN MEDICAL ASSOCIATION. 188(8):26, 1964.

"Factors leading to drug abuse," by Demos, G.D., et al. JOURNAL OF THE AMERICAN COLLEGE HEALTH ASSOCIATION. 16:345-347, Apr., 1968.

"Facts against free narcotic clinics for addicts," by Cleveland, G.W. TEXAS JOURNAL OF MEDICINE. 59:309-310, 1963.

"Failure of permissiveness; addiction increasing in Great Britain." TIME. 89:76, Feb. 17, 1967.

"Features of drug addiction in Geneva," by Haenni, M. BULLETIN ON NARCOTICS. 16:7-16, July-Sept., 1964.

"The female drug addict: a profile," by Boothroyd, W.E. ADDICTIONS. 10:36-40, 1963.

"Finding the real answer," by Gardner, R. LISTEN. 14:20-23, Jan.-Feb., 1961.

"First memories of drug addicts," by Lombardi. D.N., and Angers, P. INDIVIDUAL PSYCHOLOGIST. 5(1):7-13, 1967.

"Fix in the igloo," by Klein, M. NATION. 190:361-364, Apr. 23, 1960.

"Flight from violence: hippies and the green rebellion," by Allen, J.R., et al. AMERICAN JOURNAL OF PSYCHIATRY. 125:364-370, Sept., 1968.

"The fog keeps rolling in," by Nowlis, H.H. JOURNAL OF THE AMERICAN PHARMACEUTICAL ASSOCIATION. 8:117-119, Mar., 1968.

"Four cases of progressive drug abuse," by Bartholomew, A.A., et al. MEDICAL JOURNAL OF AUSTRALIA. 1:653-657, Apr. 1, 1967.

"Four hundred years of 'witchcraft', 'projection' and 'delusion'," by Meerloo, J.A.M. AMERICAN JOURNAL OF PSYCHIATRY. 120:83-86, 1963.

"From hard to soft drugs: temporal and substantive changes in drug usage among gangs in a working class community," by Klein, J., and Phillips, D.L. JOURNAL OF HEALTH AND SOCIAL BEHAVIOR. 9(2):139-145, 1968.

"Gambling and drugs in the plant." FACTORY. 126:88-89, Feb., 1968; also SUPERVISORY MANAGEMENT. 13:34-35, May, 1968.

"Gasoline addiction in children," by Lawton, J.J., and Malmquist, C.P. PSYCHIATRIC QUARTERLY. 35:555-561, 1961.

"Gasoline inhalation," by Brown, N.W. JOURNAL OF THE MEDICAL ASSOCIATION OF GEORGIA. 57:217-221, May, 1968.

"Gasoline-sniffing by an adult. Report of a case with the unusual complication of lead encephalopathy," by Law, W.R., et al. JOURNAL OF THE AMERICAN MEDICAL ASSOCIATION. 204:1002-1004, June 10, 1968.

"Gasoline sniffing complicated by acute carbon tetrachloride poisoning," by Durden, W.D., Jr., and Chapman, D.W. ARCHIVES OF INTERNAL MEDICINE. 119(4):371-374, 1967.

"A genetic trip." JOURNAL OF THE AMERICAN MEDICAL ASSOCIATION. 204:328-329, Apr. 22, 1968.

"Generations and drugs." NEW STATESMAN. 74:1, July 7, 1967.

"Giver of delight or liberator of sin: drug use and 'addiction' in Asia," by Fort, J. BULLETIN ON NARCOTICS. 17(3):1-11, July-Sept., 1965.

"Giver of delight or liberator of sin: drug use and 'addiction' in Asia - chapters 5-10," by Fort, J. BULLETIN ON NARCOTICS. 17(4):13-19, 1965.

"Glue sniffing and heroin abuse," by Merry, J. BRITISH MEDICAL JOURNAL. 2:360, May 6, 1967.

"Goal behavior of adolescent addicts and delinquent nonadict peers," by Laskowitz, D., and Einstein, S. PSYCHOLOGICAL REPORTS. 17(1):102, 1965.

"Goof-ball set: addiction in the suburbs; problem in Long Island," by Schram, M. NATION. 203:242-245, 1966.

"The great narcotics muddle," by DeMott, B. HARPER'S MAGAZINE. 224:46-50, 1962.

"Great Neck North Senior High School; Guide Post narcotics survey results." GUIDE POST. Feb. 15, 1967.

"The Greenwich Village addicts," by Walsh, G. COSMOPOLITAN. 155(6):81, 1963.

"Greenwich Village: life in a coffeehouse," by Krim, S. COSMOPOLITAN. 155(6):58-65, 1963.

"Group hypnotherapy techniques with drug addicts," by Ludwig, A.M., et al. INTERNATIONAL JOURNAL OF CLINICAL AND EXPERIMENTAL HYPNOSIS. 12:53-66, 1964.

"Group therapy with young drug addicts - the addicts' point of view," by Glatt, M.M. NURSING TIMES. 63:519-520, 1967.

"Growing drive against drugs." U.S. NEWS AND WORLD REPORT. 67(24):38-40, Dec. 15, 1969.
"Growing peril: teenage use of drugs for kicks." GOOD HOUSEKEEPING. 162:168, May, 1966.
"Habituation and addiction," by Macdonald, A.D. INDIAN JOURNAL OF PHYSIOLOGY AND PHARMACOLOGY. 6:165-173, 1962.
"A halfway house for narcotic addicts," by Geis, G. BRITISH JOURNAL OF ADDICTION. 61:79-89, Nov., 1965.
"The 'hang-loose' ethic and the sprit of drug use," by Suchman, E.A. JOURNAL OF HEALTH AND SOCIAL BEHAVIOR. 9(2): 146-155, June, 1968.
"Harlem diary," by Edmon, L. RAMPARTS. 3:12 passim, 1964.
"The Harrison act and drug addiction: scientific treatment of this disease, not criminal prosecution, is the answer," by Gassman, B. BAR BULLETIN. 22(1):22-27, 1964.
"Haverford policy on drug use," by Borton, H. SCHOOL AND SOCIETY. 95:250 passim, Apr. 15, 1967.
"He turned disaster into triumph," by Abramson, M. READER'S DIGEST. 77:64-68, Dec., 1960.
"Head nurse on a drug addiction ward," by Bell, M JOURNAL OF PSYCHIATRIC NURSING. 4(6):546-562, 1966.
"Heads and freaks: patterns and meanings of drug use among hippies," by Davis, F., and Munoz, L. JOURNAL OF HEALTH AND SOCIAL BEHAVIOR. 9:156-164, 1968.
"Help for the addict," by Ramirez, E. AMERICAN JOURNAL OF NURSING. 67:2348-2353, 1967.
"The helping process in a hospital for narcotic addicts," by Berliner, A.K. FEDERAL PROBATION. 26(3):57-62, 1962.
"Heroin." THE ATTACK ON NARCOTIC ADDICTION AND DRUG ABUSE. 3:3, Spring, 1969.
"Heroin addiction, a case history." NURSING TIMES. 64: 79-81, Jan. 19, 1968.
"Heroin addiction - a metabolic disease," by Dole, V.P., et al. ARCHIVES OF INTERNAL MEDICINE. 120:19-24, July, 1967.
"Heroin addiction and the Fifth Estate," by Casselman, B.W. JOURNAL OF THE AMERICAN MEDICAL ASSOCIATION. 194(6): 680, 1965.
"Heroin addiction in the United Kingdom (1954-64)," by Bewley, T. BRITISH MEDICAL JOURNAL. 27(2):1284-1286, Nov., 1965.
"Heroin addiction: some of its problems," by Merry J. NURSING TIMES. 64:77-78, Jan. 19, 1968
"The heroin addict's pseudoassertive behavior and family dynamics," by Ganger, R., and Shugart, G. SOCIAL CASEWORK. 47(10):643-649, 1966.
"Heroin and cocaine addiction," by Bewley, T. LANCET. 1:808-810, Mar. 6, 1965.
"Heroin and cocaine addiction," by Glatt, M.M. LANCET. 1:910-911, 1965.
"Heroin dependence in Britain and the U.S.A.," by Cherubin, C. BRITISH MEDICAL JOURNAL. 2:489-490, May 25, 1968.
"High inhibitor: cyclazocine." TIME. 87:85, Mar. 18, 1966.
"The hill tribes of northern Thailand and the opium problem,"

by Saihoo, P. BULLETIN ON NARCOTICS. 15(2):35-45, Apr.-
June, 1963.
"Historical aspects of narcotics addiction," by Distler,
M.D. LISTEN. 15:8-9 passim, May-June, 1962.
"History, culture and subjective experience: an exploration
of the social bases of drug-induced experience," by Beck-
er, Howard S. JOURNAL OF HEALTH AND SOCIAL BEHAVIOR.
8:163-176, Sept., 1967.
"A history of drug abuse." JOURNAL OF THE AMERICAN PHARMA-
CEUTICAL ASSOCIATION. 8:16-21 passim, Jan., 1968.
"History of legal and medical roles in narcotic abuse in
the United States," by Simrell, E.V. PUBLIC HEALTH RE-
PORTS. 83:587-593, July, 1968.
"The history of the abuse of narcotic drugs in Czechoslova-
kia," by Matousék, Miloslav. BULLETIN ON NARCOTICS.
18(3):1-2, July-Sept., 1966.
"Hong Kong: its many splendored face," by Boal, S. DINER'S
CLUB MAGAZINE. 14:28-35, Oct., 1963.
"Hong Kong's prison for drug addicts." BULLETIN ON NARCOT-
ICS. 13(1):13-20, Jan.-Mar., 1961.
"The horrors of heroin," by Severs, R. READER'S DIGEST.
96(573):72-75, Jan., 1970.
"Hospital pharmacist speaks to his community on drug abuse,"
by Grancey, T. HOSPITAL PHARMACIST. 2:25-27, 1967.
"The hospitalized narcotic addict," by Gorwitz, K. MARY-
LAND STATE MEDICAL JOURNAL. 14:143, 1965.
"Houston's halfway house." REHABILITATION RECORD. 7:22-
23, 1966.
"How Bill Eppridge photographed the world of junkies," by
Eppridge, B. MODERN PHOTOGRAPHY. 29:22, June, 1965.
"How California is licking drug addiction," by Ross, I.
READER'S DIGEST. 91:138-142, Sept., 1967.
"How can we teach adolescents about smoking, drinking and
drug abuse?" by Hochbaum, G.M. JOURNAL OF HEALTH, PHY-
SICAL EDUCATION AND RECREATION. 39:34-38, Oct., 1968;
also EDUCATION DIGEST. 34:28-31, Jan., 1969.
"How drugs act - second series. II. Drugs and addiction,"
by Smith, S.E. NURSING TIMES. 63:388-389, 1967.
"How high the moon - jazz and drugs," by Winick, C. ANTIOCH
REVIEW. 21:53-68, Spring, 1961.
"How is addiction spreading?" by Chapple, P. MENTAL HEALTH.
25(3):21-23, 1966.
"How needy doctors get that way," by Carlova, J. MEDICAL
ECONOMICS. 42:108-119, 1965.
"How opiates change behavior," by Nichols, J.R. SCIENTIFIC
AMERICAN. 212(2):80-88, 1965.
"How to handle a dope scandal: candor clears the air," by
Goben, R.D. SCHOOL MANAGEMENT. 10:106-107, June, 1966.
"How to handle temptation," by Blonton, S. READER'S DIGEST.
p. 188, May, 1960.
"How we faced up to student drug abuse; Mamaroneck, N.Y.,"
by Haake, B.F. NATION'S SCHOOLS. 81:62-64, May, 1968.
"Hypnosis and addiction," by Black, S. BRITISH JOURNAL OF
ADDICTION. 58(2):61-64, 1962.

"I played Sir Galahad," by Goldberg, S.J. LISTEN. 14:17
passim, May-June, 1961.
"Identification and the sociopathic personality," by Dia-
mond, B.L. ARCHIVES OF CRIMINAL PSYCHODYNAMICS (Special
psychopathy issue). 1961.
"Identification processes in hospitalized narcotic drug
addicts," by Monroe, J.J., and Astim, A.W. JOURNAL OF
ABNORMAL AND SOCIAL PSYCHOLOGY. 63:215-218, 1961.
"Ideological supports to becoming and remaining a heroin
addict," by Feldman, H. JOURNAL OF HEALTH AND SOCIAL
BEHAVIOR. 9(2):131-139, 1968.
"Ill-advised medication with drugs leading to habituation
and addiction," by Myerson, C. BRITISH JOURNAL OF AD-
DICTION. 59:11-14, 1963.
"Ill-advised medication with drugs leading to habituation
and addiction. An interpretation: using drimanyl and
dextromoramide as examples," by Wilson, C.W.M. BRITISH
JOURNAL OF ADDICTION. 59(2):14-23, 1963.
"Illegal drug usage and industry," by Sweeney, F.E. AMER-
ICAN ASSOCIATION OF INDUSTRIAL NURSES JOURNAL. 15:19,
Aug., 1967.
"Illicit drug use among Canadian youth," by Unwin, J.R.
CANADIAN MEDICAL ASSOCIATION JOURNAL. 98(8):402-407,
1968.
"Illinois Rx men help police catch addicts." AMERICAN
DRUGGIST. 154:14, Oct. 10, 1966.
"The image of man," by Chein, I. JOURNAL OF SOCIAL ISSUES.
18:1-35, 1962.
"Immediate action on young Swedish drug-takers," by Burke,
P.E. TIMES (London) EDUCATIONAL SUPPLEMENT. 2712:1602,
May 12, 1967.
"In defense of youth," by Fiedler, L. HUMANIST. 27:117ff,
1967.
"In search of green pastures." MEDICAL JOURNAL OF AUSTRALIA.
1:17-18, Jan. 6, 1968.
"Incidence of drug addiction." United Nations: UNITED NA-
TIONS DOCUMENT E-CN.7-439., 1963.
"Increase in drug-taking?" TIMES (London) EDUCATIONAL SUP-
PLEMENT. 2670:211, July 22, 1966.
"Inside dope." NEWSWEEK. 60:62, Oct. 1, 1962.
"Instant happiness," by Goldman, R.P. LADIES HOME JOURNAL.
80(8), Oct., 1963.
"The institutional treatment of the narcotic addict," by
Rasor, R.W. JOURNAL OF THE MISSISSIPPI MEDICAL ASSOCIA-
TION. 6:11-14, 1965.
"Interference with family relationships," by Cahal, M.F.,
and Cady, E.L. GP. 27:174-175, 1963.
"Intoxication, addiction possible with non-barbiturate
drugs." JOURNAL OF THE AMERICAN MEDICAL ASSOCIATION.
187:33, 1964.
"Is narcotic addiction a chronic disease?" by Lasagna, L.
JOURNAL OF CHRONIC DISEASES. 19:949-951, Sept., 1966.
"It couldn't happen to us!" by Abramson, M. GOOD HOUSE-
KEEPING. 151:102, Sept., 1960; same abreviated with

title "He turned disaster into triumph." READER'S DIGEST. 77:64-68, Dec., 1960.
"It's no use telling an addict he needs a cure," by Wansell, G. TIMES (London) EDUCATIONAL SUPPLEMENT. 2764:1564, may 10, 1968.
"Job placement of addicts through a half-way house," by Wiener, F., and Turkington, K. REHABILITATION RECORD. 8:12-15, 1967.
"Joint statement on narcotic addiction in the United States by the American Medical Association and the National Research Council of the National Academy of Sciences." NEW YORK MEDICINE. 18:561, Aug. 20, 1962; also CHRISTIAN CENTURY. 80:140, Jan. 30, 1963.
"A junior high school seminar on dangerous drugs and narcotics," by Johnson, B.B. JOURNAL OF SCHOOL HEALTH. 38:84-76, Feb., 1968.
"Junkies give best advice on drugs," by Luckin, W. TIMES (London) EDUCATIONAL SUPPLEMENT. 2759:1154, Apr. 5, 1968.
"Junkie's life." NEWSWEEK. 65:63, Mar. 8, 1965.
"Junkies'world." NEWSWEEK. 58:56, Dec. 4, 1961.
"The juvenile narcotics addict: a profile," by Brown, E.M. PASTORAL COUNSELOR. 1:26-30, Fall, 1963.
"The 'kick' hang-up," by Verhulst, H.L., et al. NATIONAL CLEARINGHOUSE FOR POISON CONTROL CENTERS BULLETIN. pp. 1-2, Nov.-Dec., 1967.
"Kicking drugs: a very personal story," by Burroughs, W.S. HARPER'S MAGAZINE. 235:39-42, July, 1967.
"Laboratory control in the treatment of the narcotic addict," by Kurland, A.A. CURRENT PSYCHIATRIC THERAPIES. 6:243-246, 1966.
"A layman's notes on addiction," by Carnahan, P.M. PENNSYLVANIA MEDICINE. 70:73-76, June, 1967.
"The legistator looks at addiction," by Moran, J.B. ILLINOIS MEDICAL JOURNAL. 130:524-529, 1966.
"Less dangerous substitutes urged for addictive drugs," by Cass, L.J. HARVARD LAW RECORD. 40(6):1-2, 1965.
"Let's think twice about free narcotics." GENERAL PRACTITIONER. 21:156-162, May, 1960.
"Letter from the Berkeley underground," by Miller M. ESQUIRE. 64:3, 85-87 passim, 1965.
"Letter to the editor: drug abuse," by Pruden, E. AMERICAN JOURNAL OF MEDICAL TECHNOLOGY. 34:369-370, June, 1968.
"The Lexington program for narcotic addicts," by O'Donnell, J.A. FEDERAL PROBATION. 26(1):55-60, 1962.
"The life cycle of the narcotic addict and of addiction," by Winick, C. BULLETIN ON NARCOTICS. 16:1-11, Jan.-Mar., 1964.
"Lighter fluid 'sniffing'," by Acjerktm, W.C. AMERICAN JOURNAL OF PSYCHIATRY. 120:1056-1061, 1964.
"Lindensmith proposes general theory to explain addict's craving for drugs." JAPAN NEWSLETTER. 1(6):2, 1963.
"Living death, the truth about drug addiction," by Giordano, H.L. THE UNION SIGNAL. 92(6), Mar. 26, 1966.
"Loas: the boys at the snow leopard." TIME. 73:35, Feb. 29, 1960.

138

"A lobby for people?" by Blum, R.H., and Funkhouser, M.L.
AMERICAN PSYCHOLOGIST. 20(3):208-210, 1965.
"Locating and interviewing narcotic addicts in Puerto Rico,"
by Ball, J.C., and Pabon, D.O. SOCIOLOGY AND SOCIAL RE-
SEARCH. 49:401-411, July, 1965.
"Logistics of junk," by Lyle, D. ESQUIRE. 65:59-67 passim,
Mar., 1966.
"A loser all the way," by Willis, J.H. MENTAL HEALTH. 25
(3):31-32, 1966.
"Love on Haight; Haight-Ashbury district of San Francisco."
TIME. 89:27, Mar. 17, 1967.
"MD's as addicts." SCIENCE DIGEST. 62:72-73, Oct., 1967.
"Mainliners and blue velvet," by Wetherall, J.F., et al.
JOURNAL OF FORENSIC SCIENCES. 10:466-472, 1965.
"Making of a hippie; with study-discussion guide," by Smal-
lenburg, C., and Smallenburg, H. PTA MAGAZINE. 63:6-9
passim, Jan., 1969; also EDUCATION DIGEST. 34:32-34,
Apr., 1969.
"Management of drug habituation," by Tingle, D. JOURNAL OF
THE FLORIDA MEDICAL ASSOCIATION. 55:32-36, Jan., 1968.
"Marital history of narcotic addicts," by O'Donnell, J.A.,
et al. INTERNATIONAL JOURNAL OF THE ADDICTIONS. 2(1):
21-38, 1967.
"Masturbation and its relation to addiction," by Laten-
dresse, J.D. REVIEW OF EXISTENTIAL PSYCHOLOGY AND PSY-
CHIATRY. 8(1):16-27, 1968.
"Maturing out of narcotic addiction," by Winick, C. BUL-
LETIN ON NARCOTICS. 14:1-7, Jan.-Mar., 1962.
"Medical and social problems of drug addiction in West Af-
rica," by Lambo, T.A. BULLETIN ON NARCOTICS. 17(1):
3-13, Jan.-Mar., 1965.
"Medical deontology and the reporting of drug addicts," by
Muller, Prof. M., and Muller, Dr. P. BULLETIN ON NAR-
COTICS. 13(1):7-11, Jan.-Mar., 1961.
"Medical ethics, narcotics, and addiction." JOURNAL OF THE
AMERICAN MEDICAL ASSOCIATION. 185(12):962-963, 1963.
"Medical perspectives on habituation and addiction," by See-
vers, M.H. JOURNAL OF THE AMERICAN MEDICAL ASSOCIATION.
181(2):92-98, 1962.
"Medical responsibility and drug addiction," by Eisenberg,
L. PEDIATRICS. 34:155-156, 1964.
"Medicine and law in the treatment of drug addiction," by
Lowry, J.V., and Simrell, E.V. BULLETIN ON NARCOTICS.
15(3-4):9-16, July-Dec., 1963.
"The medico-legal conflict," by Ostrow, S. AMERICAN JOUR-
NAL OF NURSING. 63:67-71, July, 1963.
"Medico-legal conflict in drug usage," by Bowen, O.K.
JOURNAL OF SCHOOL HEALTH. 39:165-172, Mar., 1969.
"Medicolegal issues in the care of addicts," by Cameron,
D.C. ANNALS OF INTERNAL MEDICINE. 67:209-210, 1967.
"Menace of dope," by Silverman, B.M. PARENTS MAGAZINE.
37:82-83 passim, Oct., 1962.
"The menace of drug abuse," by Goddard, J. AMERICAN EDU-
CATION. 2(5):4-7, 1966.

"Mental illness, alcoholism, and drug dependence," by De-
mone, H.W., Jr. ANNALS OF THE AMERICAN ACADEMY OF POLI-
TICAL AND SOCIAL SCIENCE. 378:22-33, July, 1968.
"Migration and residential mobility of narcotic drug ad-
dicts," by Ball, J.C., and Bates, W.M. SOCIAL PROBLEMS.
14(1):56-69, 1966.
"A million pipelines from afar to dope addict's mainline,"
by Ehrlich, D.A. NEW YORK JOURNAL AMERICAN. June 10,
1965.
"Misapprehensions about drug addiction: some origins and
repercussions," by Brill, H. COMPREHENSIVE PSYCHIATRY.
4:150-159, June, 1963.
"Mischievous drugs," by Rossi, G. AMERICAN JOURNAL OF
PHARMACY. 140:38-43, Mar.-Apr., 1968.
"The misuse of drugs," by Gibbens, T.C.N. THE HOWARD JOUR-
NAL OF PENOLOGY AND CRIME PREVENTION. 11(4):257-261,
1965.
"Misuse of drugs: some facts." Royal Bank of Canada MONTH-
LY NEWSLETTER. Sept., 1968.
"The misuse of narcotics by patients suffering from cancer,"
by Callaway, E. CANCER. 10:33-36, 1960.
"Mix-up on drugs," by Coles, R. NEW REPUBLIC. 155:23-25,
Sept. 17, 1966.
"Modern threats to health. 8. Some other diseases of in-
creasing incidence," by Burn, J.L. NURSING TIMES. 58:
1548-1550, 1962.
"Monkeys with men on their backs," by McCann, H.W. SCIENCE
DIGEST. 49:6, June, 1961.
"Morbidity and mortality from heroin dependence." BULLETIN
ON NARCOTICS. 21(1):39, Jan.-Mar., 1969.
"Martality among young narcotic addicts," by Mason, P.
JOURNAL OF THE MOUNT SINAI HOSPITAL, NEW YORK. 34:4-10,
Jan.-Feb., 1967.
"Mothers of addiction," by Sayre, N. NEW STATESMAN. 69:
716, May 7, 1965.
"Multiple-drug addiction in New York City in a selected
population group," by Abeles, H., et al. PUBLIC HEALTH
REPORTS. 81:685-690, Aug., 1966.
"My biggest professional mistake," by Clarey, A. MEDICAL
ECONOMICS. Mar., 1960.
"My birthday is not the day I was born," by Jones, A. AMER-
ICAN JOURNAL OF NURSING. 67:1434-1438, 1967.
"My life with juvenile gangs; excerpt from 'All the way
down'," ed. B. Slocum, and V. Riccio. SATURDAY EVENING
POST. 235:72-75, Sept. 29, 1962.
"My son is a dope addict," by Carlson, B. as told to P.
Young. CHATELAINE MAGAZINE. 37:29 passim, 1964.
"My son was a drug addict," by David, L. GOOD HOUSEKEEP-
ING. 160:53, Jan., 1965.
"My son was caught using narcotics," ed. H. Spence. SAT-
URDAY EVENING POST. 233:32-33 passim, Dec. 10, 1960.
"The narcotic addict and 'the street'," by Weech, A.A., Jr.
ARCHIVES OF GENERAL PSYCHIATRY. 14(3):299-306, 1966.
"The narcotic addict as a medical patient," by Sapira, J.D.

AMERICAN JOURNAL OF MEDICINE. 45:555-588, Oct., 1968.
"The narcotic addict in the general hospital," by Freedman,
A.M. MENTAL HOSPITALS. 16:230-232, 1965.
"Narcotic-addict prisoners in Japan," by Hemmi, Takemitsu.
CORRECTIVE PSYCHIATRY AND JOURNAL OF SOCIAL THERAPY.
11(2):87-89, 1965.
"Narcotic addict rehabilitation," by Rubin, M.M. ILLINOIS
MEDICAL JOURNAL. 130:494-499, 1966.
"The narcotic addict. Some reflections on treatment," by
Kurland, A.A. MARYLAND MEDICAL JOURNAL. 15:37-39, 1966.
"Narcotic addiction." NEW YORK MEDICINE. 21(2):3-8, 1965.
"Narcotic addiction," by O'Donnell, J.A. ENCYCLOPEDIA OF
SOCIAL WORK. 15:522-526, 1965.
"Narcotic addiction: a clinical approach," by Myerson, D.J.
PSYCHIATRIC OPINION. 11:31-33, 1965.
"Narcotic addiction: a public health approach," by Michael,
G.A. PSYCHIATRIC OPINION. 11:33-34, 1965.
"Narcotic addiction, a social scotoma." AMERICAN JOURNAL
OF PSYCHOTHERAPY. 15:337-340, 1961.
"Narcotic addiction among physicians: a ten-year follow-
up," by Putnam, P.L., and Ellinwood, E.H. AMERICAN JOUR-
NAL OF PSYCHIATRY. 122(7):745-748, 1966.
"Narcotic addiction and crime," by O'Donnell, J.A. SOCIAL
PROBLEMS. 13:374-385, Spring, 1966.
"Narcotic addiction and criminal responsibility under Dur-
ham," by Bowman, A.M. GEORGETOWN LAW JOURNAL. 53:1017-
1048, 1965.
"Narcotic addiction and the teenager. Summary report of
a 3-day conference of the In-service Training Department.
New York City Youth Board." AMERICAN JOURNAL OF CORREC-
TION. 24:8-12, 1962.
"Narcotic addiction as viewed by a federal narcotic agent,"
by Levine, S FEDERAL PROBATION. 28(4):30-34, Dec., 1964.
"Narcotic addiction in males and females: a comparison," by
Ellingwood, E.H., Jr., et al. INTERNATIONAL JOURNAL OF
THE ADDICTIONS. 1(2):33-45, 1966.
"Narcotic addiction in nurses and doctors," by Farb, S.
NURSING OUTLOOK. 13:30-34, 1965.
"Narcotic addiction in physicians; medical and legal as-
pects of rehabilitation," by Quinn, W.F. BULLETIN ON
NARCOTICS. 15(1):11-13, Jan.-Mar., 1963.
"Narcotic addiction in the pain-prone female patient. I.
A comparison with addict controls," by Glaser, F.B.
INTERNATIONAL JOURNAL OF THE ADDICTIONS. 1(2):47-59,
1966.
"Narcotic addiction is reversible," by Antell, M.J. ST.
VINCENT'S HOSPITAL MEDICAL BULLETIN. 6:37-40, 1964.
"Narcotic addiction of physicians," by Jones C.H. NORTH-
WEST MEDICINE. 66:559-564, June, 1967.
"Narcotic addiction - pattern of U.K. narcotic problems
said to be trending toward young." MEDICAL TRIBUNE AND
MEDICAL NEWS. Oct. 6, 1965.
"Narcotic addiction - some thoughts on present programs,
and future needs," by Holmes, S.J. PAPERS ON DRUGS -

ADDICTION, ALCOHOLISM AND DRUG ADDICTION RESEARCH FOUNDA-
TION, Toronto, 1965, pp. 21-31, also PROGRESS. 5:2-10.
June, 1963.
"Narcotic addiction, the institution and the community,"
by Berliner, A.K. INTERNATIONAL JOURNAL OF THE ADDIC-
TIONS. 1(1):74-85, 1966.
"Narcotic addiction -- the neglect of research," by Marcus,
R.L. SCIENCE. 144:144, 1964.
"Narcotic addiction - wholly new approach urged to solving
problem of abuse," by Goshen, C.E. MEDICAL TRIBUNE AND
MEDICAL NEWS. 6(128):1-24, 1965.
"Narcotic addicts in the mid-1960's," by Smith, W.G., et al.
PUBLIC HEALTH REPORTS. 81:403-412, May, 1966.
"Narcotic addicts - patients or criminals?" by Schur, E.M.
TUFTS FOLIA MEDICA. 9:41-48, 1963.
"Narcotic and dangerous drug problems. Current status of
legislation, control and rehabilitation," by Quinn, W.F.
CALIFORNIA MEDICINE. 106(2):108-111, 1967.
"Narcotic and drug abuse: report of Advisory Commission
prescribes for old problems, new dangers," by Walsh, J.
SCIENCE. 143:662-666, Feb. 14, 1964.
"Narcotic and methamphetamine use during pregnancy," by
Sussman, S. AMERICAN JOURNAL OF DISEASES OF CHILDREN.
106:325-330, 1963.
↙"Narcotic drug addiction," by Cameron, D.C. AMERICAN JOUR-
NAL OF PSYCHIATRY. 119(8):793-794, 1963.
"Narcotic drug addiction in Canada," by MacDonald, R. St. J.
CURRENT LAW AND SOCIAL PROBLEMS. pp. 162-204, 1960.
"Narcotic drug addiction: one year's experiences at Pilgrim
State Hospital," by Rice, J., and Cohen, L. PSYCHIATRIC
QUARTERLY. 39:457-465, 1965.
"Narcotic drug addiction problems," by Livingston, R.B., ed.
PUBLIC HEALTH SERVICE PUBLICATION No. 1050, 1963.
"The narcotic problem," by Schwartz, G. WESTERN MEDICINE.
6:335-338, 1965.
"The narcotic problem. A challenge to physicians," by Mil-
ler, H.B. JOURNAL OF THE MEDICAL SOCIETY OF NEW JERSEY.
61:378-379, 1964.
"Narcotic tools of addiction ... of control," by Giordano,
H.L. AMERICAN PROFESSIONAL PHARMACIST. 33:30-35, 1967.
"Narcotics addiction," by The Medical Society of the County
of New York. NEW YORK MEDICINE. 21:2, Jan., 1965.
"Narcotics addiction, a hazard to physicians." SCIENCE
DIGEST. 48:50-51, Dec., 1960.
"Narcotics addiction -- a unique challenge," by New York
State Department of Mental Hygiene. MENTAL HYGIENE NEWS.
35:4-5 passim, 1965.
"Narcotics addiction and teenagers." CURRICULUM AND MATER-
IALS. 19(3):10-11, 1965.
"Narcotics addiction and the 'American system'," by Hausman,
R. TEXAS STATE JOURNAL OF MEDICINE. 60:335-336, 1964.
"Narcotics addiction and the physician," by Miller, D.E.
JOURNAL OF THE AMERICAN OSTEOPATHIC ASSOCIATION. 66:
1232-1236, July, 1967.

142

"Narcotics addiction in physicians," by Modlin, H.S., and
Montes, A. AMERICAN JOURNAL OF PSYCHIATRY. 121(4):
358-365, 1964.
"Narcotics addiction: punishment or treatment," by Shaffer,
H.B. EDITORIAL RESEARCH REPORTS. pp. 519-536, July 18,
1962.
"Narcotics and crime; why our cities are taking a new look."
SENIOR SCHOLASTIC. 81:16-19, Nov. 14, 1962.
"Narcotics and drug abuse: the federal response," by Walsh,
J. SCIENCE. 162:1254 passim, Dec. 13, 1968.
"Narcotics bugaboo. TODAY'S HEALTH. 38(3):62-63, Mar.,
1960.
"Narcotics dilemma: crime or disease?" by Kobler, J. SAT-
URDAY EVENING POST. 235:64-66 passim, Sept. 8, 1962.
"Narcotics, negroes and the South," by Bates, W.M. SOCIAL
FORCES. 45:61-67, Sept., 1966.
"Narcotics on campus," by Beall, L.L. JOURNAL OF SECONDARY
EDUCATION. 43:233-235, May, 1968.
"Narcotics problem." COMMONWEAL. 77:61, Oct. 12, 1962.
"Narcotics: the international picture," by Fort, J. CAL-
IFORNIA YOUTH AUTHORITY QUARTERLY. 14:3-17, Summer, 1961.
"Narcotics use and abuse," by Trellis, E.S. PENNSYLVANIA
MEDICINE. 69:50-52, 1966.
"The negro drug addict as an offender type," by Roebuck,
J.B. JOURNAL OF CRIMINAL LAW, CRIMINOLOGY AND POLICE
SCIENCE. 53(1):36-43, 1962.
"Neonatal narcotic addiction," by Vincow, A., and Hackel,
A. GP. 22:90-93, 1960.
"New addicts; teen-agers hooked on goof balls, glue, and
cough medicine." NEWSWEEK. 60:42, Aug. 13, 1962.
"New approach; more humane treatment." NEWSWEEK. 61:94,
Apr. 15, 1963.
"New approaches to the narcotic problem. Summary and dis-
cussion," by Wortis, S.B. BULLETIN OF THE NEW YORK ACAD-
EMY OF MEDICINE. 40:314-318, 1964.
"New approaches to the treatment of drug addiction," by
Jones, G.L. JOURNAL OF THE MEDICAL SOCIETY OF NEW JER-
SEY. 64:85-88, 1967.
"New hope for drug addicts," by Schreiber, F.R., and Herman,
M. SCIENCE DIGEST. 60:15-17, July, 1966.
"New improved drug scene," by Larner, J. NATION. 201:120-
124, Sept. 20, 1965.
"New York's dope nostrum," by Prisendorf, A. NATION. 204
(16):486-490, 1967.
"No drug-takers reported." TIMES (London) EDUCATIONAL SUP-
PLEMENT. 2721:84, July 14, 1967.
"No mercy, no haven for addicts." CHRISTIAN CENTURY. 83:
577, May 4, 1966
"No way out? drugs and therapeutic community programs."
NEWSWEEK. 68:77-78, Oct. 10, 1966.
"Nonnarcotic addiction. Incidence in a university hospital
psychiatric ward," by Bakewell, W.E., and Wikler, A.
JOURNAL OF THE AMERICAN MEDICAL ASSOCIATION. 196:710-
713, May, 1966

"Nonnarcotic addiction. Size and extent of the problem,"
by Sadusk, F.J., Jr. JOURNAL OF THE AMERICAN MEDICAL
ASSOCIATION. 196:707-709, May 23, 1966.
"Notification of drug addicts in the United Kingdom."
BULLETIN ON NARCOTICS. 20(3):40, July-Sept., 1968.
"Nurses relieved of narcotic record keeping," by Hambright,
J.B. HOSPITAL MANAGEMENT. 101:52-58, 1965.
"Oberlin's revised policy; student use and provision of
drugs." SCHOOL AND SOCIETY. 96:167, Mar. 16, 1968.
"Object; kill the habit." NEWSWEEK. 57:52, Jan. 23, 1961.
"On drug addiction," by Rosenfeld, H. INTERNATIONAL JOUR-
NAL OF PSYCHOANALYSIS. 41:467-475, 1960.
"On getting busted at fifty," by Fiedler, L.A. NEW YORK
REVIEW. pp. 8 passim, July 13, 1967.
"On the nature of addiction and habituation," by Wikler, A.
BRITISH JOURNAL OF ADDICTION. 57:73, 1961.
"Once you get hooked;...addicts trace path to tragedy," by
Sims, P. NEW ORLEANS STATES-ITEM. Oct., 1965.
"One wrong to justify another," by Alden, J.D. SCIENCE.
160:604-605, May 10, 1968.
"Opiate addiction." LANCET. 1:649-650, 1964.
"Opiate addiction," by Bewley, T.H. LANCET. 1:938, 1964.
"Opiate addiction," by Clark, J.A. PROCEEDINGS OF THE
ROYAL SOCIETY OF MEDICINE. 58(6):412-414, 1965.
"Opiate addiction of Marcus Aurelius," by Africa, T.W.
JOURNAL OF THE HISTORY OF IDEAS. 22:97-102, Jan., 1961.
"Opiate use, addiction and relapse," by Akers, R.L., et al.
SOCIAL PROBLEMS. 15(4):459-469, 1968.
"The orbiting teenager - a seminar. Problems with smoking,
alcohol and drug abuse," by Offord, D.R. MEDICAL TIMES.
93:207-208, 1965.
"Our new drug addicts," by Grafton, S. MCCALLS. 92:112-
113, Apr., 1965.
"Ours is the addicted society," by Farber, L.H. NEW YORK
TIMES MAGAZINE. p. 43 passim, Dec. 11, 1966.
"Outpatient treatment for narcotic addicts will get its
test." NEW YORK MEDICINE. 19:635-636, 1963.
"Pain tolerance and narcotic addiction," by Martin, J.E.,
et al. BRITISH JOURNAL OF SOCIAL AND CLINICAL PSYCHOLOGY.
4:224-229, Sept., 1965.
"Paregoric and triplennamine (blue velvet) addiction in-
creasing, claims Detroit pathologist." JOURNAL OF THE
AMERICAN MEDICAL ASSOCIATION. 188(suppl.):34, 1964.
"Parent-child cultural disparity and drug addiction," by
Vaillant, G.E. JOURNAL OF NERVOUS AND MENTAL DISEASE.
142:534-539, June, 1966.
"Parental deprivation in psychiatric conditions: III. In
personality disorders and other conditions," by Oltman,
J.E., and Friedman, S. DISEASES OF THE NERVOUS SYSTEM.
28(5):298-303, 1967.
"Parents to act on drugs." TIMES (London) EDUCATIONAL SUP-
PLEMENT. 2807:737, Mar. 7, 1969.
"Past, present and future in the treatment of drug addic-
tion," by Bowman, K.M. COMPREHENSIVE PSYCHIATRY. 4:145-

149, June, 1963.
"Patterns and profiles of addiction and drug abuse," by
Scher, J. INTERNATIONAL JOURNAL OF ADDICTIONS. 2:171-
190, Fall, 1967; also ARCHIVES OF GENERAL PSYCHIATRY.
15:539-551, 1966.
"Pennsylvania Department of Health notes dangers of con-
junctive use of alcohol and drugs." MARYLAND STATE MED-
ICAL JOURNAL. 16:134-136, May, 1967.
"Pentecostals and drug addiction; teen challenge centers,"
by McDonnell, K. AMERICA. 118:402-406, Mar. 30, 1968.
"People get hooked," by Baker, R.S. COMMENTARY. 35:243-
246, Mar., 1963.
"People in search of dreams," by MacInnes, C. MENTAL HEALTH.
25(3):24-25, 1966.
"People versus Baby," by Samuels, G. NEW YORK TIMES MAGA-
ZINE. pp. 40-41 passim, Jan. 17, 1965.
"The pharmacist's role in drug abuse education," by Chal-
mers, R.K. JOURNAL OF THE AMERICAN PHARMACEUTICAL ASSOC-
IATION. 8:30-34, Jan., 1968.
"Physician narcotic addicts," by Winick, C. SOCIAL PROBLEMS.
9:174-186, Fall, 1961.
"The physician's role in abating drug addiction," by Myers,
I.L. JOURNAL OF THE MEDICAL ASSOCIATION OF THE STATE OF
ALABAMA. 36:565, 1966.
"Pills and Olympians." SCIENCE NEWS. 91:353, Apr. 15, 1967.
"Pills, glue and kids: an American tragedy," by Selby, E.,
and Selby, A. READER'S DIGEST. 88:66-70, June, 1966.
"Playmates in the narcotics game," by Barnes, H.E. SATUR-
DAY REVIEW. 48:25, Mar. 6, 1965.
"Preaching the monkey off their backs: teen challenge cen-
ters." TIME. 84:43, Aug. 14, 1964.
"Preliminary experiences of a pilot project in drug addic-
tion," by Brill, L. SOCIAL CASEWORK. 42:28-32, Jan,
1961.
"Preliminary observations on patterns of drug consumption
among medical students," by Blaine, J.D., et al. INTER-
NATIONAL JOURNAL OF THE ADDICTIONS. 3:389-396, Spring,
1968.
"Present state of the coca-leaf habit in Colombia," by Be-
jarano, J. BULLETIN ON NARCOTICS. 13(1):1-5, Jan.-Mar.,
1961.
"Preventing drug addiction through education," by Esty, G.W.
PUBLIC HEALTH NEWS (New Jersey State Health Department).
47:87-90, 1966.
"The problem of addiction," by Chessick, R.D. MEDICAL TIMES.
90:247-252, 1962.
"The problem of drug addiction." SCOTTISH MEDICAL JOURNAL.
11:340-342, Sept., 1966.
"Problem of drug addiction: an overview," by Gubar, G.
PENNSYLVANIA PSYCHIATRIC QUARTERLY. 7(2):10-20, 1967.
"The problem of drug dependencies: some general perspec-
tives," by Brill, H. JOURNAL OF THE HILLSIDE HOSPITAL.
16(2):108-110, 1967.
"Problem of narcotic addiction," by Cameron, D.C. CHRIST-

IAN CENTURY. 80:138-141, Jan. 30, 1963.
"Problem of neonatal narcotic addiction," by Yerby, A.S.
NEW YORK STATE JOURNAL OF MEDICINE. 66(10):1248-1249,
1966.
"Problems and pseudo-problems," by Trocchi, A. MENTAL
HEALTH. 25(3):29-30, 1966.
"Problems common to alcoholism and drug dependence," by
Glatt, M.M. WHO CHRONICLE. 21:293-303, July, 1967.
"Problems of addiction," by Bartholomew, A.A. MEDICAL
JOURNAL OF AUSTRALIA. 50(1):315-318, 1963.
"Problems of drug addiction and drug abuse in surgical pa-
tients," by Morton, R.C., et al. JOURNAL OF THE LOUISI-
ANA STATE MEDICAL SOCIETY. 119:475-481, Dec., 1967.
"The problems of drug addicts," by Christophers, B.E. MED-
ICAL JOURNAL OF AUSTRALIA. 1:188, Jan. 28, 1967.
"Problems of inpatient treatment of addiction," by Jurgen-
sen, W.P. INTERNATIONAL JOURNAL OF THE ADDICTIONS.
1:62-73, 1966.
"The prognosis in drug addiction," by Clark, J.A. JOURNAL
OF MENTAL SCIENCE. 108:411-418, 1962.
"A prosecutor's thoughts concerning addiction," by Kuh, R.H.
JOURNAL OF CRIMINAL LAW. 52:321-327, Sept.-Oct., 1961.
"Psychedelic sentence; T.F. Leary and daughter." NEWSWEEK.
67:35, Mar. 21, 1966.
"Psychosocial aspects of drug addiction," by Radin, S.S.
JOURNAL OF SCHOOL HEALTH. 36:481-487, Dec., 1966.
"Psychotherapy of successful musicians who are drug addicts,"
by Winick, C., and Nyswander, M. AMERICAN JOURNAL OF
ORTHOPSYCHIATRY. 31:622-636, 1961.
"Public health aspects of maternal and neonatal narcotic
addiction," by Oettinger, K.B. BOSTON MEDICAL QUARTERLY.
17:38-40, 1966.
"Public health aspects of narcotic addiction," by Freedman,
A.M. NEW YORK STATE JOURNAL OF MEDICINE. 63(11):1656-
1665, June 1, 1963.
"Public health laboratory in the fight against narcotic ad-
diction in Iran," by Olszyna-Marzys, A.E. BULLETIN ON
NARCOTICS. 15(2):27-34, Apr.-June, 1963.
"Puffy-hand sign of drug addiction (correspondence)," by
Abeles, H. NEW ENGLAND JOURNAL OF MEDICINE. 273(21):
1167, 1965.
"Purely medical approach to addiction proposed." SCIENCE
NEWS LETTER. 82:272, Oct. 27, 1962.
"Queen Anne's lace." BULLETIN ON NARCOTICS. 20(3):18,
July-Sept., 1968.
"Question of drug abuse," by Ledger, L. THE TEXAS OUTLOOK.
51:26-27, Sept., 1967.
"Quick Watson, the needle," by Bigelow, N. PSYCHIATRIC
QUARTERLY. 37:355-365, 1963.
"The quiet revolution," by Uhr, L., and Uhr, E. PSYCHOLOGY
TODAY. 1:40-43, 1967.
"Rapid habituation to chlordiazepoxide (librium)," by Guile,
L.A. MEDICAL JOURNAL OF AUSTRALIA. 2:56-57, 1963.
"Realism and addicts." BRITISH MEDICAL JOURNAL. 4:436-437,

Nov. 25, 1967.
"Reappraisal of the concept of drug addiction," by Goshen,
C.E. MEDICAL ANNALS OF THE DISTRICT OF COLUMBIA. 29:
493-495, 1960.
"Reassuring report." ECONOMIST. 199:988, June 3, 1961.
"Rebels - with a cause. A report on synanon," by Mueller,
E.E. AMERICAN JOURNAL OF PSYCHOTHERAPY. 18:272-284,
Apr., 1964.
"Rebels without a cause," by Holden, H.M. MENTAL HEALTH.
25(3):33-35, 1966.
"Recent changes in the incidence in all types of drug de-
pendence in Great Britain," by Bewley, T.H. PROCEED-
INGS OF THE ROYAL SOCIETY OF MEDICINE. 61:175-177, Feb.,
1968.
"Recent changes in the pattern of drug abuse in the United
Kingdom," by Bewley, T. BULLETIN ON NARCOTICS. 18(4):
1-13, Oct.-Dec., 1966.
"Recent patterns of addiction in Czechoslovakia," by Von-
dracek, V., et al. BRITISH JOURNAL OF PSYCHIATRY. 114
(508):285-292, Mar., 1968.
"Recognizing the newborn addict," by Fleming, J.W. AMER-
ICAN JOURNAL OF NURSING. 65:83, 1965.
"Reflections on heroin and cocaine addiction," by Glatt,
M.M. LANCET. 2(7404):171-172, 1965.
"Reflections on narcotics addiction," by Hoffman, M. YALE
REVIEW. 54:17-30, Autumn, 1964.
"Rehabilitation of the street addict," by Dole, V.P., et
al. ARCHIVES OF ENVIRONMENTAL HEALTH. 14:477-480, 1967.
"The rehabilitative effectiveness of a community correction-
al residence for narcotic users," by Fisher, S. JOURNAL
OF CRIMINAL LAW, CRIMINOLOGY, AND POLICE SCIENCE. 56
(2):190-196, 1965.
"Relationships of social activity, work capacity, responsi-
bility, and competence to drug effects," by Goldman, D.
JOURNAL OF FORENSIC SCIENCES. 12:431-443, Oct., 1967.
"Relevance of American experience of narcotics addiction
to the British scene," by Edwards, G. BRITISH MEDICAL
JOURNAL. 3:425-429, Aug, 12, 1967.
"The reliability and validity of interview data obtained
from 59 narcotic drug addicts," by Ball, J.C. AMERICAN
JOURNAL OF SOCIOLOGY. 72:650-654, May, 1967.
"Ren tutor section winter conference: drugs and addiction."
NURSING TIMES. 63:161, 1967.
"Report of a conference on narcotic addiction," by Maddux,
J.F. REHABILITATION RECORD. 7:7-15, 1966.
"Report on drug addiction." NEW YORK STATE JOURNAL OF
MEDICINE. 63(13):1977-2000, July, 1963.
"Report on the current status of cocaism in Colombia," by
Bejarano, J. REVISTA COLOMBIABA DE PEDIATRIA Y PUERI-
CUTURA. 20:174-178, 1962.
"Required reading. The panic in needle park," by Quinn,
W.F. WESTERN MEDICINE. 7:140, 1966.
"Requirements and evaluations of narcotics tests," by Man-
nering, G.J. PSYCHOPHARMACOLOGY BULLETIN; NATIONAL

147

CLEARINGHOUSE FOR MENTAL HEALTH INFORMATION. 3:27-29, 1966.
"Responsibility and addiction," by Armstrong, J.D. CANADIAN PSYCHIATRY ASSOCIATION JOURNAL. 11:116-122, Apr., 1966.
"Responsibility and addiction: a psychiatric approach," by Armstrong, J.D. ADDICTIONS. 13(4):1-10, 1966.
"Retailers to teach kids re drug evils." AMERICAN DRUGGIST. 156:24, Sept. 25, 1967.
"A review of some significant phases of the addiction problem," by Fuller, J.K. CALIFORNIA YOUTH AUTHORITY QUARTERLY. 5:22-23, Fall, 1962.
"A review of the second report of the Interdepartmental Committee on Addiction," by Glatt, M.M. BULLETIN ON NARCOTICS. 18(2):29-42, Apr.-June, 1966.
"Rimbaud in a raincoat," by Allsop, K. SPECTATOR. 205: 176-177, July 29, 1960.
"Rise and decline of a subculture," by O'Donnell, J.A. SOCIAL PROBLEMS. 15:73-84, Summer, 1967.
"Rituals of addiction," by Sayre, N. NEW STATESMAN. 70: 248, Aug. 20, 1965.
"Rockefeller and the drug plan," by Buckley, W.F., Jr. NATIONAL REVIEW. 18:257, Mar. 22, 1966.
"The rush to combine: sociological dissimilarities of alcoholism and drug abuse," by Pittman, D.J. BRITISH JOURNAL OF ADDICTION. 62:337-343, Dec., 1967.
"Rx for the ill and handicapped," by Hill, B., and Young, E. RECREATION. 54:155, Mar., 1961.
"S.S. hang tough; synanon system," by Schneider, J. TIME. 77:72+, Apr. 7, 1961; also PROGRESSIVE. 28:32-34, Feb., 1964.
"Science, drugs, students," by Beecher, H.K. HARVARD ALUMNI BULLETIN. 65:338, 1963.
"A second look at the New York State parole drug experiment," by Diskind, M.H., and Klonsky, G. FEDERAL PROBATION. 28:34-41, Dec., 1964.
"The second report of the Interdepartmental Committee on Drug Addiction," by Matthew, H. BRITISH JOURNAL OF ADDICTION. 61:169-179, Aug., 1966.
"Selected social characteristics of consecutive admissions to Lexington in 1965," by Ball, J., et al. CRIMINOLOGICA. 4:13-16, Aug., 1966.
"Self-poisoning." BRITISH MEDICAL JOURNAL. 5474:1323-1324, 1965.
"Sex drawn first and sex drawn larger by opiate addict and non-addict inmates on the Draw-A-Person Test." by Kurtzberg, R.L., et al. JOURNAL OF PROJECTIVE TECHNIQUES AND PERSONALITY ASSESSMENT. 30:55-58, Feb., 1966.
"Side effects: a new worry for doctors," by Hunt, M.M. . LOOK. 27(26):24-26 passim, 1963.
"Signs of heroin usage detected by drug users and their parents," by Rathod, N.H., et al. LANCET. 2:1411-1414, Dec. 30, 1967.
"Sins of the mothers; withdrawal babies." NEWSWEEK. 59:

84, May 7, 1962.
"60-member team at center probes drug addiction," LEXING-
TON HERALD. May 23, 1965.
"Slanguage of the addict." ANNALS OF INTERNAL MEDICINE.
67:217-218, July, 1967.
"Social and cultural factors related to narcotic use among
Puerto Ricans in New York City," by Preble, E. INTER-
NATIONAL JOURNAL OF THE ADDICTIONS. 1(1):30-41, 1966.
"Social considerations of drug taking," by Holden, H.M.
NURSING TIMES. 63:476-478, Apr. 14, 1967.
"The social deviant and initial addiction to narcotics and
alcohol," by Hill, H.E. QUARTERLY JOURNAL OF STUDIES
ON ALCOHOL. 23(4):562-582, 1962.
"Social disease." TIMES (London) EDUCATIONAL SUPPLEMENT.
2813:1257, Apr. 18, 1969.
"Social reactions to 'crimes without victims'," by Ronney,
E.A., and Gibbons, D.C. SOCIAL PROBLEMS. 13(4):400-
410, 1966.
"Sociology of addiction," by Lindesmith, A.R. ILLINOIS
MEDICAL JOURNAL. 130:447-450, Oct., 1966.
"Some cases of addiction to new drugs among the Paris 'beat-
nik'." BULLETIN ON NARCOTICS. 21(1):31, Jan.-Mar., 1969.
"Some future directions for research in adolescent drug
addiction," by Ausubel, D.P. ADOLESCENCE. 1:70-78, 1966.
"Some medical aspects of the life of Dante Gabriel Rosset-
ti," by Dyke, S.C. PROCEEDINGS OF THE ROYAL SOCIETY OF
MEDICINE. 56:1089-1093, 1963.
"Some questions concerning illicit use of drugs on the cam-
pus," by Pervin, L.A. AMERICAN JOURNAL OF ORTHOPSYCHI-
ATRY. 37:299, Mar., 1967.
"Some thoughts on narcotics problems in Africa," by Gard-
iner, R.K.A. BULLETIN ON NARCOTICS. 20(1):39-40, Jan.-
Mar., 1968.
"Some trends in the treatment and epidemiology of drug ad-
diction: psychotherapy and synanon," by Sabath, G. PSY-
CHOTHERAPY: THEORY, RESEARCH AND PRACTICE. 4(2):92-96,
1967.
"The soprano on West 15th Street," by Marine, G. RAMPARTS.
p. 41, Aug., 1966.
"Speaking out; give drugs to addicts," by Straus, N. SAT-
URDAY EVENING POST. 237:6+, Aug. 8, 1964.
"Speaking out; give drugs to addicts so we can be safe,"
by Goldstein, J.J. SATURDAY EVENING POST. 239:12 pas-
sim, July 30, 1966.
"Special island; Palisades high school students and narcot-
ics." NEWSWEEK. 67:40, Apr. 11, 1966.
"Special issue on drug addiction." COMPREHENSIVE PSYCHIA-
TRY. 4:3, 1963.
"Special symposium on drug abuse; with introduction by
Feinglass, S.J. JOURNAL OF SECONDARY EDUCATION. 43:
196-235, May, 1968.
"Sports shadow." THE ATTACK ON NARCOTIC ADDICTION AND DRUG
ABUSE. 3:4, Summer, 1969.
"The spread of heroin abuse in a community," by deAlarcon,

R. BULLETIN ON NARCOTICS. 21(3):17-22, July-Sept., 1969.
"Start on narcotics." AMERICA. 107:915-916, Oct. 20, 1962.
"Statistical study of criminal drug addicts," by Messinger,
   E., and Zitrin, A. CRIME AND DELINQUENCY. 11(3):283-
   292, 1965.
"Stealing and addiction are linked problems." SCIENCE NEWS
   LETTER. 84:3, July 6, 1963.
"Stoned age?" by Oliphant, H.N. EDUCATION DIGEST. 34:32-
   35, May, 1969; also EDUCATION AGE. 5:2-5, Jan.-Feb.,
   1969.
"Stony Brook," by Glass, B. SCIENCE. 159:919, Mar. 1, 1968.
"Stony Brook," by Pond, T.A. SCIENCE. 159:920, Mar. 1,
   1968.
"Straight talk about the drug problem." SCHOOL MANAGEMENT.
   12:52-56 passim, Feb., 1968.
"The strange case of the Harvard drug scandal," by Weil,
   A.T. LOOK. 27(22):38 passim, 1963.
"Students and drug abuse." TODAY'S EDUCATION. 58:35-50,
   Mar., 1969.
"A study of employee attitudes toward patients in a hos-
   pital for the treatment of drug addiction," by Levitt,
   L.I., et al. PSYCHIATRIC QUARTERLY. 37(2):210-219, 1963.
"Successful treatment of a case of drinamyl addiction," by
   Kraft, T. BRITISH JOURNAL OF PSYCHIATRY. 114(516):
   1363-1364, 1968.
"Suicide and mortality amongst heroin addicts in Britain,"
   by Pierce, J.I. BRITISH JOURNAL OF ADDICTION. 62:391-
   398, Dec., 1967.
"Suicide in the United States." BULLETIN ON NARCOTICS.
   20(2):56, Apr.-June, 1968.
"A survey of drug use at Ithaca College," by Rand, M.E.,
   et al. JOURNAL OF THE COLLEGE HEALTH ASSOCIATION. 17:
   43-51, Oct., 1968.
"A survey of procurers in Israel, 1961-1963," by Horowitz,
   M. THE ISRAEL ANNALS OF PSYCHIATRY. 4(2):219-227, Aut-
   umn, 1966.
"Symposium -- non-narcotic addiction. Size and extent of
   the problem," by Sadusk, J.R., and Joseph, F. JOURNAL
   OF THE AMERICAN MEDICAL ASSOCIATION. 196:707-709, 1966.
"Synanon and eupsychia," by Maslow, A.H." JOURNAL OF HU-
   MANISTIC PSYCHOLOGY. 7(1):28-35, 1967.
"Synanon and the learning process: a critique of attack
   therapy," by Walder, E. CORRECTIVE PSYCHIATRY AND JOUR-
   NAL OF SOCIAL THERAPY. 11(6):299-304, 1965.
"Synanon foundation: a radical approach to the problem of
   addiction," by Cherkas, M. AMERICAN JOURNAL OF PSYCHI-
   ATRY. 121(11):1065-1068, 1965.
"Synanon House where drug addicts join to salvage their
   lives." LIFE. 52:52-65, Mar. 9, 1962.
"Systemic infections in heroin addicts." BULLETIN ON NAR-
   COTICS. 20(4):2, Oct.-Dec., 1968.
"Systemic infections in heroin addicts," by Beckett, H.D.
   LANCET. 1:48, Jan. 6, 1968.
"Systemic infections in heroin addicts," by Cherubin, C.E.,

et al. LANCET. 1:298-299, Feb. 10, 1968.
"Systemic infections in heroin addicts," by Willis, J.
LANCET. 1:361, Feb. 17, 1968.
"Talking about addiction." LANCET. 2:672, Sept. 21, 1968.
"Task force looks at drug abuse," by Shipp, B., and Hurt, B.
ATLANTA CONSTITUTION. Sept. 20, 1965.
"A technique for self-injection of drugs in the study of
reinforcement," by Davis, W.M., and Nichols, J.R. JOUR-
NAL OF EXPERIMENTAL ANALYSIS OF BEHAVIOR. 6(2):233-235,
1963.
"Teen-age drinking and drug addiction," by Pollack, J.H.
NEA JOURNAL. 55:8-12, May, 1966.
"Teenager and drug abuse," by Johnson, F.K., and Westman,
J.C. JOURNAL OF SCHOOL HEALTH. 38:645-654, Dec., 1968.
"Teen-agers and the dope hazard," by Millet, G.H. PARENTS
MAGAZINE. 39:46-47+, May, 1964.
"Teen-agers and the use of drugs: reflections on the emo-
tional setting," by Pollard, J.C. CLINICAL PEDIATRICS.
6:613-620, Nov., 1967.
"Tendency systems and the effects of a movie dealing with
a social problem," by Winick, C. JOURNAL OF GENERAL
PSYCHOLOGY. 68:298-305, 1963.
"Tests for addiction (chronic intoxication) of morphine
type," by Halbach, H., and Eddy, N.B. BULLETIN OF THE
WORLD HEALTH ORGANIZATION. 28:139-173, 1963.
"Therapist bias and student use of illegal drugs," by Wal-
ters, P.A. JOURNAL OF THE AMERICAN COLLEGE HEALTH ASSOC-
IATION. 16:30-34, Oct., 1967.
"There's no hiding place down there," by Janowitz, J.F.
AMERICAN JOURNAL OF ORTHOPSYCHIATRY. 37:296, Mar., 1967.
"Thoughts on narcotics addiction," by Dole, V.P. BULLETIN
OF THE NEW YORK ACADEMY OF MEDICINE. 41(2):211-213, 1965.
"The thrill-pill menace," by Davidson, B. SATURDAY EVENING
POST. 24:23 passim, 1965.
"The thrill seekers," by Leighton, F.S. THIS WEEK MAGAZINE.
pp. 4-7, Aug. 22, 1965.
"Time for decision on narcotics addiction,' by Javits, J.K.
COMPREHENSIVE PSYCHIATRY. 4:137-139, 1963.
"To drug or not to drug; Britain." NATIONAL REVIEW. 20:
536, June 4, 1968.
"Today's drug addicts." SCIENCE NEWS LETTER. 89:432,
June 4, 1966.
"Toughness to the task; Federal Bureau of Narcotics and
The Bureau of Drug Abuse Control combined." NEW REPUB-
LIC. 159:10-11, Nov. 2, 1968.
"Treating young drug users: a casework approach," by Fra-
zier, T.L. SOCIAL WORK. 7:94-101, July, 1962.
"Treatment of alcoholics and drug addicts by verbal aver-
sion technique," by Anant, S.S. PSYCHOTHERAPY AND PSY-
CHOSOMATICS. 15(1):6, 1967.
"The treatment of drug addiction," by Vogel, V.H. JOURNAL
OF THE AMERICAN MEDICAL ASSOCIATION. 194(6):680-681,
1965.
"Treatment of drug addiction in a community general hospi-

tal," by Freedman, A.M. COMPREHENSIVE PSYCHIATRY. 4(3):199-207, 1963.

"The treatment of drug addiction: private practice experience with 84 addicts," by Pearson, M.M., and Little, R.B. AMERICAN JOURNAL OF PSYCHIATRY. 122:164-169, 1965.

"The treatment of drug addicts in Switzerland," by Kielholz, P., and Battegay, R. COMPREHENSIVE PSYCHIATRY. 4(3):225-235, 1963.

"The treatment of hard-core voluntary drug addict patients," by Sabath, G. INTERNATIONAL JOURNAL OF GROUP PSYCHOTHERAPY. 14(3):307-317, 1964.

"Treatment of narcotic addicts." by Cameron, D.C. TODAY'S HEALTH. 41:12+, Oct., 1963.

"The truth about drug addiction," by Kane, J.J. U.S. CATHOLIC. 31:11-16, 1966.

"Turned-on way of life." NEWSWEEK. p. 72, Nov. 28, 1966.

"Twenty years of drug addiction," by Oltman, J.E., and Friedman, S. DISEASES OF THE NERVOUS SYSTEM. 25(2):90-96, 1964.

"Two cases of addiction to heroin by smoking," by Bartholomew, A.A., and Bruce, D.W. MEDICINE, SCIENCE AND THE LAW. 4(2):108-111, 1964.

"Two patterns of narcotic addiction in the United States," by Ball, J.C. JOURNAL OF CRIMINAL LAW, CRIMINOLOGY AND POLICE SCIENCE. 56(2):203-211, June, 1965.

"Two types of drug use," by Rubington, Earl. INTERNATIONAL JOURNAL OF THE ADDICTIONS. 3:301-318, Spring, 1968.

"Uncharted terrain," by Sanders, M.K. HARPERS. 235:42, July, 1967.

"Underground, the lost and the lonely play the glue game." LIFE. 67:44, Sept. 5, 1969.

"Untouchables." TIME. 80:20-21, 1962.

"Use and abuse of drugs," by Rapp, M.S. CANADIAN MEDICAL ASSOCIATION JOURNAL. 98:922, May 11, 1968.

"The use and abuse of mixtures of active drugs. Requirements of modern drug therapy," by Starr, I. JOURNAL OF THE AMERICAN MEDICAL ASSOCIATION. 181(2):106-110, 1962.

"Use computer to spot repeat buyer of exempts, New Jersey pharmaceutical association urges." AMERICAN DRUGGIST. 155:26, Feb. 27, 1967.

"The use of barbiturates by heroin addicts," by Cumberlidge, M.C. CANADIAN MEDICAL ASSOCIATION JOURNAL. 98:1045-1049, June 1, 1968.

"Use of drugs by jazz musicians," by Winick, C. SOCIAL PROBLEMS. 7:240-253, 1960.

"The use of drugs by teenagers for sanctuary and illusion," by Levy, N.J. AMERICAN JOURNAL OF PSYCHOANALYSIS. 28 (1):48-58, 1968.

"The use of drugs in the management of drug dependence," by Eddy, N.B. JOURNAL OF THE TENNESSEE MEDICAL ASSOCIATION. 60:269-273, 1967.

"Vague and nebulous life of a heroin addict," by Wansell, G. TIMES (London) EDUCATIONAL SUPPLEMENT. 2763:1470, May 3, 1968.

"Varieties of drug experience." TRANS-ACTION. 5:5-6, Oct., 1968.

"Victorian oblivion," by Pearsall, R. ADDICTIONS. 12:20-23, 1965.

"Viewpoints on addiction: the narcotics user as seen by the physician, law enforcer, legislator, sociologist, psychiatrist." JOURNAL OF THE AMERICAN MEDICAL ASSOCIATION. 184(10):30-37, 1964.

"The village beat scene," by Polsky, N. DISSENT. 8:3-23, 1961.

"Wages of addiction." LANCET. 2:818, Oct. 14, 1967.

"Waging a war on drug abuse." BUSINESS WEEK. pp. 106-107, Jan. 20, 1968.

"The waltzing or skating sign," by Arieff, A.J., et al. TRANSACTIONS OF THE AMERICAN NEUROLOGICAL ASSOCIATION. 90:222, 1965.

"Warning on drugs; London secondary schools. TIMES (London) EDUCATIONAL SUPPLEMENT. 2711:1514, May 5, 1967.

"Was Plotinus influenced by opium?" by Jevons, F.R. MEDICAL HISTORY. 9:374-380, 1965.

"What makes teens try dope?" by Bloomquist, E.R. PARENTS MAGAZINE. 35:42-44+, Feb., 1960.

"What the surgeon should know about the narcotic addict," by Felder, M.E. AMERICAN JOURNAL OF SURGERY. 104:560-563, 1962.

"What you should know about the drug problem: interview with J.L. Goddard. SCHOOL MANAGEMENT. 10:96-99, June, 1966.

"What's happening?" by Honn, F.R. JOURNAL OF SECONDARY EDUCATION. 42:45-48, Jan., 1967.

"Where we stand on drug abuse," by California Medical Association. BULLETIN OF THE LOS ANGELES MEDICAL ASSOCIATION. 97:20-22, 1967.

"White-collar pill party," by Jackson, B. ATLANTIC MONTHLY. 218:35-40, Aug., 1966.

"Who is vulnerable?" by Glatt, M. MENTAL HEALTH. 25(3):26-28, 1966.

"Why addicts relapse." SCIENCE NEWS. 93:425-426, May 4, 1968.

"Why adolescents drink and use drugs; with study-discussion guide," by Smallenburg, C., et al. PTA MAGAZINE. 63:2-5 passim, Mar., 1969.

"Why compulsory closed-ward treatment of narcotic addicts?" by Ausubel, D.P. ILLINOIS MEDICAL JOURNAL. 130:474-485, 1966; also PSYCHIATRIC QUARTERLY SUPPLEMENT. 40(2):225-243, 1966.

"Why kids take drugs." SCIENCE DIGEST. 63:69-70, June, 1968.

"Why students turn to drugs." READER'S DIGEST. 92:173-174 passim, Apr., 1968.

"Why students use drugs," by Nowlis, H.H. AMERICAN JOURNAL OF NURSING. 68(8):1680-1685, Aug., 1968.

"Wikler offers 'two factors' theory to explain relapse in addiction." NAPAN NEWSLETTER. 1(7):2-3, 1963

"William Burroughs and the literature of addiction," by
McConnell, F.D. MASSACHUSETTS REVIEW. 8:665-680, Aut-
umn, 1967.
"Withdrawal from drugs." SCIENCE NEWS LETTER. 84:4, July
6, 1963.
"The wives of drug addicts," by Taylor, S.D., et al. AMER-
ICAN JOURNAL OF PSYCHIATRY. 123:585-591, 1966.
"The world of the righteous dope fiend," by Sutter, A.G.
ISSUES IN CRIMINOLOGY. 2:177-222, Fall, 1966.
"You can't even step in the same river once," by Lettvin, J.
NATURAL HISTORY. 76:6-12 passim, Oct., 1967.
"You cannot be a drug addict without really trying," by
Casselman, B.W. DISEASES OF THE NERVOUS SYSTEM. 25:
161-163, 1964.
"Young addicts." NEWSWEEK. 59:78, Jan. 22, 1962.
"Young drug addict: can we help him?" by Larner, J. ATLAN-
TIC MONTHLY. 215:75-80, Feb., 1965.
"Young drug addicts: addiction and its consequences," by
Rosenberg, C.M. MEDICAL JOURNAL OF AUSTRALIA. 1(26):
1031-1033, 1968.
"Your adolescent's health; drug abuse among teenagers," by
Sauer, L.W. PTA MAGAZINE. 63:25-26, Feb., 1969.
"Youth and drug abuse," by De-Boskey, R. CLINICAL TOXICOL-
OGY. 1:187-193.
"Youth and the drug problem," by Nowlis, H.H. NEW YORK
STATE EDUCATION. 56:10-13+, Dec., 1968.
"Youth: the voice of prophecy," by Leary, J.P. AMERICA.
121:190-192, Sept. 20, 1969.
"Zombie and son," by Brien, A. NEW STATESMAN. 73:291,
Mar. 3, 1967.

NARCOTIC ADDICTION: Periodical Literature

Scientific Publications

"Abnormal emotional reactions to hospitalization jeopardiz-
ing medical treatment," by Freemon, F.R., et al. PSYCHO-
SOMATICS. 8:150-155, May-June, 1967.
"Absence of anemia in hepatitis due to heroin addiction.
Evidence for tendency to erythrocytosis among heroin ad-
dicts," by Schoenfeld, M.R., and Samala, R. JOURNAL
OF NEW DRUGS. 6(3):149-152, 1966.
"Acute myeloblastic leukemia in a benzedrine addict," by
Berry, J.N. SOUTHERN MEDICAL JOURNAL. 59:1169-1170,
Oct., 1966.
"The adjustment of drug addicts as measured by the sentence
completion test," by Gardner, J.M. JOURNAL OF PROJECTIVE
TECHNIQUES AND PERSONALITY ASSESSMENT. 31(3):28-29, 1967.
"Alcoholism and reliance upon drugs as depressive equiva-

lents," by Fox, R. AMERICAN JOURNAL OF PSYCHOTHERAPY.
21(3):585-596, 1967.
"Amiphenazole in the treatment of morphine and opium addiction," by Bruce, D.W. LANCET. 7341:1010-1012, 1964.
"Angiothrombotic pulmonary hypertension in addicts. 'Blue
Velvet' addiction," by Wendt, V.E., et al. JOURNAL OF
THE AMERICAN MEDICAL ASSOCIATION. 188(8):755-757, 1964.
"An approach to testing narcotic addicts based on community
mental health diagnosis," by Brotman, R., et al. COMPRE-
HENSIVE PSYCHIATRY. 6(2):104-118, 1965.
"Assessing subjective effects of drugs: an index of care-
lessness and confusion for use with the Addiction Re-
search Center Inventory (ARCI)," by Haertzen, C.A., and
Hill, H.E. JOURNAL OF CLINICAL PSYCHOLOGY. 19(4):
407-412, 1963.
"An assessment of inhalation as a mode of administration
of heroin by addicts," by Mo, B.P., and Way, E.L. JOUR-
NAL OF PHARMACOLOGY AND EXPERIMENTAL THERAPEUTICS. 154
(1):142-151, 1966.
"Asymptomatic pulmonary atelectasis in drug addicts," by
Gelfand, M.L., et al. DISEASES OF THE CHEST. 52:782-
787, Dec., 1967.
"'Bad habits' and social deviation: a proposed revision in
conflict theory," by Austin, A.W. JOURNAL OF CLINICAL
PSYCHOLOGY. 18(2):227-231, 1962.
"Biochemical aspects of drug addiction," by Knox, S.C.
BULLETIN OF THE LOS ANGELES NEUROLOGICAL SOCIETY. 28:
165-166, 1963.
"Biochemical aspects of psychotomimetic drug addiction,"
by Giarman, N.J., et al. PHARMACOLOGICAL REVIEWS. 17:
1, 1965.
"Blood rheology: effect of fibrinogen deduced by addiction,"
by Merrill, E.W., et al. CIRCULATION RESEARCH. 18:
437-446, 1966.
"Cardiac valve replacement for the narcotic addict," by
Carey, J.S., et al. JOURNAL OF THORACIC AND CARDIOVAS-
CULAR SURGERY. 53:663-667, May, 1967.
"The case of the tremulous man, addiction to sedatives and
hypnotics," by Storrow, H.A. JOURNAL OF THE KENTUCKY
STATE MEDICAL ASSOCIATION. 63:112-113, 1965.
"Changes in correlation between responses to items of the
Addiction Research Center Inventory produced by LSD-25,"
by Haertzen, C.A. JOURNAL OF PSYCHOPHARMACOLOGY. 1(1):
27-36, 1966.
"Character problems and their relationship to drug abuse,"
by Sharoff, R.L. AMERICAN JOURNAL OF PSYCHOANALYSIS.
29(2):186-193, 1969.
"Characteristics and sequelae of paregoric abuse," by Lerner, A.M., et al. ANNALS OF INTERNAL MEDICINE. 65:
1019-1030, Nov., 1966.
"Characteristics of drug abusers admitted to a psychiatric
hospital," by Hekimian, L.J., and Gershon, S. JOURNAL
OF THE AMERICAN MEDICAL ASSOCIATION. 205(3):125-130,
1968.

"The chemopharmacological approach to the addiction problem," by Eddy, N.B. PUBLIC HEALTH REPORTS. 78:673-680, 1963.

"Chronic liver disease in narcotics addicts," by Kaplan, K. AMERICAN JOURNAL OF DIGESTIVE DISEASES. 8:402-410, 1963.

"Chronic pulmonary disease in a morphine addict. A clinicopathologic conference." PENNAYLVANIA MEDICAL JOURNAL. 69:45-49, 1966.

"Classical conditioning of a morphine abstinence phenomenon, reinforcement of opioid-drinking behavior and 'relapse' in morphine-addicted rats," by Wikler, A., and Pescor, F.T. PSYCHOPHARMACOLOGIA. 10(3):255-284, 1967.

"Clinical and psychological observation on narcotic drug addiction," by Mason, P. ISRAEL MEDICAL JOURNAL. 19:19-26, 1960.

"The clinical aspects of drug addiction," by Partridge, M. PROCEEDINGS OF THE ROYAL SOCIETY OF MEDICINE. 53:919-921, 1960.

"Clinical experiences with hypnosis in psychiatric treatment," by Alexander, L. INTERNATIONAL JOURNAL OF NEURO-PSYCHIATRY. 3:118-124, 1967.

"Clinical severity of tetanus in narcotic addicts in New York City," by Cherubin, C.E. ARCHIVES OF INTERNAL MEDICINE (Chicago). 121:156-158, Feb., 1968.

"Clinical studies on the pathogenesis and personality structure of the male narcotic addicts," by Easton, K. JOURNAL OF THE HILLSIDE HOSPITAL. 14(1-2):36-53, Jan., 1965.

"Colonic fecal impaction in a young drug addict," by Fetterman, L.E. JOURNAL OF THE AMERICAN MEDICAL ASSOCIATION. 202:1056, Dec. 11, 1967.

"Comments on the character structure and psychodynamic processes of heroin addicts," by Torda, C. PERCEPTUAL AND MOTOR SKILLS. 27(1):143-146, 1968.

"A comparison between acute and chronic physical dependence in the chronic spinal dog," by Martin, W.R., and Eades, C.G. JOURNAL OF PHARMACOLOGY AND EXPERIMENTAL THERAPEUTICS. 146(3):385-394, 1964.

"A comparison of the intellectual performance of the juvenile addict with standardization norms," by Laskowitz, D. JOURNAL OF CORRECTIONAL EDUCATION. 14:31-32, 1962.

"Compliance and improvement in drug-treated and placebo-treated neurotic outpatients," by Rickels, K., and Downing, R. ARCHIVES OF GENERAL PSYCHIATRY. 14(6):631-633, 1966.

"Conditioned inhibition of craving in drug addiction: a pilot experiment," by Wolpe, J. BEHAVIOR RESEARCH AND THERAPY. 2:285-288, 1965.

"Conditioning processes in opiate addiction and relapse," by Wikler, A. JOURNAL OF THE HILLSIDE HOSPITAL. 16(2):141-149, 1967.

"'Consciousness-limiting' side effects of 'consciousness-expanding' drugs," by Mamlet, L.N. AMERICAN JOURNAL OF ORTHOPSYCHIATRY. 37:296-297, Mar., 1967.

"Crucial factors in the treatment of narcotic addiction,"
by Freedman, A.M., and Sharoff, R.L. AMERICAN JOURNAL
OF PSYCHOTHERAPY. 19(3):397-407, 1965.
"Cyclazocine and methadone in narcotic addiction," by Freedman, A.M., et al. JOURNAL OF THE AMERICAN MEDICAL ASSOC-
IATION. 202(3):191-194, 1967.
"Cyclazocine in the treatment of narcotic addiction," by
Jaffe, J.H. CURRENT PSYCHIATRIC THERAPIES. 7:147-156,
1967.
"Dermatologic complications of heroin addiction," by Min-
kin, W., et al. NEW ENGLAND JOURNAL OF MEDICINE. 277:
473-475, Aug. 31, 1967.
"Description of psychologic, demographic, addiction history,
and treatment related variables employed in the screen-
ing of addict patients," by Monroe, J.J., et al. EXPER-
IMENTAL TEST MANUAL, UNITED STATES PUBLIC HEALTH SERVICE
HOSPITAL, 1963.
"Despair, trifluoperazine, exercise, and temperature of
108 degrees F.," by Shapiro, M.F. AMERICAN JOURNAL OF
PSYCHIATRY. 124:705-707, Nov., 1967.
"Differential responses of addicts and nonaddicts on the
MMPI," by Lombardi, D.N., et al. JOURNAL OF PROJECTIVE
TECHNIQUES AND PERSONALITY ASSESSMENT. 32(5):479-482,
1968.
"Diffuse myopathy related to meperidine addiction in a mo-
ther and daughter," by Aberfeld, D.C., et al. ARCHIVES
OF NEUROLOGY. 19:384-389, Oct., 1968.
"Diseases of therapeutic origin; analytical study," by Pe-
quignot, H. CONCOURS MEDICAL. 85:6027-6032, 1963.
"Drug addiction and gynecomastia," by Camiel, M.R., et al.
NEW YORK JOURNAL OF MEDICINE. 67:2494-2495, Sept. 15,
1967.
"Drug addiction and habit formation: an attempted integra-
tion," by Walton, D. JOURNAL OF MENTAL SCIENCE. 106:
1195-1229, 1960.
"Drug addiction and habituation," by Rettersol, N., and
Sund, A. ACTA PSYCHIATRICA SCANDINAVICA. 40(suppl.
179):120, 1964.
"Drug addiction and logic," by Hoffman, F. JOURNAL OF THE
AMERICAN MEDICAL ASSOCIATION. 201:491-492, Aug. 7, 1967.
"Drug addiction, pharmacological aspects of addiction to
morphine and other drugs," by Wilson, C.W.M. PROCEED-
INGS OF THE ROYAL SOCIETY OF MEDICINE. 58(6):405-409,
1965.
"Drug dependence as a criterion for differentiation of
psychotropic drugs," by Battegay, R. COMPREHENSIVE PSY-
CHIATRY. 7:501-509, 1966.
"Drug dependence: important considerations from the anes-
thesiologist's viewpoint," by Adriana, J., et al. ANES-
THESIA AND ANALGESIA; CURRENT RESEARCH. 47:472-482,
Sept.-Oct., 1968.
"Drug dependence: its significance and characteristics,"
by Eddy, N.B., et al. PSYCHOPHARMACOLOGY BULLETIN; NA-
TIONAL CLEARINGHOUSE FOR MENTAL HEALTH INFORMATION. 3:

1-12, July, 1966; also BULLETIN OF THE WORLD HEALTH OR-
GANIZATION. 32:721-733, 1965.
"Drug dependence of the morphine type and the evolution of
totally synthetic morphine-like analgesics," by May,
E.L. JOURNAL OF THE WASHINGTON ACADEMY OF SCIENCES.
57(3):53-60, 1967.
"Drug use: symptom, disease or adolescent experimentation -
the task of therapy," by Liebert, R.S. JOURNAL OF THE
AMERICAN COLLEGE HEALTH ASSOCIATION. 16:25-29, Oct.,
1967.
"Drug withdrawal and fighting in rats," by Florea, J., and
Thor, D.H. PSYCHONOMIC SCIENCE. 12(1):33, 1968.
"Drug-withdrawal psychoses," by James, I.P. AMERICAN JOUR-
NAL OF PSYCHIATRY. 119:880-881, 1963.
"Drugs and doctors. Problem in the production of certain
behavioral disorders," by Hagedorn, A.B., and Steinbil-
der, R.M. MINNESOTA MEDICINE. 50:1187-1189, 1967.
"Effect of a cycle of addiction to intravenous heroin on
certain physiological measurements," by Fraser, H.F.,
et al. BULLETIN ON NARCOTICS. 16:17-23, July-Sept.,
1964.
"The effect of age on four scales of the California Psy-
chological Inventory," by Grupp, S., et al. JOURNAL
OF GENERAL PSYCHOLOGY. 78(2):183-187, 1968.
"The effect of the addition of a narcotic antagonist on
the rate of development of tolerance and physical de-
pendence to morphine," by Eddy, N.B., et al. BULLETIN
ON NARCOTICS. 12(4):1-16, Oct.-Dec., 1960.
"Electro-clinical study of a case of addiction to merinax,"
by Utrilla-Robles, M. ELECTROENCEPHALOGRAPHY AND CLIN-
ICAL NEUROPHYSIOLOGY. 22:391, Apr., 1967.
"The epidemiologic aspects of tetanus in narcotic addicts
in New York City," by Cherubin, C.E. ARCHIVES OF EN-
VIRONMENTAL HEALTH. 14(6):802-808, 1967.
"Epidemiologic factors in drug addiction in England and the
United States," by Larimore, G.W., and Brill, H. PUB-
LIC HEALTH REPORTS. 77:555-560, 1962.
"Evaluation of dependence-producing drugs: report of a WHO
scientific group." WORLD HEALTH ORGANIZATION TECHNICAL
REPORT SERIES. 287:1-25, 1964.
"Evaluation of narcotics treatment programs," by Dole, V.P.,
and Warner, A. AMERICAN JOURNAL OF PUBLIC HEALTH AND
THE NATION'S HEALTH. 57:2000-2005, 1967.
"Evaluation of the nalorphine pupil diagnostic test for
narcotic usage in long-term heroin and opium addicts,"
by Way, E.L., et al. CLINICAL PHARMACOLOGY AND THERA-
PEUTICS. 7(3):311, May-June, 1966.
"Evolution of group therapy policies with hospitalized
drug addicts in the narcotic unit at Central Islip State
Hospital," by Brett, S.R., and Villeneuve, A. PSYCHI-
ATRIC QUARTERLY. 37:666-670, 1963.
"The existential approach to the management of character
disorders with special reference to narcotic drug addiction," by Ramirez, E. REVIEW OF EXISTENTIAL PSYCHOLOGY

AND PSYCHIATRY. 8(1):43-53, 1968.
"Experiences from an outpatient department for drug addicts in Goteborg," by Holmberg, Maj. B., and Jannson, B. ACTA PSYCHIATRICA SCANDINAVICA. 44(2):172-189, 1968.
"Experimental morphine addiction: method for automatic intravenous injections in unrestrained rats," by Weeks, J.R. SCIENCE. 138(whole no. 3537), 1962.
"Experimental narcotic addiction," by Weeks, J.R. SCIENTIFIC AMERICAN. 210:46-52, Mar., 1964.
"Experimental production of human 'blue velvet' and 'red devil' lesions," by Puro, H.E., et al. JOURNAL OF THE AMERICAN MEDICAL ASSOCIATION. 197:1100-1102, Sept. 26, 1966.
"An exploratory examination of the social and psychological characteristics of 100 Pennsylvania drug addicts," by Royfe, E.H. PENNSYLVANIA PSYCHIATRIC QUARTERLY. 5(4): 38-47, 1966.
"Extension of psychopathic deviancy scales for the screening of addict patients," by Monroe, J.J., et al. EDUCATIONAL AND PSYCHOLOGICAL MEASUREMENT. 24:47-56, Spring, 1964.
"A factorial study of sexuality in adult males," by Thorne, F.C. JOURNAL OF CLINICAL PSYCHOLOGY. 22:378-386, Oct., 1966.
"Fighting narcotic bondage and other forms of narcotic disorders," by Rado, S. COMPREHENSIVE PSYCHIATRY. 4(3): 160-167, 1963.
"Follow-up of criminal narcotic addicts," by Richman, A. CANADIAN PSYCHIATRIC ASSOCIATION JOURNAL. 11:107-115, Apr., 1966.
"A follow-up of narcotic addicts. Mortality, relapse and abstinence," by O'Donnell, J.A. AMERICAN JOURNAL OF ORTHOPSYCHIATRY. 34(5):948-954, 1964.
"Follow-up of narcotic drug addicts after hospitalization," by Hunt, G.H., and Odoroff, M.E. PUBLIC HEALTH REPORTS. 77:41-54, 1962.
"Follow-up studies on previously hospitalized narcotic addicts," by Lieberman, D. AMERICAN JOURNAL OF ORTHOPSYCHIATRY. 35:601-604, 1965.
"Follow-up study of narcotic drug addicts five years after hospitalization," by Duvall, H.J., et al. PUBLIC HEALTH REPORTS. 78(3):185-194, Mar., 1963.
"A general theory of the genesis of drug dependence by induction of receptors," by Collier, H.O. NATURE. 205: 181-182, 1965.
"Group hypnotherapy techniques with drug addicts," by Ludwig, A.M., et al. INTERNATIONAL JOURNAL OF CLINICAL AND EXPERIMENTAL HYPNOSIS. 12(2):53-66, 1964.
"A gynecologic study of drug addicts," by Stoffer, S.S. AMERICAN JOURNAL OF OBSTETRICS AND GYNECOLOGY. 101: 779-783, July 15, 1968.
"Hepatic dysfunction in heroin and cocaine users," by Marks, V., et al. BRITISH JOURNAL OF ADDICTION. 62:189-195, Mar., 1967.

159

"Hepatic inflammation in narcotic addicts," by Norris, R.F. ARCHIVES OF ENVIRONMENTAL HEALTH. 11:622, 1965.
"Hepatic inflammation in narcotic addicts. Viral hepatitus a possible cause," by Norris, R.F., and Potter, H.P., Jr. ARCHIVES OF ENVIRONMENTAL HEALTH. 11(5):662-668, 1965.
"Hypotension during anesthesia in narcotic addicts." NEW YORK STATE JOURNAL OF MEDICINE. 66:2685-2686, Oct. 15, 1966.
"The imagery of visual hallucinations," by Horowitz, M.J. JOURNAL OF NERVOUS AND MENTAL DISEASE. 138(6):513-523, 1964.
"Inducing a preference for morphine in rats without premedication," by Kuman, R., et al. NATURE. 218(5141):564-565, 1968.
"Infections in paregoric addicts," by Oerther, F.J. et al. THE JOURNAL OF THE AMERICAN MEDICAL ASSOCIATION. 190(7):683-686, 1964.
"Inhalation psychosis and related states. A review," by Glaser, F.B. ARCHIVES OF GENERAL PSYCHIATRY. 14(3):315-322, 1966.
"Interaction testing: an engaged couple of drug addicts tested separately and together," by Kaldegg, A. JOURNAL OF PROJECTIVE TECHNIQUES AND PERSONALITY ASSESSMENT. 30:77-87, Feb., 1966.
"Irreversible effects of Glutethimide addiction," by Lingl, F.A. AMERICAN JOURNAL OF PSYCHIATRY. 123:349-351, Sept., 1966.
"Laboratory investigation of drug addiction," by Marks, V. BRITISH JOURNAL OF ADDICTION. 61:291-294, Aug., 1966.
"Liver function tests in morphine-addicted and in nonaddicted rhesus monkeys," by Brooks, F.P., et al. GASTROENTEROLOGY. 44:287-290, 1963.
"Liver lesions in narcotic addicts." JOURNAL OF THE AMERICAN MEDICAL ASSOCIATION. 194:158-159, 1965.
"An MMPI factor analytic study of alcoholics, narcotic addicts, and criminals," by Hill, H.E., et al. QUARTERLY JOURNAL OF STUDIES ON ALCOHOL. 23:411-431, 1962.
"MMPI sex differences in narcotic addicts," by Olson, R.W. JOURNAL OF GENETIC PSYCHOLOGY. 71(2):257-266, 1964.
"The major medical complications of heroin addiction," by Louria, D.B., et al. ANNALS OF INTERNAL MEDICINE. 67:1-22, July, 1967.
"Management of narcotic-drug dependence by high-dosage methadone HCl technique; Dole-Nyswander program." JOURNAL OF THE AMERICAN MEDICAL ASSOCIATION. 201:956-957, Sept. 18, 1967.
"Management of the narcotic withdrawal syndrome in the neonate," by Hill, R.M., and Desmond, M.M. PEDIATRIC CLINICS OF NORTH AMERICA. 10:67-86, 1963.
"The management of pathologic interdependency in drug addiction," by Little, R.B., and Pearson, M.M. AMERICAN JOURNAL OF PSYCHIATRY. 123(5):554-560, 1966.
"Mania associated with the use of I.N.H. and cocaine," by Kane, F.J., and Taylor, T.W. AMERICAN JOURNAL OF PSY-

CHIATRY. 119:1098-1099, 1963.
"Medical correlation clinics, 12: drug addiction," by
Schmidt, C.R., et al. AMERICAN PRACTITIONER. 12:863-877, 1961.
"The medical sequelae of narcotic addiction," by Cherubin,
C.E. ANNALS OF INTERNAL MEDICINE. 67:23-33, July, 1967.
"Medical testimony in a schizophrenia and heroin addiction
case, showing the direct examination of the chemist, and
direct and cross-examination of the psychiatrists."
MEDICAL TRIAL TECHNIQUE QUARTERLY. 10:89-116, 1964.
"A medical treatment of diacetylmorphine (heroin) addiction.
A clinical trial with methadone hydrochloride," by Dole,
V.P., and Nyswander, M. JOURNAL OF THE AMERICAN MEDICAL
ASSOCIATION. 193(8):646-650, 1965.
"Menstrual abnormalities associated with heroin addiction,"
By Gauldin, E.C., et al. AMERICAN JOURNAL OF OBSTETRICS
AND GYNECOLOGY. 90:155-160, 1964.
"Mental illness due to the voluntary inhalation of petrol
vapour," by Black, P.D. MEDICAL JOURNAL OF AUSTRALIA.
2:70-71, July 8, 1967.
"Methaqualone addiction and delirium tremens," by Ewart,
R.B., et al. BRITISH MEDICAL JOURNAL. 3:92-93, July 8,
1967.
"Methods for assessing the addiction liability of opioids
and opioid antagonists in man," by Fraser, H. RESEARCH
PUBLICATIONS ASSOCIATION FOR RESEARCH IN NERVOUS AND
MENTAL DISEASE. 46:176-187, 1968.
"The mind-altering drug ('M.A.D.') world: the social and
public health perspective," by Fort, J. AMERICAN JOUR-
NAL OF ORTHOPSYCHIATRY. 37(2):338-339, 1967.
"Morbidity and mortality from heroin dependence: study of
100 consecutive inpatients," by Bewley, T.H., and Ben-
Arie, O. BRITISH MEDICAL JOURNAL. 1(5594):727-730, 1968.
"Morbidity and mortality from heroin dependence: survey of
heroin addicts known to home office," by Bewley, T.H.,
et al. BRITISH MEDICAL JOURNAL. 1(5594):725-726, 1968.
"Morbidity and mortality from heroin dependence: relation
of hepatitis to self-injection techniques," by Bewley,
T.H., et al. BRITISH MEDICAL JOURNAL. 1:730-732, Mar.
23, 1968.
"Narcotic addiction and BFP reactions in tests for syphilis,"
by Harris, A., et al. PUBLIC HEALTH REPORTS. 77:537-543, 1962.
"Narcotic addiction and cervical carcinoma," by Weaver,
J.M., et al. ACTA CYTOLOGICA. 10:154-155, May-June,
1966.
"Narcotic addiction - the neglect of research," by Blachly,
P.H. SCIENCE. 144:135-136, 1964.
"Narcotic antagonists in the detection of narcotic use,"
by Elliott, H.W., and Way, E.L. PROCEEDINGS OF THE WEST-
ERN PHARMACOLOGY SOCIETY. 4:42-43, 1961.
"Narcotic blockade - a medical technique for stopping her-
oin use by addicts," by Dole, V.P., et al. TRANSACTIONS
OF THE ASSOCIATION OF AMERICAN PHYSICIANS. 79:112-136,
1966.

"Narcotic drug addiction: one year's experience at Pilgrim state hospital," by Rice, J., and Cohen, L. PSYCHIATRIC QUARTERLY. 39(3):457-465, 1965.

"Narcotic septal perforations due to drug addiction," by Messinger, E. JOURNAL OF THE AMERICAN MEDICAL ASSOCIA-TION. 179:964-965, 1962.

"Narcotic usage. I. A spectrum of a difficult medical problem," by Zinberg, N.E., and Lewis, D.C. NEW ENGLAND JOURNAL OF MEDICINE. 270(19):989-993, 1964.

"Narcotic usage. II. A historical perspective on a difficult medical problem," by Lewis, D.C., and Zinberg, N.E. NEW ENGLAND JOURNAL OF MEDICINE. 270(20):1045-1050, 1964.

"Narcotic withdrawal reaction in a newborn infant due to codeine," by Van Leeuwen, G., et al. PEDIATRICS. 36 (4):635-636, 1965.

"Narcotic withdrawal syndrome. Suppression of by means of electric convulsive therapy," by Kelman, H. MINNESOTA MEDICINE. 47:525-527, 1964.

"A new test for morphine-like physical dependence (addiction liability) in rats," by Buckett, W.R. PSYCHOPHAR-MACOLOGIA. 6(6):410-416, 1964.

"Newborn narcotic withdrawal associated with regional enteritis in pregnancy," by Henley, W.L., and Fisch, G.R. NEW YORK STATE JOURNAL OF MEDICINE. 66(19):2565-2567, 1966.

"Nicotinamide metabolism in schizophrenics, drug addicts, and normals: the effect of psychotropic drugs and hormones," by Heyman, J.J. TRANSACTIONS OF THE NEW YORK ACADEMY OF SCIENCES. 26(3):354-360, 1964.

"Observations in the Haight-Ashbury medical clinic of San Francisco: health problems in a 'hippie' subculture," by Smith, D., and Rose, A. CLINICAL PEDIATRICS. 7:313-316, 1968.

"Observations on euphomania in general practice," by Wiingaard, P. MAANEDSSKRIFT FOR PRAKTISK LAEGEGERNING OG SOCIAL MEDICIN. 41:402-405, 1963.

"Obstetric and gynecologic aspects of heroin addiction," by Claman, A.D., and Strang, R.I. AMERICAN JOURNAL OF OBSTETRICS AND GYNECOLOGY. 83:252-257, 1962.

"On Addiction Research Center Inventory scores of former addicts receiving LSD and untreated schizophrenics," by Haertzen, C.H. PSYCHOLOGICAL REPORTS. 14(2):483-488, 1964.

"On narcomania-euphomania," by Frey, T.S. SVENSKA LAKARE-SALLSKAPET IN NORDISK MEDICIN. 57:3391-3408, 1960.

"On the anthropology of addiction," by Sattes, H. NERVEN-AERZT. 33:184-187, 1962.

"On the severity of hepatitis among heroin addicts," by Schoenfeld, M.R., et al. JOURNAL OF NEW DRUGS. 4(2): 79-81, 1964.

"Opium addiction in the dog," by Segall, S. JOURNAL OF THE AMERICAN VETERINARY MEDICAL ASSOCIATION. 144(6): 603+, 1964.

"Opiate addiction. I. The nalorphine test. II. Current

concepts of treatment," by Poze, R.S. STANFORD MEDICAL
BULLETIN. 20:1-23, 1962.
"Opiate withdrawal as measured by the Addiction Research
Center Inventory (ARCI)," by Haertzen, C.A., and Meketon,
M.J. DISEASES OF THE NERVOUS SYSTEM. 29(7):450-455,
1968.
"The opiate-withdrawal syndrome as a state of stress, by
Krystal, H. PSYCHIATRIC QUARTERLY. 36(1):53-65, 1962.
"An overview of the problem of drug abuse: as a clinical
entity," by Cameron, D.C. JOURNAL OF THE HILLSIDE HOS-
PITAL. 16(2):120-127, 1967.
"Pentazocine and its relation to drug addiction," by Eddy,
N.B. JOURNAL OF THE AMERICAN MEDICAL ASSOCIATION. 195
(5):322-323, 1966.
"Performance as a function of drug, dose, and level of train-
ing," by Ray, O.S., and Bivens, L.W. PSYCHOPHARMACOLO-
GIA. 10(2):103-109, 1966.
"Personality characteristics of adolescent addicts: mani-
fest rigidity," by Laskowitz, D., and Einstein, S. COR-
RECTIVE PSYCHIATRY AND JOURNAL OF SOCIAL THERAPY. 9(4):
215-218, 1963.
"Personality characteristics of drug addicts," by Muhlen-
camp, A.F. PERSPECTIVES IN PSYCHIATRIC CARE. 6(5):113-
129, Sept.-Oct., 1968.
"Personality characteristics of narcotic addicts as indi-
cated by the MMPI," by Hill, H.E., et al. JOURNAL OF
GENERAL PSYCHOLOGY. 62:127-139, 1960.
"Personality characteristics of young male narcotic addicts,"
by Gilbert, J.G., et al. JOURNAL OF CONSULTING PSYCHOL-
OGY. 31:536-538, Oct., 1967.
"Personality patterns in narcotic addiction," by Regal, L.H.
DISSERTATION ABSTRACTS. 23(10):3982-3983, 1963.
"The pharmacogenic orgasm in drug addiction," by Chessick,
R.D. AMERICAN MEDICAL ASSOCIATION ARCHIVES OF GENERAL
PSYCHIATRY. 3:545-556, 1960.
"Pharmacologic factors in relapse and the possible use of
the narcotic antagonists in treatment," by Martin, W.R.
ILLINOIS MEDICAL JOURNAL. 130:489-494, 1966.
"Pharmacological aspects of drug dependence," by Deneau,
G.A., and Seevers, M.H. ADVANCES IN PHARMACOLOGY. 3:
267-283, 1964.
"The pharmacology and physiology of drug addiction," by
Sherrod, T.M. ILLINOIS MEDICAL JOURNAL. 130:453-456,
Oct., 1966.
"The phenomena of drug dependence and drug abuse (sympos-
ium of the Pharmaceutical section, American Association
for the Advancement of Science," by Eddy, N.B. AMERICAN
JOURNAL OF HOSPITAL PHARMACY. 22(3):131-132, 1965.
"Phenomenology and pathology of addiction," by Lehmann,
H.E. COMPREHENSIVE PSYCHIATRY. 4:168-180, June, 1963.
"The phenomenology of doriden (glutethimide) dependence
among drug addicts," by Laskowitz, D. INTERNATIONAL
JOURNAL OF THE ADDICTION. 2(1):39-52, 1967.
"Philosophy of narcotic addiction," by Lowry, J.T. MEDICAL

RECORDS AND ANNALS. 55:24, 1962.
"Physical dependence on heroin and pentobarbitone," by Bew-
ley, T.H., et al. PRACTITIONER. 200:251-253, Feb., 1968.
"Plasma catecholamine levels and urinary excretion of cate-
cholamines and metabolites in two human subjects during
a cycle of morphine addiction and withdrawal," by Weil-
Malherbe, H., et al. BIOCHEMICAL PHARMACOLOGY. 14(11):
1621-1633, 1965.
"A post-hospital study of Kentucky addicts, a preliminary
report," by O'Donnell, J.A. JOURNAL OF THE KENTUCKY
MEDICAL ASSOCIATION. 61:573-577, 1963.
"Preference for human or animal drawings among normal and
addicted males," by Wisotsky, M., and Birner, L. PER-
CEPTUAL AND MOTOR SKILLS. 10:43-45, 1960.
"Pregnancy outcomes of diagnosed addicts," by Rosenthal,
T., et al. AMERICAN JOURNAL OF PUBLIC HEALTH. 54:1252-
1262, 1964.
"The pregnant addict. A study of 66 case histories, 1950-
1959," by Stern, R. AMERICAN JOURNAL OF OBSTETRICS AND
GYNECOLOGY. 94:253-257, Jan. 15, 1966.
"Prevalence and early detection of heroin abuse,: by de Al-
arcón, R., and Rathod, N.H. BRITISH MEDICAL JOURNAL.
2(5604):549-553, 1968.
"Primary and secondary addiction," by Booij, J. NEDERLANDS
TIJDSCHRIFT VOOR GENEESKUNDE. 104:57-59, 1960.
"Problem of neonatal narcotic addiction," by Yerby, A.S.
NEW YORK JOURNAL OF MEDICINE. 66:1248-1249, 1966.
"A procedure which produces sustained opiate-directed be-
havior (morphine addiction) in the rat," by Nichols, J.R.
PSYCHOLOGICAL REPORTS. 13(3):895-904, 1963.
"The prognosis in drug addiction," by Clark, J.A. JOURNAL
OF MENTAL SCIENCE. 108(455):411-418, 1962.
"The prognosis of kidney damage and anemia in the analgesic
abuser," by Kasanen, A. ANNALES MEDICINAE INTERNAE FEN-
NIAE. 56:93-97, 1967.
"Prolonged adverse reactions from unsupervised use of hal-
lucinogenic drugs," by Kleber, H.D. JOURNAL OF NERVOUS
AND MENTAL DISEASE. 144(4):308-319, 1967.
"Psychiatric illness in the medical profession," by A'Brook,
M.F., et al. BRITISH JOURNAL OF PSYCHIATRY. 113(502):
1013-1023, 1967.
"Psychiatry in drug dependence." BRITISH MEDICAL JOURNAL.
2(5603):486-487, 1968.
"Psychic dependence in addiction," by Holloway, I. AUS-
TRALIAN PSYCHOLOGIST. 2(1); 1967.
"Psychoanalytic studies on addiction: ego structure in nar-
cotic addiction," by Savitt, R.A. PSYCHOANALYTIC QUAR-
TERLY. 32:43-57, 1963.
"Psychodynamic factors in the mother-child relationship in
adolescent drug addiction: a comparison of mothers of
schyzophrenics and mothers of normal adolescent sons,"
by Accardo, N. PSYCHOTHERAPY AND PSYCHOSOMATICS. 13:
249-255, 1965.
"The psychodynamics of a drug addict. A three-year study,"

by Guttman, O. AMERICAN JOURNAL OF PSYCHOTHERAPY. 19 (4):653-665, 1965.
"Psychodynamics of narcotic addiction," by Barnard, G.W., et al. JOURNAL OF THE FLORIDA MEDICAL ASSOCIATION. 55: 831-834, Sept., 1968.
"Psychogenic dependence to a variety of drugs in the monkey," by Deneau, G.A., et al. PHARMACOLOGIST. p. 182, Fall, 1964.
"Psychological deficit in chewers of coca leaf," by Negrete, J.C., and Murphy, H.B.M. BULLETIN ON NARCOTICS. 19(4): 11-18, Oct.-Dec., 1967.
"The psychology of drug addiction: some literature reviewed," by Shooter, A. RORSCHACH NEWSLETTER. 10:3-11, 1965.
"Psychosis, psychoneurosis, mental deficiency, and personality type in criminal drug addicts," by Messinger, E., and Zitrin, A. QUADERNI DI CRIMINOLOGIA CLINICA. 7(2): 137-154, 1965.
"Pulmonary edema accompanying heroin intoxication," by Selzman, H.M., et al. CARDIOVASCULAR RESEARCH CENTER BULLETIN. 6:77-79, Oct.-Dec., 1967.
"Pulmonary valve regurgitation secondary to bacterial endocarditis in heroin addicts," by Massumi, R.A., et al. AMERICAN HEART JOURNAL. 73:308-316, Mar., 1967.
"The pupil test for diagnosing narcotic usage," by Way, E.L. TRIANGLE. 7:152-156, 1965.
"Recent advances in research on drug addiction," by Aoki, Y. MEDICINE (Tokyo). 20:82-85, 1963.
"The relationship between future time perspective, time estimation, and impulse control in a group of young offenders and in a control group," by Siegman, A.W. JOURNAL OF CONSULTING PSYCHOLOGY. 25:470-476, 1961.
"Renal papillary necrosis and abuse of analgesics," by Koch, B., et al. CANADIAN MEDICAL ASSOCIATION JOURNAL. 98: 8-15, Jan. 6, 1968.
"Response of adult heroin addicts to a total therapeutic program," by Freedman, A.M., et al. AMERICAN JOURNAL OF ORTHOPSYCHIATRY. 33(5):890-899, 1963.
"Rhinitis medicamentosa," by Blue, J.A. ANNALS OF ALLERGY. 26:425-429, Aug., 1968.
"Rorschach study of adolescent addicts who died of an overdose: a sign approach," by Jones, F., and Laskowitz, D. PSYCHIATRIC DIGEST. 25:21-30, May, 1964.
"Serologic tests for syphilis among narcotic addicts," by Harris, W.D., et al. NEW YORK JOURNAL OF MEDICINE. 67:2967-2974, Nov. 15, 1967.
"Severe systemic infections complicating 'mainline' heroin addiction," by Briggs, J.H., et al. LANCET. 2:1227-1231, Dec. 9, 1967.
"Socioeconomic affluence as a factor," by Schonfeld, W.A. NEW YORK STATE JOURNAL OF MEDICINE. 67(14):1981-1990, 1967.
"Some abstinence syndromes." BRITISH MEDICAL JOURNAL. 5422:1412-1413, 1964.
"Spontaneous opiate addiction in Rhesus monkeys," by Clag-

horn, J.L., et al. SCIENCE. 149(3):440-441, 1965.
"Staphylococcal endocarditis in narcotic addict with Mar-
fan's Syndrome," by Cohen, D.N., et al. NEW YORK JOUR-
NAL OF MEDICINE. 67:2362-2367, Sept.1, 1967.
"Steroids are drugs of addiction," by Kelly, M. RHEUMATISM.
21(2):50-54, 1965.
"Studies on the effects of drugs on performance of a delayed
discrimination," by Roberts, M.H.T., and Bradley, P.B.
PHYSIOLOGY AND BEHAVIOR. 2(4):389-397, 1967.
"Studies on 300 Indian addicts with special reference to
psychosociological aspects, etiology and treatment," by
Chopra, G.S., and Chopra, P.S. BULLETIN ON NARCOTICS.
17(2):1-9, Apr.-June, 1965.
"Study of mathadone as an adjunct in rehabilitation of her-
oin addicts," by Dole, V.P., et al. ILLINOIS MEDICAL
JOURNAL. 130:487-489, Oct., 1966.
"Subculture identification of hospitalized male drug ad-
dicts: a further examination," by Retting, S., and Pas-
amanick, B. JOURNAL OF NERVOUS AND MENTAL DISEASE.
139(1):83-86, 1964.
"Subjective drug effects: a factorial representation of
subjective drug effects on the Addiction Research Cen-
ter Inventory," by Haertzen, C.A. JOURNAL OF NERVOUS
AND MENTAL DISEASE. 140(4):280-289, 1965.
"Surgery on the narcotic addict," by Eisenman, B., et al.
ANNALS OF SURGERY. 159:748-757, 1964.
"A survey of the experience of tension in alcoholics and
other diagnostic groups," by Cheek. F.E., et al. INTER-
NATIONAL JOURNAL OF NEUROPSYCHIATRY. 3:477-488, Dec.,
1967.
"Susceptibility to readdiction as a function of the addic-
tion and withdrawal environments," by Thompson, T., and
Ostlund, W. JOURNAL OF COMPARATIVE AND PHYSIOLOGICAL
PSYCHOLOGY. 60(3):388-392, 1965.
"Symposium: nonnarcotic addiction. Clinical manifestations
and treatment of amphetamine type of dependence," by
Connell, P.H. JOURNAL OF THE AMERICAN MEDICAL ASSOCIA-
TION. 196(8):718-722, 1966.
"Symposium: nonnarcotic addiction. Incidence in a univer-
sity hospital psychiatric ward," by Bakewell, W.E., and
Wikler, A. JOURNAL OF THE AMERICAN MEDICAL ASSOCIATION.
196(8):710-713, 1966.
"Synaptic and behavioral correlates of psychotherapeutic
and related drug actions," by Marrazzi, A.S. ANNALS OF
THE NEW YORK ACADEMY OF SCIENCE. 96:211, 1962.
"Tetanus in addicts." JOURNAL OF THE AMERICAN MEDICAL ASSOC-
IATION. 205:584-585, Aug. 19, 1968.
"Tetanus in drug addicts," by Mason, P. JOURNAL OF THE
AMERICAN MEDICAL ASSOCIATION. 205:188, July 15, 1968.
"A thin-layer chromatographic screening test for the detec-
tion of users of morphine or heroin," by Davidow, B.,
et al. AMERICAN JOURNAL OF CLINICAL PATHOLOGY. 46:
58-62, 1966.
"Tolerance and dependence in the planarian after continuous

exposure to morphine," by Needleman, H.L. NATURE. 215 (5102):784-785, 1967.

"Toxicomania. Situations and conditions," by Balduzzi, E. RASSEGNA DI NEUROPSICHIATRIA. 19:137-146, 1965.

"Toxicomanias and drug abuse in general practice," by Schulte, W. FOLIA CLINICA INTERNACIONAL. 16:3-11, 1966.

"A twelve-year follow-up of New York narcotic addicts: I. The relation of treatment to outcome," by Vaillant, G.E. AMERICAN JOURNAL OF PSYCHIATRY. 122(7):727-737, 1966.

"A 12-year follow-up of New York narcotic addicts. III. Some social and psychiatric characteristics," by Vaillant, G.E. ARCHIVES OF GENERAL PSYCHIATRY. 15:599-609, Dec., 1966.

"A twelve-year follow-up of New York narcotic addicts. IV. Some characteristics and determinants of abstinence," by Vaillant, G.E. AMERICAN JOURNAL OF PSYCHIATRY. 123:573-585, 1966.

"Two cases of altered consciousness with amnesia apparently telepathically induced," by Paul, M.A. PSYCHEDELIC REVIEW. No. 8:4-8, 1966.

"Urban tetanus. The epidemiologic aspects of tetanus in narcotic addicts in New York City," by Cherubin, C.E. ARCHIVES OF ENVIRONMENTAL HEALTH. 14:802-808, June, 1967.

"Urine detection tests in the management of the narcotic addict," by Kurland, A.A., et al. AMERICAN JOURNAL OF PSYCHIATRY. 122:737-742, 1966.

"Viral hepatitis in a group of Boston hospitals. 3. Importance of exposure to shellfish in a nonepidemic period," by Koff, R.S., et al. NEW ENGLAND JOURNAL OF MEDICINE. 276:703-710, Mar. 30, 1967.

"Viral hepatitis in narcotic users. An outbreak in Rhode Island," by Rosenstein, B.J. JOURNAL OF THE AMERICAN MEDICAL ASSOCIATION. 199:696-700, Mar. 6, 1967.

"Visual recognition thresholds for narcotic argot in post-addicts," by Jones, B.E. PERCEPTUAL AND MOTOR SKILLS. 20(3, pt.2):1065-1069, 1965.

"Von Recklinghausen's neurofibromatosis with longstanding pelvic lesions, drug addiction, and mental sequelae," by Sloan, W.R., and Nabney, J.B. JOURNAL OF OBSTETRICS AND GYNAECOLOGY OF THE BRITISH COMMONWEALTH. 70:523-524, 1963.

"Wechsler-Bellevue performance of adolescent heroin addicts," by Laskowitz, D. JOURNAL OF PSYCHOLOGICAL STUDIES. 13(1):49-59, 1962.

"Withdrawal reactions from chlordiazepoxide (librium)," by Hollister, L.E., et al. PSYCHOPHARMACOLOGIA. 2:63-68, 1961.

"Womb fantasies in heroin addiction: a Rorschach study," by Silverman, L.H., and Silverman, D.K. JOURNAL OF PROJECTIVE TECHNIQUES. 24:52-63, 1960.

NARCOTIC REHABILITATION: Books and Essays

American Bar Association and the American Medical Association. Joint Committee on Narcotic Drugs. DRUG ADDICTION: crime or disease? Bloomington, Indiana: Indiana University Press, 1961.
Brill, Henry, and Larimore, G.W. ON-THE-SITE STUDY OF THE BRITISH NARCOTIC SYSTEM. Albany: Department of Mental Hygiene, 1965.
Brill, Leon. "Community approaches in the addiction problem," CHATHAM CONFERENCE ON PERSPECTIVES ON NARCOTIC ADDICTION. Chatham, Massacusetts, Sept. 9-11, 1963, pp. 45-57.
Brotman, R., and Freedman, A. A COMMUNITY MENTAL HEALTH APPROACH TO DRUG ADDICTION. Office of Juvenile Delinquency and Youth Development. Department of Health, Education and Welfare. Juvenile Delinquency Publication no.9005. Washington: Government Printing Office, 1968.
Brotman, R., et al. HOSPITAL STAFF ATTITUDES AND ADJUSTMENTS TO WORKING WITH NARCOTIC ADDICTS, presented at the 40th Annual Meeting of the American Orthopsychiatric Association. Washington, D.C., Mar. 8, 1963.
Burkhart, W.R., and Sathmary, A. CALIFORNIA NARCOTIC TREATMENT - CONTROL PROJECT, phase I and II. Sacramento: Department of Corrections, May, 1963.
California. Department of Corrections. Research Division. SUMMARY STATISTICS: CIVIL COMMITMENT PROGRAM FOR NARCOTIC ADDICTS, 1961 through 1966. Sacramento, California: California Rehabilitation Center Program, 1968.
CALIFORNIA NARCOTICS ADDICT CONTROL AND REHABILITATION PROGRAM: SPECIAL REPORT. Sacramento: California Department of Corrections, 1962.
Calof, Judith. STUDY OF VOLUNTARY TREATMENT PROGRAMS FOR NARCOTIC ADDICTS. New York: Community Service Society, 1969.
Casriel, Daniel. SO FAIR A HOUSE: the story of Synanon. Englewood Cliffs, New Jersey: Prentice-Hall, 1963.
Castle Peak Drug Addiction Treatment Centre. ANNUAL REPORT (various years).
Cattell, S.H. HEALTH, WELFARE AND SOCIAL ORGANIZATION IN CHINATOWN, NEW YORK CITY. New York: Community Service Society, 1962.
Chien, M.N., and Lawn, J. THE PROCESS OF INTAKE, REHABILITATION AND DISCHARGE OF TREATED ADDICTS. Hong Kong: SARDA, 1963.
Diamond, M.A. "Treatment of the narcotic addict: physical facilities," PROCEEDINGS: WHITE HOUSE CONFERENCE ON NARCOTIC AND DRUG ABUSE. Washington: Government Printing Office, 1962, pp. 74-77.
Diehl, H.S., et al. HEALTH AND SAFETY FOR YOU, 2nd edition. New York: McGraw-Hill, 1961.
Diskind, M.H., et al. AN EXPERIMENT IN THE SUPERVISION OF PAROLED OFFENDERS ADDICTED TO NARCOTIC DRUGS. Albany:

168

New York State Division of Parole, 1960.

Diskind, M.H., and Klonsky, G. RECENT DEVELOPMENTS IN THE TREATMENT OF PAROLED OFFENDERS ADDICTED TO NARCOTIC DRUGS. Albany: New York State Division of Parole, 1964.

Duncan, T.L. UNDERSTANDING AND HELPING THE NARCOTIC HABIT. Philadelphia: Fortress Press, 1968.

Duster, Troy. THE LEGISTATION OF MORALITY; LAW, DRUGS, AND MORAL JUDGEMENT. New York: Free Press, 1969.

Eichlenlaub, J.E. COLLEGE HEALTH. New York: Macmillan, 1962, pp. 42-73.

Einstein, S., and Jones, F. "Group therapy with adolescent addicts," DRUG ADDICTION IN YOUTH, ed. E. Harms. New York: Pergamon Press, 1965, pp. 132-147.

Endore, Guy. SYNANON: CONTROVERSIAL DRUG ADDICTION CURE. New York: Doubleday, 1968.

Fairweather, G.W. SOCIAL PSYCHOLOGY IN TREATING MENTAL ILL-NESS: an experimental approach. New York: John Wiley and Sons, Inc., 1964.

Felix, R.H. PROCEEDINGS OF CONFERENCE ON POST-HOSPITAL CARE AND REHABILITATION OF ADOLESCENT NARCOTIC ADDICTS. Albany, 1960.

Glaser, D., and O'Leary, V. THE CONTROL AND TREATMENT OF NARCOTIC USE. Washington: United States Department of Health, Education and Welfare, Office of Juvenile Delinquency and Youth Development, 1966.

Grossberg, L. DOPE ADDICTS DISCOVER A CURE FOR THEMSELVES. Los Angeles: Synanon, 1961.

Harms, E. DRUG ADDICTION IN YOUTH. New York: Pergamon Press, 1965.

HONG KONG DRUG ADDICTS TREATMENT AND REHABILITATION ORDI-NANCE No. 34 of 1960. Hong Kong: Gevernment Printer, c. 1960.

Humphrey, James. READING IN HEALTH EDUCATION. Dubuque, Iowa: Wm. C. Brown, 1964.

Illinois. Department of Public Instruction. PROGRAM DE-VELOPMENT FOR FOUNDATIONS IN ALCOHOL AND NARCOTIC IN-STRUCTION. Springfield: [author], 1963.

Jeffee, Saul. NARCOTICS: AN AMERICAN PLAN. New York: P.S. Eriksson, 1966.

Jurgensen, W.P. "Inpatient treatment of the narcotic ad-dict," THE CHATHAM CONFERENCE ON PERSPECTIVES ON NAR-COTIC ADDICTION. Chatham, Massachusetts, Sept. 9-11, 1963, pp. 34-44.

Land, Herman W. WHAT YOU CAN DO ABOUT DRUGS AND YOUR CHILD. New York: Hart Pub., 1969.

Listen (Washington, D.C.). NOW YOU'RE LIVING! Basic in-formation for scientific education for prevention of alcoholism and drug addiction, revised edition. Wash-inton: Published for Narcotics Education, 1964.

Listen (Washington, D.C.). REALLY LIVING; basic informa-tion for scientific education for the prevention of al-colholism and drug addiction, revised edition. Wash-ington: Published for Narcotic Education, Inc., 1960.

Lutheran World Service. PROJECT FOR THE AFTER-CARE OF NAR-

COTIC ADDICTS. Hong Kong, 1962.
Martin, W.R., et al. A PROPOSED METHOD OF AMBULATORY TREAT-
MENT OF NARCOTIC ADDICTS USING A LONG-ACTIVE ORALLY EF-
FECTIVE NARCOTIC ANTAGONIST, CYCLAZOCINE-- an experiment-
al study, presented before the Committee on Drug Addic-
tion and Narcotics, minutes of the 27th meeting of Na-
tional Academy of Sciences and National Research Council,
Houston, Texas, Feb., 1965.
Masserman, J.H., ed. CURRENT PSYCHIATRIC THERAPIES. Vol.
7. New York: Grune and Stratton, 1967.
Miller, B., and Miller, Z. GOOD HEALTH - PERSONAL AND COM-
MUNITY. Philadelphia: W.B. Saunders Co., 1960.
Society for the Aid and Rehabilitation of Drug Addicts.
SHEK KWU CHAU CANTRE OPENED BY H. E. THE GOVERNOR... on
23rd April, 1963. Hong Kong, 1963.
Society for the Aid and Rehabilitation of Drug Addicts.
Aftercare Service. FOLLOW UP AND AFTERCARE REPORT NO. I.
Hong Kong, 1964.
Stoller, F.H. ACCELERATED INTERACTION: a time-limited ap-
proach based on the brief, intensive group. California
Department of Mental Hygiene, Bureau of Research. Pre-
publication copy no. 352, 1966.
Texas Alcohol Narcotics Education. THE ALCOHOL-NARCOTICS
PROBLEM; a handbook for teachers, revised edition. Dade
County, Florida, public schools edition. Dallas: Tane
Press, 1964.
United States Bureau of Narcotics. CONTROL AND REHABILITA-
TION OF THE NARCOTIC ADDICT; a symposium. Washington:
Government Printing Office, 1961.
United States. Congress. Senate Committee on the Judic-
iary. JUVENILE DELINQUENCY: treatment and rehabilita-
tion of juvenile drug addicts. Washington: Government
Printing Office, 1968.
United States. Department of Health, Education and Wel-
fare. REHABILITATING THE NARCOTIC ADDICT. Washington:
Vocational Rehabilitation Administration, 1967.
United States. National Institute of Mental Health. NAR-
COTIC DRUG ADDICTION. Mental Health Monograph no. 2.
Washington: Government Pringing Office, 1963.
United States. National Institute of Mental Health. De-
monstration Center, New York. REHABILITATION IN DRUG
ADDICTION; a report on a five-year community experiment
of the New York Demonstration Center; Leon Brill, project director. Mental Health Monograph no. 3. Wash-
ington: Government Printing Office, 1963.
United States. National Institute of Mental Health Services. NARCOTIC ADDICT REHABILITATION ACT OF 1966 (revised May, 1969). Washington: Government Printing Office, 1969.
United States. Senate. Labor and Public Welfare Committee.
COMPILATION OF SELECTED PUBLIC HEALTH LAWS, including
particularly Public health service act, Clean air act,
Solid waste disposal act, Mental retardation facilities
and community mental health center construction act, and

NARCOTIC ADDICT REHABILITATION ACT, prepared by Subcom-
mittee on Health, March, 1968. Washington: Government
Printing Office, 1968.
Wagner, R.F. REMARKS BY MAYOR ROBERT F. WAGNER at the White
House Conference on Narcotics. Press Release, Sept, 27,
1962.
Winick, Charles. "The drug addict and his treatment," LEGAL
AND CRIMINAL PSYCHOLOGY, by Toch, Hans. New York: Holt,
Rinehart and Winston, 1961, pp. 357-380.
Yablonsky, Lewis. TUNNEL BACK: SYNANON. New York, Mac-
millan, 1965.

NARCOTIC REHABILITATION: Periodical Literature

"AMA restates position on ambulatory clinics for addicts."
JOURNAL OF THE AMERICAN MEDICAL ASSOCIATION. 182:30,
1962.
"AMA-NRC define addict treatment." MEDICAL WORLD NEWS.
4:87, July 5, 1963.
"Accidental therapeutic drug addiction," by Friend, D.G.
CLINICAL PHARMACOLOGY AND THERAPEUTICS. 7:832-834, Nov.-
Dec., 1966.
"Action research in a treatment center," by Freedman, A.M.
AMERICAN JOURNAL OF NURSING. 7:57-60, July, 1963.
"The addict and the physician," by Berger, H. MEDICAL
TIMES. 94:710-720, 1966.
"The addict and treatment," by Raskin, H.A. ILLINOIS MED-
ICAL JOURNAL. 130:465-473, Oct., 1966.
"The addict as a rehab client," by Richman, S. REHABILI-
TATION RECORD. 7:24-26, May-June, 1966.
"Addict, heal thy self," by Champlin, C.D. ISLAND LANTERN.
pp. 20-25, June, 1965.
"Admissions of narcotic drug addicts to Public Health Ser-
vice hospitals, 1935-1963," by Ball, J.C., and Cottrell,
E.S. PUBLIC HEALTH REPORTS. 80(6):471-475, 1965.
"Aftercare: an addict's bridge to new life." THE ATTACK
ON NARCOTIC ADDICTION AND DRUG ABUSE. 2(4):2-3, Nov.,
1968.
"Aftercare and follow-up, part of N.A.C.C.programs," THE
ATTACK ON NARCOTIC ADDICTION AND DRUG ABUSE. 3:8,
Spring, 1969.
"Aftercare of drug addicts: the missing link in rehabili-
tation," by Egan, D. ILLINOIS MEDICAL JOURNAL. 130:
500-512, 1966.
"After the cure what?" JOURNAL OF THE AMERICAN MEDICAL
ASSOCIATION. 186(6):26-28, 1963.
"Aid for the addicted," by Fry, J.R. PRESBYTERIAN LIFE.
16(14):11-15, 1963.
"Aiding drug addicts," by Goldman, J.J. WALL STREET JOUR-
NAL. 163:1+, Jan. 17, 1964.

"Alcohol-narcotics education," by Keeler, O. ILLINOIS ED-
UCATION. 54:314-315, Mar., 1966.
"Alcoholic and drug addiction units." NURSING TIMES. 64:
111, Jan. 26, 1968.
"Alcoholics anonymous imitated by gamblers and narcotics
addicts," by McGuinness, G. WALL STREET JOURNAL. 158:
1+, Dec. 29, 1961.
"An alternative proposal for dealing with drug addiction,"
by Celler, Emanuel. FEDERAL PROBATION. 27:24-26, June,
1963.
"Ambulatory treatment of drug addiction," by Wong, P.C.
BRITISH JOURNAL OF ADDICTION. 61:101-114, 1965.
"Ambulatory withdrawal treatment of heroin addicts," by
Berle, B.B., and Nyswander, M. NEW YORK STATE JOURNAL
OF MEDICINE. 64:1846-1848, 1964.
"Amiphenazole in the treatment of morphine and opium ad-
diction," by Bruce, D.W. LANCET. 7341:1010-1012, 1964.
"Analgesic drugs and drug dependence," by May, E.L. BRI-
TISH JOURNAL OF ADDICTION. 62:197-202, Mar., 1967.
"The anticriminal society: Synanon," by Yablonsky, L. FED-
ERAL PROBATION. 26(3):50-57, 1962.
"Anti-heroin's methadone." SCIENTIFIC AMERICAN. 212:62,
Apr., 1965.
"Anti-narcotic testing: a physician's point of view," by
Hurley, C.T. FEDERAL PROBATION. 27(2):32-41, 1963.
"An approach to treating narcotic addicts based on commun-
ity mental health diagnosis," by Brotman, R., et al.
COMPREHENSIVE PSYCHIATRY. 6:104-118, 1965.
"Approaches to narcotic addiction in private practice," by
Wilson, N.J. SOUTHERN MEDICAL JOURNAL. 60:583-587,
June, 1967.
"Are there special programs of medical treatment for alco-
holics, drug addicts, and agressive sex offenders?"
CORRECTIONAL RESEARCH. 12:19-28, 1962.
"Assessment: 1968. New York State Welfare Conference, Nov.
19-22, 1968." THE ATTACK ON NARCOTIC ADDICTION AND DRUG
ABUSE. 3:5, Winter, 1969.
"Assessment of the dependence-producing properties of dihy-
drocodeinone and codoxime," by Jasinski, D.R., et al.
CLINICAL PHARMACOLOGY AND THERAPEUTICS. 8:266-270, Mar.-
Apr., 1967.
"Aversive conditioning of drug addicts: a pilot study," by
Liberman, R. BEHAVIOUR RESEARCH AND THERAPY. 6(2):
229-231, 1968.
"Basic purpose of U.S. hospital hasn't changed," by Vaughn,
N. LEXINGTON HERALD. May 23, 1965.
"Behavior therapy with a narcotics user: a case report,"
by Lesser, E. BEHAVIOUR RESEARCH AND THERAPY. 5(3):
251-252, 1967.
"Breaking the habit." NEWSWEEK. 65:60, June 21, 1965.
"Bridging the gap between institution and community in the
treatment of narcotic addicts," by Berliner, A.K. MEN-
TAL HYGIENE. 52:263-271, Apr., 1968.
"Bureaucracy and morality: an organizational perspective

on a moral crusade," by Dickson, D.T. SOCIAL PROBLEMS. 16(2):143-156, 1968.
"California's attack on narcotics addiction," by Haines, A.B. CHRISTIAN CENTURY. 85:1549-1550, Dec. 4, 1968.
"A Canadian programme of voluntary treatment of drug dependence - the work of the Narcotic Addiction Foundation of British Columbia," by Hoskin, H.F. BULLETIN ON NARCOTICS. 20(2):45-48, Apr.-June, 1968.
"Care and treatment of the addict," by Scaduto, A. NEW YORK POST. Nov. 12, 1965.
"Care of patients addicted to non-narcotic drugs," by Epp, M.L. CANADIAN NURSE. 63:42-44, Mar., 1967.
"Carl Koller and cocaine," by Becker, H.G. PSYCHOANALYTIC QUARTERLY. 32:309-373, 1963.
"The centre for treatment and rehabilitation of narcotic addicts in Macau," by Reves, S., and Guerra, A.C. BULLETIN ON NARCOTICS. 15(1):1-10, Jan.-Mar., 1963.
"Centres for treatment of drug addiction. Advantages of special centres," by Bewley, T.H. BRITISH MEDICAL JOURNAL. 2:498-499, May 20, 1967.
"Centres for treatment of drug addiction. Importance of research," by Connell, P.H. BRITISH MEDICAL JOURNAL. 2:499-500, May 20, 1967.
"Centres for treatment of drug addiction. Integrated approach," by Owens, J. BRITISH MEDICAL JOURNAL. 2:501-502, May 20. 1967.
"Centres for treatment of drug addiction. Treatment in the community," by Chapple, P.A. BRITISH MEDICAL JOURNAL. 2:500-501, May 20, 1967.
"Centres for the treatment of addiction." LANCET. 1:288-289, Feb. 10, 1968.
"Characteristics of hospitalized narcotic addicts," by Ball, J., et al. HEALTH, EDUCATION AND WELFARE INDICATORS. Mar., 1966.
"The chemotherapy of drug dependence," by Eddy, N.B. BRITISH JOURNAL OF ADDICTION. 61:155-167, Aug., 1966.
"Chlormethiazole treatment of abstinence symptoms after drug withdrawal. Preliminary reports. I.," by Sattes, H. ACTA PSYCHIATRICA SCANDINAVICA. 42(suppl. 192):191, 1966.
"Chlormethiazole treatment of abstinence symptoms after drug withdrawal. Preliminary report. II.," by Glatt, M.M. ACTA PSYCHIATRICA SCANDINAVICA. 42(suppl. 192): 192, 1966.
"Chlormethiazole treatment of abstinence symptoms after drug withdrawal. Preliminary reports. III.," by Gastager, H. ACTA PSYCHIATRICA SCANDINAVICA. 42(suppl. 192):193+, 1966.
"Civil commitment for narcotic addicts," by Kuh, R.H. FEDERAL PROBATION. 27:21-23, June, 1963.
"A clergyman looks at drug abuse," by Starkey, L.M. JOURNAL OF SCHOOL HEALTH. 39:478-486, Sept., 1969.
"A clinical comparison of the analgesic effects of methadone and morphine administered intramuscularly, and of orally

and parenterally administered methadone," by Beaver,
W.T., et al. CLINICAL PHARMACOLOGY AND THERAPEUTICS.
8(3):415-426, 1967.
"Clinical experiences with hypnosis in psychiatric treat-
ment," by Alexander, L. INTERNATIONAL JOURNAL OF NEURO-
PSYCHIATRY. 3:118-124, Apr., 1967.
"Clinical studies of cyclazocine in the treatment of nar-
cotic addiction," by Freedman, A.M., et al. AMERICAN
JOURNAL OF PSYCHIATRY. 124(11):1499-1504, 1968.
"Coma center in New York." LISTEN. 13:15, Nov.-Dec., 1960.
"Commentary on the above paper: why compulsory closed-ward
treatment of narcotic addicts?" by Schlich, R. ILLINOIS
MEDICAL JOURNAL. 130:485-487, Oct., 1966.
"Communities help to open doors for treatment." THE ATTACK
ON NARCOTIC ADDICTION AND DRUG ABUSE. 2(4):14-15, Nov.,
1968.
"A community counseling center for addicts," by Osnos, R.
NURSING OUTLOOK. 13:38-40, 1965.
"Comparative effects of (1) chronic administration of cy-
clazocine (arc II-C-3). (II) substitution of nalorphine
for cyclazocine and (III) chronic administration of
morphine. Pilot crossover study," by Fraser, H.F., and
Rosenberg, D.E. INTERNATIONAL JOURNAL OF THE ADDICTIONS.
1:86-98, 1966.
"Control of opiate abstinence syndrome with meclofenoxate
(ludicril, ANP235). A report of two cases," by Goward-
man, M.G. NEW ZEALAND MEDICAL JOURNAL. 66:174-176, Mar.,
1967.
"A correctional dilemma: the narcotics addict," by Nahren-
dorf, R.O. SOCIOLOGY AND SOCIAL RESEARCH. 53:21-33,
Oct., 1968.
"Correctional problems the court can help solve," by Ben-
nett, J.V. CRIME AND DELINQUENCY. 7:1-8, Jan., 1961.
"A counseling center for drug addicts," by Osnos, R., and
Laskowitz, D. BULLETIN ON NARCOTICS. 18(4):31-46,
Oct.-Dec., 1966.
"Counseling the adolescent addict," by Telson, S. JOUR-
NAL OF REHABILITATION. 30:10-12, 1964.
"Court steps for addicts explained." THE ATTACK ON NARCOT-
IC ADDICTION AND DRUG ABUSE. 2(4):4, Nov., 1968.
"Crash program on drug abuse," by Pinkerton, P.B. JOURNAL
OF SECONDARY EDUCATION. 43:228-232, May, 1968.
"Crucial factors in the treatment of narcotic addiction,"
by Freedman, A.M., and Sharoff, R.L. AMERICAN JOURNAL
OF PSYCHOTHERAPY. 19:397-407, 1965.
"Cured addict." JOURNAL OF THE AMERICAN MEDICAL ASSOCIA-
TION. 185(6), Aug. 10, 1963.
"Curing the heroin addict," by Campbell, J. NEW STATESMAN.
70:866+, Dec. 3, 1965.
"Current provision and practice in U.S. relating to the
commitment of opiate addicts," by Harney, M. BULLETIN
ON NARCOTICS. 3:11-23, 1962.
"Current trends in the rehabilitation of narcotics addicts,"
by Lieberman, L. SOCIAL WORK. 12:53-59, Apr., 1967.

"Cyclazocine, a long acting narcotic antagonist: its voluntary acceptance as a treatment modality by narcotic abusers," by Jaffe, J.H., and Brill, L. INTERNATIONAL JOURNAL OF THE ADDICTIONS. 1(1):99-123, Jan., 1966.

"Cyclazocine and methadone in narcotic addictions," by Freedman, A.M., et al. JOURNAL OF THE AMERICAN MEDICAL ASSOCIATION. 202(3):191-194, 1967.

"Cyclazocine in the treatment of narcotic addiction," by Jaffe, J.H. CURRENT PSYCHIATRIC THERAPIES. 7:147-156, 1967.

"The cycle of abstinence and relapse among heroin addicts," by Ray, M.B. SOCIAL PROBLEMS. 9:9, Fall, 1961.

"Daytop Lodge - halfway house for addicts on probation," by Shelly, J.A. REHABILITATION RECORD. 7:19-21, 1966.

"Daytop Lodge: halfway house for drug addicts." FEDERAL PROBATION. 28:46-54, Dec., 1964.

"Delaware's mental health plan," by Lieberman, D. DELAWARE MEDICAL JOURNAL. 37:251-253, 1965.

"The determination of cocaine HCL," by Deltombe, J., and Dutrieux, F. JOURNAL DE PHARMACIE DE BELGIQUE. 17: 331-334, 1962.

"Diagnosis and management of depressant drug dependence," by Ewing, J.A., et al. AMERICAN JOURNAL OF PSYCHIATRY. 123:909-917, Feb., 1967.

"Diagnosis and treatment of drug dependence of the barbiturate type," by Wikler, A. AMERICAN JOURNAL OF PSYCHIATRY. 125:758-765, Dec., 1968.

"Differential association and the rehabilitation of drug addicts," by Volkman, R. BRITISH JOURNAL OF ADDICTION. 61:91-100, Nov., 1965; also AMERICAN JOURNAL OF SOCIOLOGY. 69(2):129-142, 1963.

"Diphosphopyridine nucleotide in the prevention, diagnosis and treatment of drug addiction," by)'Hallaren, P. WESTERN JOURNAL OF SURGERY. 69:213-215, 1961.

"Discharge of narcotic drug addicts against medical advice," by Levine, J., and Monroe, J.J. PUBLIC HEALTH REPORTS. 79:13-18, 1964.

"The Dole-Nyswander treatment of heroin addiction," by Ausubel, D.P. JOURNAL OF THE AMERICAN MEDICAL ASSOCIATION. 195(11):949-950, 1966.

"Dope addicts discover a cure for themselves." SEPIA MAGAZINE. Aug., 1961.

"Dope cure has not affected singer's piano, vocal talents (II)," by Brown, C.E. JET. 29:62-63, 1965.

"Drug abuse as a social problem," by Brill, L. INTERNATIONAL JOURNAL OF THE ADDICTIONS. 1(2):7-21, 1966.

"Drug abuse education," by Weinswig, M.H., et al. PHI DELTA KAPPAN. 50:222, Dec., 1968.

"Drug abuse education program," by Barr, M. SCHOOL AND SOCIETY. 97:273, Summer, 1969.

"Drug abuse project, Coronado, California," by Jordan, C.W. JOURNAL OF SCHOOL HEALTH. 38:692-695, Dec., 1968.

"Drug addiction: a way back," by McCarrick, H. NURSING TIMES. 63:569-570, Apr. 28, 1967.

"Drug addiction. Action research in a treatment center," by Freedman, A.M. AMERICAN JOURNAL OF NURSING. 63: 57-60, 1963.
"Drug addiction: an eclectic view," by Freedman, A.M. JOURNAL OF THE AMERICAN MEDICAL ASSOCIATION. 197:878-882, 1966.
"Drug addiction, psychotic illness and brain self-stimulation: effective treatment and explanatory hypothesis," by Roper, P. CANADIAN MEDICAL ASSOCIATION JOURNAL. 95: 1080-1086, Nov. 19, 1966.
"Drug addiction. The addict as an inpatient," by Rohde, I.M. AMERICAN JOURNAL OF NURSING. 63:61-66, 1963.
"Drug addicts in a therapeutic community. Outline on the California Rehabilitation Center Program, Corona," by Fischmann, V.S. INTERNATIONAL JOURNAL OF THE ADDICTIONS. 3:351-359, Spring, 1968; also PSYCHOTHERAPY AND PSYCHOSOMATICS. 15(1):21, 1967.
"Drug addicts need medicine not punishment." SCIENCE NEWS LETTER. 84:4, July 6, 1963.
"Drug dependency research--expensive luxury or necessary commodity?" by Paulus, I. CANADIAN NURSE. 63:36-38, Mar., 1967.
"Drug dependency units." NURSING TIMES. 64:1145-1146, Aug. 23, 1968.
"Drug treatment centres." BRITISH MEDICAL JOURNAL. 2: 455-456, May 20, 1967.
"Drug withdrawal with promazine hydrochloride," by Rolo, A. NEW YORK STATE JOURNAL OF MEDICINE. 62:1429-1431, 1962.
"Drugs for curing drug addicts," by Vaishnav, J.N. PHARMACEUTIST. 7(4):44-48, 1961.
"An eclectic approach with hypnosis in the therapy of a drug addict," by Goldburgh, S.J. PSYCHOTHERAPY: THEORY, RESEARCH AND PRACTICE. 5(3):189-192, 1968.
"Education is the answer to drug abuse by our young people," by Goddard, J.L. JUNIOR COLLEGE JOURNAL. 38:8-9, Sept., 1967.
"An effective therapeutic procedure for the heroin addict," by Torda, C. PERCEPTUAL AND MOTOR SKILLS. 26(3, pt.1): 753-754, 1968.
"The effects of abstinence and re-training on the chewer of coca-leaf," by Murphy, H.B.M., et al. BULLETIN ON NARCOTICS. 21(2):41-47, Apr.-June, 1969.
"Electric compulsive therapy and the narcotic withdrawal syndrome," by Litwin, E.M. MINNESOTA MEDICINE. 47: 547, 1964.
"Employment status of narcotic addicts one year after hospital discharge," by Baganz, P.C., and Maddux, J.F. PUBLIC HEALTH REPORTS. 80:615-621, 1965.
"Evaluation of narcotics treatment programs," by Dole, V.P., et al. AMERICAN JOURNAL OF PUBLIC HEALTH. 57:2000-2005, Nov., 1967.
"Evolution of group therapy policies with hospitalized drug addicts in the narcotic unit at Central Islip State Hospital," by Brett, S.R., and Villeneuve, A. PSYCHI-

ATRIC QUARTERLY. 37:666-670, 1963.
"The experimental production of narcotic drug effects and
withdrawal symptoms through hypnosis," by Ludwig, A.M.
INTERNATIONAL JOURNAL OF CLINICAL AND EXPERIMENTAL HYP-
NOSIS. 12:1-17, 1964.
"An experimental study in the treatment of narcotic addicts
with cyclazocine, by Martin, W.R., et al. CLINICAL
PHARMACOLOGY AND THERAPEUTICS. 7:455-465, 1966.
"Extended supervision for discharged addict-parolees," by
Konsky, G. FEDERAL PROBATION. 29(1):39-44, 1965.
"Face to face with the drug addict: an account of an inten-
sive group experience," by Kruschke, D., and Stoller,
F.H. FEDERAL PROBATION. 31:47-52, June, 1967.
"Facilities for treatment and rehabilitation of narcotic
drug users and addicts," by Winick, C., et al. AMERI-
CAN JOURNAL OF PUBLIC HEALTH. 57:1025-1033, June, 1967.
"Facts against free narcotic clinics for addicts," by Cleve-
land, G.W. TEXAS JOURNAL OF MEDICINE. 59:309-310, 1963.
"The Federal Bureau of Prisons treatment program for narcot-
ic addicts," by Petersen, M., et al. FEDERAL PROBATION.
33:35-40, June, 1969.
"Few return from drug hell," by Hockman, W.S. EDUCATIONAL
SCREEN AV GUIDE. 46:26-27, Feb., 1967.
"Fighting narcotic bondage and other forms of narcotic dis-
orders," by Rado, S. COMPREHENSIVE PSYCHIATRY. 4:160-
167, 1963.
"Follow-up study of narcotic drug addicts after hospitali-
zation," by Hunt, G.H., and Odoroff, M.E. PUBLIC HEALTH
REPORTS. 77:41-54, Jan., 1962.
"Follow-up study of narcotic drug addicts five years after
hospitalization," by Duvall, H., et al. PUBLIC HEALTH
REPORTS. 78:185-193, Mar., 1963.
"Forty years of the campaign against narcotic drugs in the
United Arab Republic," by Hadka, A. BULLETIN ON NARCOT-
ICS. 17(4):1-12, 1965.
"Good medical practice in the care of the narcotic addict:
a report prepared by a special committee appointed by
the Executive Committee of the Canadian Medical Associa-
tion," by Ferguson, D.K., et al. CANADIAN MEDICAL AS-
SOCIATION JOURNAL. 92:1040-1043, 1965.
"Group hypnotherapy techniques with drug addicts," by Lud-
wig, A.M., et al. INTERNATIONAL JOURNAL OF CLINICAL AND
EXPERIMENTAL HYPNOSIS. 12:53-66, 1964.
"Group psychotherapy and the nature of drug addiction," by
Zucker, A.H. INTERNATIONAL JOURNAL OF GROUP PSYCHOTHER-
APY. 11:209-218, 1961.
"Group therapy and hospitalization of narcotic addicts,"
by Blachly, P.H., et al. ARCHIVES OF GENERAL PSYCHIATRY.
5:393-396, 1961.
"Group therapy with parents of adolescent drug addicts,"
by Hirsch, R. PSYCHIATRIC QUARTERLY. 35:702-710, 1961.
"Group therapy with young drug addicts--the addicts' point
of view," by Glatt, M.M. NURSING TIMES. 63:519-520,
Apr. 21, 1967.

177

"Growing drive against drugs. U.S. NEWS AND WORLD REPORT. 67(24):38-40, Dec. 15, 1969.
"Halfway house and mental hospital: some comparisons," by Rothwell, N.D., and Doniger, J. PSYCHIATRY. 26(3): 281-288, 1963.
"Halfway house for narcotic addicts," by Geis, G. BRITISH JOURNAL OF ADDICTION. 61(1):79-89, 1965.
"The Harrison act and drug addiction: scientific treatment of this disease, not criminal prosecution, is the answer," by Gassman, B. BAR BULLETIN. 22(1):22-27, 1964.
"Help for the addict," by Ramirez, E. AMERICAN JOURNAL OF NURSING. 67(11):2348-2353, Nov., 1967.
"The helping process in a hospital for narcotic addicts," by Berliner, A.K. FEDERAL PROBATION. 26:57-62, Sept., 1962.
"Heroin dependence. A community experiment in therapeutics," by Myers, K. LANCET. 1:805-806, Apr. 13, 1968.
"Hong Kong's prison for drug addicts." BULLETIN ON NARCOTICS. 13:13-20, Jan.-Mar., 1961.
"Hospital treated adolescent drug users: a follow-up study," by Alksne, H. HEALTH NEWS. 37:10-19, Aug., 1960.
"The hospitalized narcotic addict," by Gorwitz, K. MARYLAND MEDICAL JOURNAL. 14:143, 1965.
"Houston's halfway house." REHABILITATION RECORD. 7:22-23, May-June, 1966.
"How a health council developed a narcotics education program; Copiaque schools of Long Island, New York," by Marx, S.H. JOURNAL OF SCHOOL HEALTH. 38:243-246, Apr., 1968.
"How to cope with drug addiction in hospitals," by Krantz, J.C. MODERN HOSPITAL. 94:66-68, 1960.
"How to help an addict." THE ATTACK ON NARCOTIC ADDICTION AND DRUG ABUSE. 3:4, Winter, 1969.
"Identification of and treatment of barbiturate abusers," by Hamburger, E. JOURNAL OF THE AMERICAN MEDICAL ASSOCIATION. 193:393-394, 1965.
"Immediate action on young Swedish drug-takers," by Burke, P.E. TIMES (London) EDUCATIONAL SUPPLEMENT. 2712:1602, May 12, 1967.
"In the course of professional practice," by Dole, V. NEW YORK STATE JOURNAL OF MEDICINE. pp. 927-931, April, 1965.
"The Institute for the Study of Drug Dependence, London." BULLETIN ON NARCOTICS. 20(3):30, July-Sept., 1968.
"The institutional treatment of the narcotic addict," by Rasor, R.W. JOURNAL OF THE MISSISSIPPI STATE MEDICAL ASSOCIATION. 6:11-14, 1965.
"Institutional treatment of narcotic addiction by the U. S. Public Health Service," by Rasor, R.W., and Maddux, J.F. HEALTH, EDUCATION AND WELFARE INDICATORS. pp. 11-24, Mar., 1966.
"Job placement of addicts through a halfway house," by Wiener, F., et al. REHABILITATION RECORD. 8:12-15, Jan.-Feb., 1967.

"Kicking the habit." TIME. 93:70, Jan. 17, 1969.
"Laboratory control in the treatment of the narcotic addict," by Kurlan, A.A., et al. CURRENT PSYCHIATRIC
THERAPIES. 6:243-246, 1966.
"Less dangerous substitutes urged for addictive drugs,"
by Cass, L.J. HARVARD LAW RECORD. 40:1-2, 1965.
"Lessons from the Anti-narcotic Voluntary Treatment Programme in Hong Kong," by Yap, P.M. BULLETIN ON NARCOTICS. 19(2):35-43, Apr.-June, 1967.
"The Lexington program for narcotic addicts," by O'Donnell,
J.A. FEDERAL PROBATION. 26:55-60, Mar., 1962.
"Love needs care; clinic devoted exclusively to helping
hippies with health problems." NEWSWEEK. 70:98, July
17, 1967.
"An MMPI factor analytic study of alcoholics, narcotic addicts and criminals," by Hill, H.E., et al. QUARTERLY
JOURNAL OF STUDIES ON ALCOHOL. 23:411-431, 1962.
"Management of drug habituation," by Tingle, D. JOURNAL
OF THE FLORIDA MEDICAL ASSOCIATION. 55:32-36, Jan., 1968.
"Management of narcotic-drug dependence by high-dosage methadone HCl technique; Dole-Nyswander program." JOURNAL
OF THE AMERICAN MEDICAL ASSOCIATION. 201:956-957, Sept.
18, 1967.
"The management of pathologic interdependency in drug addiction," by Little, R.B., et al. AMERICAN JOURNAL OF
PSYCHIATRY. 123:554-560, Nov., 1966.
"Management of the opiate abstinence syndrome," by Blachly,
P.H. AMERICAN JOURNAL OF PSYCHIATRY. 122:742-744, 1966.
"The Marathon group: intensive practice of intimate interaction," by Bach, G.R. PSYCHOLOGICAL REPORTS. 18:995-
1002, 1966.
"Maturing out of narcotic addiction," by Winick, C. BULLETIN ON NARCOTICS. 14(1):1-7, 1962.
"Measures against drug addiction." BRITISH MEDICAL JOURNAL. 1:319-320, Feb. 11, 1967.
"Medic says Ray Charles has kicked dope, wife is happy (I),"
by Brown, C.E. JET. 29:60-61, 1965
"Medical perspectives on habituation and addiction," by
Seevers, M.H. JOURNAL OF THE AMERICAN MEDICAL ASSOCIATION. 181:92-98, 1962.
"Medical Society's Recommendation. Maintain addicts on
drugs if necessary, but only under proper controls."
BULLETIN (New York State District Branches, American
Psychiatric Association). 8(2):10, 1965.
"A medical treatment of diacetylmorphine (heroin) addiction. A clinical trial with methadone hydrochloride,"
by Dole, V.P., and Nyswander, M. JOURNAL OF THE AMERICAN MEDICAL ASSOCIATION. 193(8):646-650, 1965.
"Medicine and law in the treatment of drug addiction," by
Lowry, J.V., and Simrell, E.V. BULLETIN ON NARCOTICS.
15(3-4):9-16, July-Dec,, 1963.
"The medico-legal conflict," by Ostrow, S. AMERICAN JOURNAL OF NURSING. 63:67-71, July, 1963.
"Medicolegal issues in the care of addicts," by Cameron,

179

D.C. ANNALS OF INTERNAL MEDICINE. 67:209-210, July, 1967.
"Menstrual function and pregnancy in narcotics addicts treated with methadone," by Blinick, G. NATURE. 219: 180, July 13, 1968.
"Methadone blocks craving for heroin." AMERICAN DRUGGIST. 154:41, Sept. 26, 1966.
"Methadone in the relief of pain - a clinical note," by Frelick, R.W. DELAWARE MEDICAL JOURNAL. 39:297-298, 1967.
"A model continuum for a community-based program for the prevention and treatment of narcotic addiction," by Freedman, A.M., et al. AMERICAN JOURNAL OF PUBLIC HEALTH. 54:791-802, May, 1964.
"Modern treatment of drug addiction," by Maddux, J.F. CURRENT PSYCHIATRY AND THERAPEUTICS. 4:113-119, 1964.
"My birthday is not the day I was born," by Jones A. AMERICAN JOURNAL OF NURSING. 67:1434-1438, July, 1967.
"The narcotic addict in prison--aspects of compulsory treatment," by Holmes, S.J. ADDICTIONS. 11:38-45, 1964.
"Narcotic addict rehabilitation," by Rubin, M.M. ILLINOIS MEDICAL JOURNAL. 130:494-499, Oct., 1966.
"The narcotic addict. Some reflections on treatment," by Kurland, A.A. MARYLAND STATE MEDICAL JOURNAL. 15:37-39, 1966.
"Narcotic Addiction Control Commission (of New York State) guides freshman orientation on drug abuse program." THE ATTACK ON NARCOTIC ADDICTION AND DRUG ABUSE. 3(4): 9, Fall, 1969.
"Narcotic addiction in physicians; medical and legal aspects of rehabilitation," by Quinn, W.F. BULLETIN ON NARCOTICS. 15(1):11-13, Jan.-Mar., 1963.
"Narcotic addiction is reversible," by Antell, M.J. ST. VINCENT HOSPITAL MEDICAL BULLETIN. 6:37-40, 1964.
"Narcotic addiction, the institution and the community," by Berliner, A.K. INTERNATIONAL JOURNAL OF THE ADDICTIONS. 1(1):74-85, 1966.
"Narcotic addiction--theory of enforced hospitalization challenged by New York City expert," by Berger, H. MEDICAL TRIBUNE AND MEDICAL NEWS. Sept. 6, 1965.
"Narcotic and dangerous drug problems. Current status of legislation, control and rehabilitation," by Quinn, W.F. CALIFORNIA MEDICINE. 106:108-111, Feb., 1967.
"Narcotic antagonists." BULLETIN ON NARCOTICS. 20(4):8, Oct.-Dec., 1968.
"Narcotic blockade," by Dole, V.P., et al. ARCHIVES OF INTERNAL MEDICINE (Chicago). 118:304-309, Oct., 1966.
"Narcotic blockade--a medical technique for stopping heroin use by addicts," by Dole, V.P., et al. TRANSACTIONS OF THE ASSOCIATION OF AMERICAN PHYSICIANS. 79:122-136, 1966.
"Narcotic drug addiction: one year's experiences at Pilgrim State Hospital," by Rice, J., and Cohen, L. PSYCHIATRIC QUARTERLY. 39(3):457-465, 1965.
"Narcotic guidance councils move toward hundred mark." THE

ATTACK ON NARCOTIC ADDICTION AND DRUG ABUSE. 3(4):9, Fall, 1969.
"Narcotic prevention, and early treatment," by McGee, R.A. CALIFORNIA YOUTH AUTHORITY QUARTERLY. 17(4):3-11, 1964.
"Narcotic tools of addiction ... of control," by Giordano, H.L. AMERICAN PROFESSIONAL PHARMACIST. 33:30-35, 1967.
"Narcotic withdrawal reaction in a newborn infant due to codeine (experience and reason - briefly recorded)," by Van Leeuwen, G., et al. PEDIATRICS. 36(4):635-636, 1965.
"Narcotic withdrawal syndrome. Suppression of by means of electric convulsive therapy," by Kelman, H. MINNESOTA MEDICINE. 47:525-527, 1964.
"The narcotic addict in the general hospital," by Freedmam, A.M. MENTAL HOSPITALS. 16:230-232, 1965.
"Narcotics and medical practice - medical use of morphine and morphine-like drugs and management of persons dependent on them." JOURNAL OF THE AMERICAN MEDICAL ASSOCIATION. 202(3):209-212, 1967.
"Narcotics and nalline: six years of testing," by Brown, Thorvald T. FEDERAL PROBATION. 27:27-32, June, 1963.
"Narcotics, treatment and crime," by Curran, W.J. NEW ENGLAND JOURNAL OF MEDICINE. 271:309-310, 1964.
"The naval medical officer as a psychiatric patient," by Arthur, R.J. AMERICAN JOURNAL OF PSYCHIATRY. 122:290-294, 1965.
"Needed: a dose of the ABC's." NEW YORK STATE EDUCATION. 56:30-31, Dec., 1968.
"New approach to treatment of the narcotic addict," by Gutman, J.L. CORRECTIONAL REVIEW. Nov.-Dec., 1965, pp. 10-12.
"New approaches to the narcotic problem. The treatment of the addict in Britain," by Schur, E.M. BULLETIN OF THE NEW YORK ACADEMY OF MEDICINE. 40:286-291, 1964.
"New approaches to the treatment of drug addiction," by Jones, G.L. JOURNAL OF THE MEDICAL SOCIETY OF NEW JERSEY. 64:85-88, Feb., 1967.
"New developments at the Fort Worth Hospital," by Kieffer, S.N. REPORT OF THE INSTITUTE ON REHABILITATION OF THE NARCOTIC ADDICT, Feb., 1966, Washington, D.C. Government Printing Office, 1967, pp. 79-82.
"New developments at the Lexington Hospital," by Jurgensen, W.P. REPORT OF THE INSTITUTE ON REHABILITATION OF THE NARCOTIC ADDICT, Feb., 1966, Washington, D.C. Government Printing Office, 1967, pp. 83-86.
"New Hope for drug addicts," by Berg, R.H. LOOK. Nov.30, 1965, pp. 23-27.
"New horizons in the treatment of narcotic addiction," by Diskind, M.H. FEDERAL PROBATION. 24:56-63, Dec., 1960.
"A new morphine antagonist." BULLETIN ON NARCOTICS. 20 (2):55, Apr.-June, 1968.
"New penitentiary at Matsqui, B.C., for drug addicts," by Smibert, D. WESTERN PHARMACY. 35:8-10, 1966.
"New program offers hope for addicts," by Wood, R.W. FED-

ERAL PROBATION. 28(4):40-45, 1964.
"New treatments for heroin addiction." BRITISH MEDICAL
JOURNAL. 2:588, June 3, 1967.
"The Norwegian State Clinic for the Treatment of Addicts,"
by Teigen, A. BULLETIN ON NARCOTICS. 16:13-22, Oct.-
Dec., 1964.
"Nursing the drug addict," by Owens, J., et al. NURSING
TIMES. 64:584-585, May 3, 1968.
"Observations on drug addicts in a house of detention for
women," by Brummit, H. CORRECTIVE PSYCHIATRY AND JOUR-
NAL OF SOCIAL THERAPY. 9(2):62-70, 1963.
"Occupational characteristics of negro addicts," by Bates,
W.M. INTERNATIONAL JOURNAL OF THE ADDICTIONS. 3:345-
350, Spring, 1968.
"The official position of the Federal Bureau of Narcotics
on handling narcotic addicts," by Giordano, H.L. AMER-
ICAN PROFESSIONAL PHARMACIST. 30(1):24-29, 1964.
"On the fringe," by Ross, J. [interview ed. H. Frankel].
SATURDAY REVIEW OF LITERATURE. 51:23-24, July 6, 1968.
"One year's work at a centre for the treatment of addicted
patients," by Chapple, P.A., et al. LANCET. 1:908-911,
Apr. 27, 1968.
"Ontario physicians view the addict patient," by Lang, V.
ADDICTIONS. 12(3):32-33, 1965.
"Out-of-doors prison built by prisonners: reforming the
Hong Kong drug addicts." ILLUSTRATED LONDON NEWS. 245:
20-21, July 4, 1964.
"Outpatient treatment of heroin addiction," by Merry, J.
LANCET. 1:205-206, Jan. 28, 1967.
"Partner in progress." THE ATTACK ON NARCOTIC ADDICTION
AND DRUG ABUSE. 3(4):10, Fall, 1969.
"Past, present and future in the treatment of drug addic-
tion," by Bowman, K.M. COMPREHENSIVE PSYCHIATRY. 4:
145-149, June, 1963.
"The patient at Mountcollins: an institution for the treat-
ment of addiction," by Levy, A. SOUTH AFRICAN MEDICAL
JOURNAL. 37:738-740, 1963.
"Pentecostals and drug addiction; teen challenge centers,"
by McDonnell, K. AMERICA. 118:402-406, Mar. 30, 1968,
"Pharmacologic factors in relapse and the possible use of
the narcotic antagonists in treatment," by Martin, W.R.
ILLINOIS MEDICAL JOURNAL. 130:489-494, Oct., 1966.
"The Phiadelphia Parole Narcotics Project," by Konietzko,
K.C. AMERICAN JOURNAL OF CORRECTION. 28(2):12-14, 1966.
"The physician in treatment of drug addiction," by Kruse,
H.D. ARCHIVES OF GENERAL PSYCHIATRY. 10:333, 1964.
"Postwithdrawal treatment of narcotics addiction at Lex-
ington." WHAT'S NEW. 221:11-17, 1960.
"Predicting type of discharge from a narcotic detoxifica-
tion service," by Fortunado, M., et al. INTERNATIONAL
JOURNAL OF THE ADDICTIONS. 1:124-130, 1966.
"Preliminary experiences of a pilot project in drug addic-
tion," by Brill, L. SOCIAL CASEWORK. 42(1):28-32, 1961.
"The present status of methadone blockade treatment," by

Nyswander, M., and Dole, V.P. AMERICAN JOURNAL OF PSY-
CHIATRY. 123(11):1441-1442, 1967.
"Problems in the group treatment of drug addicts in the
community: observations on the formation of a group,"
by Laskowitz, D., et al. INTERNATIONAL JOURNAL OF THE
ADDICTIONS. 3:361-379, Spring, 1968.
"Problems of inpatient treatment of addiction," by Jurgen-
sen, W.P. INTERNATIONAL JOURNAL OF THE ADDICTIONS.
1(1):62-73, 1966.
"The program of the New York State Department of Mental Hygiene in the field of drug addiction," by Meiselas, H.
COMMITTEE ON DRUG ADDICTION AND NARCOTICS. Appendix 20:
4262-4266, 1965.
"A proposed method for ambulatory treatment of narcotic
addicts using a long-acting orally effective narcotic
antagonist, cyclazocine. An experimental study," by
Martin, W.R., et al. COMMITTEE ON DRUG ADDICTION AND
NARCOTICS. Appendix 25:4289-4301, 1965.
"Psychiatric treatment of the alienated college student,"
by Halleck, S.L. AMERICAN JOURNAL OF PSYCHIATRY. 124:
642, Nov., 1967.
"Psychiatry: mutual aid to prison," by Diederich, C. TIME.
82(1); March 1, 1963.
"Psychiatry -- office problems. VI. Treatment of alcoholism and drug addiction in the office," by Garner, H.H.
AMERICAN PRACTITIONER AND DIGEST OF TREATMENT. 12:21-
25, 1961.
"A psychopharmacologic experiment in a training school for
delinquent boys: methods, problems, findings," by Eisen-
bert, L., et al. AMERICAN JOURNAL OF ORTHOPSYCHIATRY.
33(3):431-447, 1963.
"The psychotherapeutic agents," by Rossi, G.V. AMERICAN
JOURNAL OF PHARMACOLOGY AND EXPERIMENTAL THERAPEUTICS.
136:6-24, 1964.
"Psychotherapy of successful musicians who are drug addicts,"
by Winick, C., and Nyswander, M. AMERICAN JOURNAL OF
ORTHOPSYCHIATRY. 31:622-636, 1961.
"Public health laboratory in the fight against narcotic ad-
diction in Iran," by Olszyna-Marzys, A.E. BULLETIN ON
NARCOTICS. 15(2):27-34, 1963.
"Rational authority and the treatment of narcotics offend-
ers," by Lieberman, L., and Brill, L. BULLETIN ON NAR-
COTICS. 20(1):33-37, Jan.-Mar., 1968.
"Rebels - with a cause; a report on synanon," by Mueller,
E.E. AMERICAN JOURNAL OF PSYCHOTHERAPY. 18:272-284,
Apr., 1964.
"Rehabilitation and the narcotic addict: results of a com-
parative methadone withdrawal program," by Paulus, I.,
et al. CANADIAN MEDICAL ASSOCIATION JOURNAL. 96:655-
659, Mar. 18, 1967.
"Rehabilitation for the addict." THE ATTACK ON NARCOTIC
ADDICTION AND DRUG ABUSE. 3:10-11, Winter, 1969.
"Rehabilitation of heroin addicts after blockade with meth-
adone," by Dole, V.P., and Nyswander, M. NEW YORK STATE

JOURNAL OF MEDICINE. 66:2011-2017, 1966.
"Rehabilitation of narcotics addicts among lower-class
teenagers," by Levitt, L. AMERICAN JOURNAL OF ORTHO-
PSYCHIATRY. 38(1):56-62, 1968.
"Rehabilitation of the narcotic addict," by Raskin, H.A.
JOURNAL OF THE AMERICAN MEDICAL ASSOCIATION. 189:956-
958, 1964.
"Rehabilitation of the street addict," by Dole, V.P., et
al. ARCHIVES OF ENVIRONMENTAL HEALTH. 14:477-480, Mar.,
1967.
"Rehabilitation on a city street." ARCHITECTURAL FORUM.
129:62-65, Oct., 1968.
"The rehabilitative effectiveness of a community correc-
tional residence for narcotic users," by Fisher, S.
JOURNAL OF CRIMINAL LAW, CRIMINOLOGY, AND POLICE SCIENCE.
56(2):190-196, 1965.
"The relevancy of some newer American treatment approaches
to England," by Brill, L., et al. BRITISH JOURNAL OF
ADDICTION. 62:375-386, Dec., 1967.
"Report of a conference on narcotic addiction,' by Maddux,
J.F. REHABILITATION RECORD. 7:7-15, 1966.
"Response of adult heroin addicts to a total therapeutic
program," by Freedman, A.M., et al. AMERICAN JOURNAL
OF ORTHOPSYCHIATRY. 33(5):890-899, 1963.
"Result of the treatment of severe forms of acute barbit-
urate poisoning," by Dobronravov, A.S., et al. KLIN-
ICHESKAYA MEDITSINA. 43:139-142, 1965.
"Return to living," by Pillai, K.S.C. FAR EASTERN ECONOM-
IC REVIEW. 42:625-627, Dec. 19, 1963.
"A review of contemporary management of narcotic addiction,"
by Martin, M., and Dancey, T.E. CANADIAN MEDICAL ASSOC-
IATION JOURNAL. 86:326-328, 1962.
"A review of pharmacologic agents used in a physical med-
icine and rehabilitation setting," by Forster, S., and
Benton, J.G. ARCHIVES OF PHYSICAL MEDICINE AND REHABIL-
ITATION. 45:277-282, 1964.
"The role of compulsory supervision in the treatment of ad-
diction," by Vaillant, G.E., and Rasor, R.W. FEDERAL
PROBATION. 30:53-59, June, 1966.
"The role of the ex-addict in treatment of addiction," by
Deitch, D., and Casriel, D. FEDERAL PROBATION. 31:
45-47, Dec., 1967.
"S.S. hang tough; synanon system," by Schneider, J. TIME.
77:72+, Apr. 7, 1961; also PROGRESSIVE. 28:32-34, Feb.,
1964.
"A second look at the New York State Parole Drug Experiment,"
by Diskind, M.H. FEDERAL PROBATION. 28:34-41, Dec.,
1964.
"Services for the prevention and treatment of dependence on
alcohol and other drugs - Fourteenth Report of the World
Health Organization Expert Committee on Mental Health."
BULLETIN ON NARCOTICS. 19(3):47-55, July-Sept., 1967.
"Some trends in the treatment and epidemiology of drug addiction: psychotherapy and synanon," by Sabath, G. PSY-

CHOTHERAPY: THEORY, RESEARCH AND PRACTICE. 4(2):92-
96, 1967.
"State Commission provides help for narcotic addicts."
THE ATTACK ON NARCOTIC ADDICTION AND DRUG ABUSE. 3:5,
Spring, 1969.
"A state hospital program for alcoholism and drug addic-
tion," by Eiden, V.M. LANCET. 82:499-502, 1962.
"Stoned on methadone; disagreement over Dole-Nyswander
treatment; with excerpts from interview with synanon
staff," by Yablonsky, L. NEW REPUBLIC. 155:14-16,
Aug. 13, 1966.
"Structural handicaps to therapeutic participation: a case
study," by Tittle, C.R., and Tittle, D.P. SOCIAL PRO-
BLEMS. 13:75-82, Summer, 1965.
"Studies on 300 Indian drug addicts with special reference
to psychosociological aspects, etiology and treatment,"
by Chopra, G.S., and Chopra, P.S. BULLETIN ON NARCOTICS.
17:1-9, 1965.
"A study of employee attitudes toward patients in a hospi-
tal for the treatment of drug addiction," by Levitt,
L.I., et al. PSYCHIATRIC QUARTERLY. 37:210-219, 1963.
"Study of methadone as an adjunct in rehabilitation of her-
oin addicts," by Dole, V.P., et al. ILLINOIS MEDICAL
JOURNAL. 130:487-489, Oct., 1966.
"Successful treatment of amphetamine addiction in a schizo-
phrenic woman," by Seelye, E.E. AMERICAN JOURNAL OF
PSYCHOTHERAPY. 21:295-301, Apr., 1967.
"Symposium: nonnarcotic addiction, clinical manifestations
and treatment of amphetamine type of dependence," by
Connell, P.H. JOURNAL OF THE AMERICAN MEDICAL ASSOCIA-
TION. 196(8):718-722, 1966.
"Synanon and eupsychia," by Maslow, A.H. JOURNAL OF HUMAN-
ISTIC PSYCHOLOGY. 7(1):28-35, 1967.
"Synanon and the learning process: a critique of attack
therapy," by Walder, E. CORRECTIVE PSYCHIATRY AND JOUR-
NAL OF SOCIAL THERAPY. 11(6):299-304, 1965.
"Synanon, Connecticut: a new way out for drug addicts," by
Anderson, C. MCCALLS. 91(1):R-16-R-18, 1963.
"Synanon Foundation," by Dederich, C. TIME. 77(15), Apr.
7, 1961.
"Synanon Foundation: a radical approach to the problem of
addiction," by Cherkas, M. AMERICAN JOURNAL OF PSYCHI-
ATRY. 121(11):1065-1068, 1965.
"Synanon House: a consideration of its implications for
American correction," by Sternberg, David. JOURNAL OF
CRIMINAL LAW, CRIMINOLOGY AND POLICE SCIENCE. 54:447
455, Dec., 1963.
"Synanon House where drug addicts join to salvage their
lives." LIFE. 52:52-65, Mar. 9, 1962.
"Synanon through the eyes of a visiting psychologist," by
Holzinger, R. QUARTERLY JOURNAL OF STUDIES ON ALCOHOL.
26:304-309, 1965.
"Ten months experience with LSD users admitted to county
psychiatric receiving hospital," by Blumenfield, M.,

and Glickman, L. NEW YORK STATE JOURNAL OF MEDICINE. 67:1849-1853, 1967.

"A therapeutic halfway hostel," by Mikels, E., and Gumrukcu, P. MENTAL HOSPITALS. 14(4):219, 1963.

"Therapeutic recreation for the narcotic addict," by Young, E. JOURNAL OF REHABILITATION. 30(1):23-24, 1964.

"A therapeutic waiting area experience for alcoholics and drug addicts," by Armstrong, J.C., and Tyndel, M. COMPREHENSIVE PSYCHIATRY. 6(2):137-138, 1965.

"Therapy of drug addiction," by Sharoff, R.L. CURRENT PSYCHIATRIC THERAPIES. 6:247-251, 1966.

"There's no hiding down there," by Janowitz, J. [from DRUGS ON CAMPUS: preventive and therapeutic approaches to illicit drug use, by J. Janowitz]. AMERICAN JOURNAL OF ORTHOPSYCHIATRY. 37:296, 1967.

"Three approaches to the casework treatment of narcotics addicts," by Brill, L. SOCIAL WORK. 13:25-35, Apr., 1968.

"3380 saw dedication of narcotics farm," by Vaughn, N. LEXINGTON HERALD. May 23, 1965.

"Treating addicts humanely," CHRISTIAN CENTURY. 83:131-132, Feb. 2, 1966.

"Treating drug-addiction," by Fink, M., et al. LANCET. 1:;256, June 8, 1968.

"Treating drug dependency." NURSING TIMES. 64:657, May 17, 1968.

"Treating narcotic addicts," by Bates, W. REIGN OF THE SACRED HEART. 36:22-26, 1964.

"Treating young drug users; a casework approach," by Frazier, T.L. SOCIAL WORK. 7:94-101, July, 1962.

"Treatment and control for narcotic addicts." CORRECTIONAL REVIEW. pp. 37-39, Sept.-Oct., 1965.

"Treatment for drug addicts in prison," by Craven, M. LANCET. 1:298, Feb. 10, 1968.

"Treatment in England of Canadian patients addicted to narcotic drugs," by Frankau, Lady. CANADIAN MEDICAL ASSOCIATION JOURNAL. 90:421-424, Feb. 8, 1964.

"The treatment of acute barbiturate poisoning," by Joran, G.E. APPLIED THERAPEUTICS. 3:452-455, 1961.

"The treatment of addiction by aversion conditioning with apomorphine," by Raymond, M.J. BEHAVIOUR RESEARCH AND THERAPY. 1:287-291, 1964.

"Treatment of addiction in British Columbia," by Halliday, R. JOURNAL OF THE AMERICAN MEDICAL ASSOCIATION. 194: 681, 1965.

"Treatment of addicts." BRITISH MEDICAL JOURNAL. 3:692-693, Sept., 16, 1967.

"Treatment of alcoholics and drug addicts by verbal aversion techniques," by Anant, S.S. INTERNATIONAL JOURNAL OF THE ADDICTIONS. 3:381-387, Spring, 1968; also PSYCHOTHERAPY AND PSYCHOSOMATICS. 15(1):6, 1967.

"Treatment of barbiturate poisoning," by Blom, P.S. NEDERLANDS TIJDSCHRIFT VOOR GENEESKUNDE. 108:2506-2510, 1964.

"Treatment of drug addiction." NEW YORK STATE JOURNAL OF MEDICINE. 63:1656-1665, June 1, 1963.
"The treatment of drug addiction," by Frankau, I.M., and Stanwell, P.M. LANCET. 2:1377-1379, 1960.
"The treatment of drug addiction," by Vogel, V.H. JOURNAL OF THE AMERICAN MEDICAL ASSOCIATION. 194:680-681, 1965.
"Treatment of drug addiction in a community general hospital," by Freedman, A.M. COMPREHENSIVE PSYCHIATRY. 4: 199-207, June, 1963.
"The treatment of drug addiction: private practice experience with 84 addicts," by Pearson, M.M., and Little, R.B. AMERICAN JOURNAL OF PSYCHIATRY. 122(2):164-169, 1965.
"Treatment of drug addicts." BRITISH MEDICAL JOURNAL. 4:627, Dec. 9, 1967.
"The treatment of drug addicts in Switzerland," by Kielholz, P., and Battegay, R. COMPREHENSIVE PSYCHIATRY. 4:225-235, June, 1963.
"Treatment of female inebriate patients at Dorothea Dix Hospital," by Rollins, R.L. NORTH CAROLINA MEDICAL JOURNAL. 22:226-227, 1961.
"The treatment of hard-core voluntary drug addict patients," by Sabath, G. INTERNATIONAL JOURNAL OF GROUP PSYCHOTHERAPY. 14(3):307-317, 1964.
"The treatment of heroin addiction," by Dole, V.P., and Nyswander, M. [Letter to the editor]. JOURNAL OF THE AMERICAN MEDICAL ASSOCIATION. 195(11):972, 1966.
"Treatment of heroin addicts in London." BULLETIN ON NARCOTICS. 21(1):29, Jan.-Mar., 1969.
"Treatment of heroin and cocaine addiction," by Frankau, L. NURSING TIMES. pp. 737-739, June 9, 1961.
"Treatment of heroin and cocaine dependence in general practice," by Hewetson, J. NURSING TIMES. 63:516-518, Apr. 21, 1967.
"Treatment of narcotic addiction." NEW ENGLAND JOURNAL OF MEDICINE. 272:693-694, 1965.
"The treatment of narcotic addiction." WESTERN MEDICINE. 6:5, 1965.
"Treatment of narcotic addiction: issues and problems," by Maddux, J.F. REPORT OF THE INSTITUTE ON REHABILITATION OF THE NARCOTIC ADDICT, Feb., 1966, Washington, D.C. Government Printing Office, 1967, pp. 11-22.
"Treatment of narcotic addicts," by Cameron, D.C. TODAY'S HEALTH. 41:12 passim, Oct., 1963.
"Treatment of narcotic addicts in private practice," by Berger, H. ARCHIVES OF INTERNATIONAL MEDICINE. 114: 59-66, 1964.
"Treatment of narcotic addicts on open wards." JOURNAL OF THE TENNESSEE MEDICAL ASSOCIATION. 60:948-952, Sept., 1967.
"The treatment of narcotic poisoning," by Clemmesen, C. MEDICAL SCIENCE. 14(6):74-82, 1963.
"Treatment of narcotic withdrawal symptoms with thioridazine," by Mulvaney, R.B. DISEASES OF THE NERVOUS SYSTEM. 27:329-330, 1966.

"The treatment of narcotics addiction," by Osnos, R.J.
NEW YORK STATE JOURNAL OF MEDICINE. 63:1182-1185, 1963.
"The treatment of narcotism in Mississippi," by Jaquith,
W.L. JOURNAL OF THE MISSISSIPPI STATE MEDICAL ASSOCIA-
TION. 6:15-17, 1965.
"Treatment of patients addicted to narcotic drugs," by
Halliday, R. CANADIAN MEDICAL ASSOCIATION JOURNAL.
90:937-938, 1964.
"Treatment of severe barbiturate poisoning by beta-ethyl-
beta-methyl-glutarimide [megimidebeme-gride]," by Alamel,
P., and Geoffroy, H. MOROCCAN MEDICINE. 42:148-149,
1963.
"A treatment program for the drug-dependent patient," by
St. Pierre, C.A. SOCIAL WORK. 14(4):98-105, Oct., 1969.
"Trends in admissions to a state hospital," by Oltman, J.E.,
and Friedman, S. ARCHIVES OF GENERAL PSYCHIATRY. 13:
544-551, 1965.
"Trial and failure of the ambulatory treatment of (opiate)
drug addiction in the United States," by Harney, M.L.
BULLETIN ON NARCOTICS. 16:29-40, Apr.-June, 1964.
"Turning off; encounter, group therapy program." TIME.
89:90-91, Mar. 31, 1967.
"A twelve-year follow-up of New York narcotic addicts: I.
The relation of treatment to outcome," by Vaillant, G.E.
AMERICAN JOURNAL OF PSYCHIATRY. 122(7):727-737, 1966.
"Twelve year follow-up of New York narcotic addicts. II.
The natural history of a chronic disease," by Vaillant,
G.E. NEW ENGLAND JOURNAL OF MEDICINE. 275:1282-1288,
Dec. 8, 1966.
"A 12-year follow-up of New York narcotic addicts. III.
Some social and psychiatric characteristics," by Vail-
lant, G.E. ARCHIVES OF GENERAL PSYCHIATRY. 15:599-609,
Dec., 1966.
"A twelve-year follow-up of New York narcotic addicts: IV.
Some characteristics and determinants of abstinence,"
by Vaillant, G.E. AMERICAN JOURNAL OF PSYCHIATRY. 123:
573-585, Nov., 1966.
"UCLA treats large number of LSD cases." SCIENCE NEWS LET-
TER. 90:117, Aug. 20, 1966.
"U.S. establishes Drug Information Center." CANADA'S MEN-
TAL HEALTH. 17:44-45, Mar.-Apr., 1969.
"United States Public Health Service Narcotic Hospital,
Lexington, Kentucky." WHAT'S NEW. 220:38-48, 1960.
"Use of diphenoxylate hydrochloride in the withdrawal per-
iod of narcotic addiction: a preliminary report," by
Goodman, A.L. SOUTHERN MEDICAL JOURNAL. 61:313-316,
Mar., 1968.
"The use of drugs in the management of drug dependence,"
by Eddy, N.B. JOURNAL OF THE TENNESSEE MEDICAL ASSOC-
IATION. 60:269-273, Mar., 1967.
"The use of high dosage deprol in alcoholic and narcotic
withdrawal," by Snowl, L., and Rickels, K. AMERICAN
JOURNAL OF PSYCHIATRY. 119:475, 1962.
"The use of narcotic drugs in medical practice and the

medical menagement of narcotic addicts," by AMA Council
on Mental Health. JOURNAL OF THE AMERICAN MEDICAL ASSOC-
IATION. 185:976-982, 1963.
"Use of narcotics in addict therapy," by Halliday, R. CAN-
ADIAN NURSE. 63:39-41, Mar., 1967.
"Utilizing drug-experienced youth in drug education programs;
Silver Lake regional high school, Kingston, Mass.," by
Freedman, M., et al. NATIONAL ASSOCIATION OF SECONDARY
SCHOOL PRINCIPALS BULLETIN. 53:45-51, Sept., 1969.
"A victory against drug addiction," by Shaw, F.H. NEW SCI-
ENTIST. 20(367):532-534, 1963.
"Visit to Narco; federal addiction treatment center, Lex-
ington, Ky," by Samuels, G. NEW YORK TIMES MAGAZINE.
pp. 32-33 passim, Apr. 10, 1966.
"What to tell young people about alcohol and narcotics,"
by Northup, D.W. WEST VIRGINIA MEDICAL JOURNAL. 59
(12):374-377, 1963.
"Why compulsory closed-ward treatment of narcotic addicts?"
by Ausubel, D.P. ILLINOIS MEDICAL JOURNAL. 130:474-
485, Oct., 1966; also PSYCHIATRIC QUARTERLY SUPPLEMENT.
40(2):225-243, 1966.
"Withdrawal from drugs." SCIENCE NEWS LETTER. 84:4, July
6, 1963.
"A word from the commissioner," by Switzer, M.E. REHABIL-
ITATION RECORD. 7:1, 1966.
"Workshop: how to make drug abuse programs more effective."
SCHOOL MANAGEMENT. 13:14+, May, 1969.
"Young drug addict: can we help him?" by Larner, J. ATLAN-
TIC MONTHLY. 215:75-80, Feb., 1965.

NARCOTIC TRADE: Books

Allen, Edward J. MERCHANT OF MENACE. Springfield, Illi-
nois: C.C. Thomas, 1962.
Buckwalter, J.A. MERCHANT OF MISERY. Mountain View, Cal-
ifornia: Pacific Press Pub. Association, 1961.
Khandelwal, I.C., compiler. DRUG AND THERAPEUTIC ENCYCLO-
PAEDIA OF INDIA. Delhi: Rajpal, 1962.
Drug News Weekly. CHANGING PATTERNS IN RETAIL DRUG DIS-
TRIBUTION. New York: Book Division, Fairchild Publi-
cations, 1962.
Harris, Richard. REAL VOICE. New York: Macmillan, 1964.
Geller, Allen, and Boas, Maxwell. DRUG BEAT; a complete
survey of the history, distribution, uses and abuses of
marijuana, LSD, and the amphetamines. New York: Cowles
Book Company, 1969.
Johns Hopkins University Conference on Drugs in Our Society,
1963. DRUGS IN OUR SOCIETY, ed Paul Talalay. Baltimore:
Johns Hopkins Press, 1964.
Moore, Robin. FRENCH CONNECTION: the world's most crucial

narcotics investigation. Boston: Little, Brown, 1969.
Moscow, Alvin. MERCHANTS OF HEROIN; an in-depth portrayal
of business in the underworld. New York: Dial Press,
1968.
New York City Community Council. RESOURCES FOR TREATMENT
OF NARCOTIC ADDICTS IN NEW YORK CITY. New York: Com-
munity Council Directory, 1961.
Olsen, Paul C. MARKETING DRUG PRODUCTS, revised edition.
New York: Topics Publishing Company, 1964.
Roy, Andrew, T. ON ASIA'S RIM. New York: Friendship Press,
1962.
Siragusa, Charles. THE TRAIL OF THE POPPY; behind the mask
of the Mafia, as told to Robert Wiedrich. Englewood
Cliffs, New Jersey: Prentice-Hall, 1966.
United Nations. AIR TRANSPORT IN THE ILLICIT TRAFFIC IN
NARCOTIC DRUGS. New York, 1961.
United Nations. REVIEW OF THE ILLICIT TRAFFIC IN NARCOTIC
DRUGS. New York, 1960.
United Nations. Commission on narcotic drugs, 20th session.
ILLICIT TRAFFIC IN BRAZIL. U.N. Document E-CN.7-R.15-
Add.55, July 30, 1965.
United States. Bureau of Narcotics. TRAFFIC IN OPIUM AND
OTHER DANGEROUS DRUGS (for the year ended Dec.31, 1961).
Washington: Government Printing Office, 1961
_____for the year ended Dec. 31, 1965. Washington:
Government Printing Office, 1966.
_____for the year ended Dec. 31, 1966. Washington:
Government Printing Office, 1967.
United States. Congress. Senate. Committee on Govern-
ment Operations. ORGANIZED CRIME AND ILLICIT TRAFFIC
IN NARCOTICS. Hearings before the Permanent Subcommit-
tee on Investigations of the Committee on Government
Operations, pursuant to Senate resolution 17, 88th Con-
gress. Washington: Government Printing Office, 1963.
United States. Congress. Senate. Committee on Govern-
ment Operations. Permanent subcommittee on Investiga-
tions. ORGANIZED CRIME AMD ILLICIT TRAFFIC IN NARCOT-
ICS; report, together with additional combined views
and individual views. Washington: Government Printing
Office, 1965.

NARCOTIC TRADE: Periodical Literature

"Alarming rise in dope traffic." U.S. NEWS AND WORLD RE-
PORT. 65:43-45, Sept. 2, 1968.
"American confrontation with opium traffic in the Philip-
pines," by Taylor, A.H. PACIFIC HISTORICAL REVIEW.
36:307-324, Aug., 1967.
"Beautiful affair; French police make largest single con-
fiscation of illegal drugs ever brought off." TIME.
84:44+, Oct. 30, 1964.

"Boom in smuggling," by Walker, D.E. NATION. 193:30-31,
July 15, 1961.
"Boys at the Snow Leopard." TIME. 75:35, Feb. 29, 1960.
"Canada: who's got it?" NEWSWEEK. 55:61, May 9, 1960.
"Cornered crook with $3 million worth of heroin." LIFE.
52:40, Jan. 26, 1962.
"Crooked, cruel traffic in drugs," by Brean, H. LIFE.
48:86-98, Jan. 25, 1960.
"Curbing the drug traffic in Britain; plans to change pre-
scription system," by Wenham, B. NEW REPUBLIC. 156:
9-10, Mar. 18, 1967.
"Data on the illicit traffic in cocaines and coca leaves
in South America, with an annex on narcotics control in
Brazil," by Parreiras, D. BULLETIN ON NARCOTICS. 13
(4):33-36, Oct.-Dec., 1961.
"D-men on the road; illegal peddling of amphetamine tablets."
TIME. 89:69, May 5, 1967.
"Dope control." U.S.NEWS AND WORLD REPORT. 67:108, Oct.
20, 1969.
"Dope smuggling diplomats," by Conniff, H.L. POPULAR SCI-
ENCE. 186:100-103, July, 1965.
"Drug addict report held for two years (record of narcotic
traffic in Chicago). EDITOR AND PUBLISHER. 98:58,
Feb. 20, 1965.
"The drug cancer and Hong Kong (sources and distribution
of opium and its derivatives and other addictive drugs),"
by Joss, F. EASTERN WORLD. 19:8-10, Jan., 1965; 19:
16-18, Feb., 1965; 19:14-15, July, 1965.
"Drug trade scores U.N.'s narcotics stand." OIL, PAINT
AND DRUG REPORT. 181:4, Feb. 12, 1962.
"Drug trafficking," by Armstrong, G. JOURNAL OF THE FOR-
ENSIC SCIENCE SOCIETY. 7:2-11, Jan., 1967.
"Drugs dilemma." ECONOMIST. 225:20-21, Oct. 7, 1967.
"Drugs: the synthetic crisis," by Page, B. NEW STATESMAN.
74:109-110, July 28, 1967.
"Fighting illegal drug traffic." WESTERN MEDICINE. 6:
123-125, 1965.
"Hong Kong: its many splendored face," by Boal, S. DINER'S
CLUB MAGAZINE. 14:28-35, Oct., 1963.
"How hazardous are drugs from abroad?" U.S. NEWS AND WORLD
REPORT. 53:4, Dec. 17, 1962.
"Illicit drug trade from North Africa." LISTEN. 13:20-
21 passim, July-Aug., 1960.
"Illicit LSD traffic hurts research efforts." SCIENCE
NEWS LETTER. 89:327, Apr. 30, 1966.
"Illicit traffic - Hong Kong: statement by the Delegation
of the United Kingdom of Great Britain and Northern Ire-
land to the United Nations for the 18th session of the
Commission on Narcotics." UN DOCUMENT E-CM.7-L.262,
1963.
"The illicit traffic in narcotic drugs in southeast asia."
UN DOCUMENT E-CN.7-440, 1963.
"In the diplomat's bags." NEWSWEEK. 41:34, Oct. 17, 1960.
"Interpol fights the narcotic traffic." LISTEN. 16(5):

191

Sept.-Oct., 1963.
"Keeping on the grass," by Coleman, Kate. NEWSWEEK. 70:
48-49, July 24, 1967.
"LBJ and drug traffic; narcotics message." NEW REPUBLIC.
158:11, Feb. 17, 1968.
"Mexicans fight drug traffic from air." AVIATION WEEK AND
SPACE TECHNOLOGY. 74:111+, Jan. 9, 1961.
"The Middle East Narcotics Survey Mission (Sept.-Oct., 1959)
of the United Nations. BULLETIN ON NARCOTICS. 12(4):
37-42, Oct.-Dec., 1960.
"Murderers: the story of the narcotic gangs," by Anslinger
and Oursler, W. [review by A.R.Lindesmith]." NATION.
194:34-35, Jan. 13, 1962.
"Narcotics victory." COMMONWEAL. 75:608, Mar. 9, 1962.
"The opium must go through," by Karnow, S. LIFE. 55:9,
Aug. 30, 1963.
"Opium trade in Szechwan, 1881 to 1911," by Adshead, S.A.M.
JOURNAL OF SOUTHEAST ASIAN HISTORY. 7:93-99, Sept., 1966.
"Pills traffic results in pelting for FDA." OIL, PAINT AND
DRUG REPORT. 187:3 passim, Feb. 15, 1965.
"Regional conferences on the illicit traffic in drugs."
BULLETIN ON NARCOTICS. 12(4):29-36, Oct.-Dec., 1960.
"Scarcity, higher prices,'crooks': effects of crackdown on
drug trade." U.S.NEWS AND WORLD REPORT. 67:48-49, Oct.
13, 1969.
"Seldom seen; illiegal narcotics." TIME. 83:19, Mar. 27,
1964.
"Smuggling: who switched the Tuna?" NEWSWEEK. 73:83-84,
May 12, 1969.
"Speed demons." TIME. 94:18, Oct. 31, 1969.
"Startling increases in drug smuggling," by Rossides, E.T.
U.S.NEWS AND WORLD REPORT. 67:50, Oct. 13, 1969.
"A study of illicit amphetamine drug traffic in Oklahoma
City," by Griffith, J. AMERICAN JOURNAL OF PSYCHIATRY.
123:560-569, Nov., 1966.
"The United Nations and the illicit traffic in narcotic
drugs," by UN Department of Social Affairs. BULLETIN
ON NARCOTICS. 12(4):21-27, 1960.
"U.S. and Mexican officials discuss control of illegal
drug traffic; joint communique, Jan. 5, 1960." UNITED
STATES DEPARTMENT OF STATE BULLETIN. 42:127, Jan. 25,
1960.

NARCOTICS: Books and Essays

Abt, Lawrence E., and Riess, B., editors. PROGRESS IN CLIN-
ICAL PSYCHOLOGY, volume 8. New York: Grune and Stratton,
1969.
Aldrich, M. DRUGS: a seminar. Buffalo: Lemar-Sunyab, 1967.

American Association for Health, Physical Education and Recreation. HOW CAN WE TEACH ADOLESCENTS ABOUT SMOKING, DRINKING, AND DRUG ABUSE? Washington: National Education Association, 1969.
Ban, Thomas A. PSYCHOPHARMACOLOGY. Baltimore: Williams and Wilkins, 1969.
Barber, Bernard. DRUGS AND SOCIETY. New York: Russell Sage Foundation, 1967.
Battista, O. MENTAL DRUGS: chemistry's challenge to psychotherapy. Philadelphia: Chilton, 1960.
Beale, M.A. DANGEROUS DOSES. Washington: Columbia, 1964.
Bill, Keith. SHOT TO HELL. Westwood, New Jersey: F.H. Revell Co., 1967.
Binns, T.B., editor. ABSORPTION AND DISTRIBUTION OF DRUGS. Baltimore: Williams and Wilkins, 1961.
Black, Perry, editor. DRUGS AND THE BRAIN: papers on the action, use and abuse of psychotropic agents. Baltimore: Hopkins, 1969.
Blum, Richard H. "A background history of drugs," SOCIETY AND DRUGS. San Francisco: Jossey-Bass, 1969, pp. 3-23.
Blum, Richard H. DRUGS AND PERSONAL VALUES [based on presentation at the NASPA Drug Education Conference]. Washington, D.C., 1966.
Blum, Richard H. "A history of opium," SOCIETY AND DRUGS. San Francisco: Jossey-Bass, 1969, pp. 45-58.
Blum, Richard H. "Social and epidemiological aspects of psychopharmacology," PSYCHOPHARMACOLOGY, ed C. Joyce. London: Tavistock, 1968, pp. 243-282.
Blum, Richard H., and Wahl, J. "Police views on drug use," UTOPIATES, by R. Blum et al. New York: Atherton Press, 1964, pp. 224-251.
Brown, William R.L., and Hadgraft, J.W. DRUG PRESENTATION AND PRESCRIBING. Oxford: Pergamon Press, 1965.
Buckwalter, J.A. MERCHANT OF MISERY. Mountain View, California: Pacific Press Pub. Association, 1961.
Burger, A.E. DRUGS AFFECTING THE CENTRAL NERVOUS SYSTEM. New York: Dekker, 1968.
Burns, Harold. DRUGS, MEDICINE, AND MAN. New York: Scribner, 1962.
Buse, Renée. THE DEADLY SILENCE. Garden City: Doubleday, 1965.
Cain, Arthur H. YOUNG PEOPLE AND DRUGS. New York: John Day Co., 1969.
California. Department of Justice. Bureau of Criminal Statistics. ADULT DRUG OFFENDERS. Sacramento, California, 1968.
California. Special Study Commission on Narcotics. FINAL REPORT. Sacramento, California, 1961.
Carey, James T. COLLEGE DRUG SCENE. Englewood Cliffs, New Jersey: Prentice-Hall, 1968.
Child Study Association of America. YOUR CHILD AND DRUGS. New York, 1969.
Cohen, Sidney. THE DRUG DILEMMA. New York: McGraw-Hill, 1968.

Cole, Jonathan O., and Wittenborn, J.R. DRUG ABUSE; social and pharmacological aspects. Springfield, Illinois: C.C. Thomas, 1969.
Cooley, Donald G. SCIENCE BOOK OF MODERN MEDICINE. New York: Watts, 1963.
Daniel, R. WOMEN, DOPE AND MURDER. London: Wright and Brown, 1962.
Deneau, G. "Pharmacologic techniques for evaluating addiction liability of drugs," ANIMAL AND CLINICAL PHARMACOLOGIC TECHNIQUES IN DRUG EVALUATION, ed J. Nodine, and P. Siegker. Chicago: Year Book Medical Publishers, 1964, pp. 406-410.
De Ropp, Robert S. DRUGS AND THE MIND. New York: Grove Press, 1960.
Downing, J. "Zihuatanejo: an experiment in trans-personative living," UTOPIATES, by R. Blum et al. New York: Atherton Press, 1964, pp. 142-177.
DRUG AND THERAPEUTIC ENCYCLOPAEDIA OF INDIA, compiled by I.C. Khandelwal. Delhi: Rajpal, 1962.
THE DRUG, THE NURSE, THE PATIENT. Philadelphia: Saunders, 1958+ [quadrennial].
DRUGS. Middletown, Connecticut: American Educational Publications, 1969.
DRUGS AND POISONS, ed William W. Turner, and the editorial staff of the Bancroft-Whitney Company. Rochester, New York: Aqueduct Books, 1965.
DRUGS AND YOUTH: proceedings of the Rutgers Symposium on drug abuse compiled and edited by J.R. Wittenborn, et al. Springfield, Illinois: C.C. Thomas, 1969.
DRUGS IN CURRENT USE, ed Walter Modell. New York: Springer Publishing Company, 1960.
DRUGS OF CHOICE, ed Walter Modell. St. Louis: Mosby, 1960.
Efron, Daniel H., et al, editors. ETHNOPHARMACOLOGIC SEARCH FOR PSYCHOACTIVE DRUGS. Public Health Service Publication no. 1645. Washington: Government Printing Office, 1967.
Eichlenlaub, John E. ALCOHOL, TRANQUILIZERS, SEDATIVES, AND NARCOTICS. New York: Macmillan, 1962.
Eldridge, W.B. NARCOTICS AND THE LAW: a critique of the American experiment in narcotic drug control. New York: New York University Press, 1962.
Evans, W.O. THE SYNERGISM OF AUTONOMIC DRUGS ON OPIATE OR OPIOID-INDUCED ANALGESIA: a discussion of its potential utility and an annotated bibliography. Washington: Unites States Army. Medical Research Laboratory Reports, 1962.
Eysenck, H.J., editor. EXPERIMENTS WITH DRUGS. New York: Pergamon Press, 1963.
Finch, Bernard. PASSPORT TO PARADISE? an account of common naturally occurring drugs and their associated synthetic compounds, some of which are erroneously considered to be a short cut to happiness. New York: Philosophical Library, 1960.
Fishman, W.H. CHEMISTRY OF DRUG METABOLISM. Springfield,

Illinois: C.C. Thomas, 1961.
Foldes, Francis F., et al. NARCOTICS AND NARCOTIC ANTAG-
ONISTS; chemistry, pharmacology, and applications in
anesthesiology and obstetrics. Springfield, Illinois:
C.C. Thomas, 1964.
Fort, J. "The semantics and logic of the drug scene,"
BACKGROUND PAPERS ON STUDENT DRUG INVOLVEMENT, ed C.
Hollander. Washington: United States National Student
Association, 1967, pp. 87-94.
Fort, J. "Social and legal response to pleasure-giving
drugs," UTOPIATES, by R. Blum et al. New York: Grove
Press, 1964, pp. 205-223.
Fort, Joel. "A world view of drugs," SOCIETY AND DRUGS,
by R.H. Blum. San Francisco: Jossey-Bass, 1969, pp.
229-243.
Gaulden, E.C., et al. THE EFFECTS OF DRUGS ON DRIVER PER-
FORMANCE. A paper given at the American Automobile As-
sociation Driver Rehabilitation Conference. Los Angeles,
June 4, 1964.
Gaulden, E.C., et al. SOME OBSERVATIONS ON THE EFFECTS OF
HEROIN ON THE FEMALE REPRODUCTIVE ORGANS. A paper pre-
sented to the American Medical Association Annual Meet-
ing. San Francisco: American Medical Association, Sec-
tion on Obstetrics and Gynecology, 1964.
Geller, Allan, and Boas, Maxwell. THE DRUG BEAT. New York:
Cowles, 1969.
Ginsberg, D. THE OPIUM ALKALOIDS. New York: Interscience
Publishers, 1962.
Glatt, M.M. THE DRUG SCENE IN GREAT BRITAIN. Baltimore:
Williams and Wilkins, 1968.
Goldberg, L, and Havard, J.D.J. RESEARCH ON THE EFFECTS
OF ALCOHOL AND DRUGS ON DRIVER BEHAVIOR AND THEIR IMPOR-
TANCE AS A CAUSE OF ROAD ACCIDENTS; a report of the
O.E.C.D. Research Group. Paris: Organization for Eco-
nomic Cooperation and Development, 1968.
Goldstein, Richard. ONE IN SEVEN: drugs on campus. New
York: Walker and Company, 1966.
Gottschalk, L. "The use of drugs in interrogation," THE
MANIPULATION OF HUMAN BEHAVIOR, ed A.Biderman and H. Zim-
mer. New York: Wiley and Sons, 1961, pp. 96-141.
Govoni, Laura E. DRUGS AND NURSING IMPLICATIONS. New York:
Appleton, 1965.
Greenblatt, Milton, et al. DRUG AND SOCIAL THERAPY IN CHRON-
IC SCHIZOPHRENIA. Springfield, Illinois: C.C. Thomas,
1965.
Gross, Jack, et al. RESPECT FOR DRUGS, COMMUNITY SERVICE
PROGRAM. Washington: United States Justice Department,
Narcotics and Dangerous Drugs Bureau, 1968.
Harvard Health Services. HARVARD REPORT ON DRUGS. Cam-
bridge, 1967.
Hayter, Alethea. OPIUM AND THE ROMANTIC IMAGINATION. Ber-
keley: University Press, 1968.
Helpern, Milton. "Deaths resulting from narcotics: yearly
incidence (Jan. 1, 1950 to Dec., 31, 1963)." Unpublish-

195

ed mimeographed report by the City of New York Chief
Medical Examiner.
Herrick, Arthur D., and Cattell, M., editors. CLINICAL
TESTING OF NEW DRUGS. New York: Revere Publishing Com-
pany, 1965.
Herxheimer, Andrew, editor. SYMPOSIUM ON DRUGS AND SEN-
SORY FUNCTIONS. London: Churchill, 1968.
Hoffman, F. G., and Southworth, H. COLUMBIA-PRESBYTERIAN
THERAPEUTIC TALKS. New York: Macmillan, 1963.
Hollander, Charles, editor. STUDENT DRUG INVOLVEMENT.
Washington: United States National Student Association,
1967.
Holmstedt, B. READINGS IN PHARMACOLOGY. New York: Mac-
millan, 1963.
Hopkins, S.I. DRUGS AND PHARMACOLOGY FOR NURSES. Balti-
more: Williams and Wilkins, 1965.
Hordern, A. "Psychopharmacology: some historical consid-
erations," PSYCHOPHARMACOLOGY: dimensions and perspec-
tives, ed C. Joyce. London: Tavistock, 1968, pp. 95-148.
Houser, Norman W. DRUGS: FACTS ON THEIR USE AND ABUSE.
Glenview, Illinois: Scott, Foresman and Company, 1969.
Hyde, Margaret O., editor. MIND DRUGS. New York: McGraw-
Hill, 1968.
IDENTIFICATION OF DRUGS AND POISONS: symposium at the School
of Pharmacy, University of London, Mar. 20, 1965. Phila-
delphia: Rittenhouse, 1965.
Illinois. Department of Public Instruction. ALCOHOLIC AND
NARCOTICS INSTRUCTION. Springfield, Illinois, 1962.
Illinois. Department of Public Instruction. PROGRAM DE-
VELOPMENT FOR FOUNDATIONS IN ALCOHOL AND NARCOTIC IN-
STRUCTION. Springfield, Illinois, 1963.
Illinois. Department of Public Instruction. SAMPLES OF
MATERIALS ON ALCOHOL AND NARCOTIC EDUCATION, RESULTING
FROM EXPLORATORY STUDIES IN SELECTED ILLINOIS SCHOOLS.
Springfield, Illinois, 1962.
Jacobsen, E. "An analysis of the gross action of drugs on
the central nervous system," MOLECULAR BASIS OF SOME AS-
PECTS OF MENTAL ACTIVITY, ed O. Walaas. London: Academic
Press, 1967, pp. 3-18.
Jeffee, Saul. NARCOTICS: AN AMERICAN PLAN. New York: Paul
S. Eriksson, 1966.
JOHNS HOPKINS UNIVERSITY CONFERENCE ON DRUGS IN OUR SOCIETY,
1963, ed Paul Talalay and J.H. Murnaghan. Baltimore:
Johns Hopkins Press, 1964.
Johnson, George. THE PILL CONSPIRACY. Los Angeles: Sher-
bourne Press, 1967.
Jones, Kenneth L., et al. DRUGS AND ALCOHOL. New York:
Harper, 1969.
Kalow, Werner. PHARMACOGENICS. Philadelphia: Saunders,
1962.
Keane, C.B., and Fletcher, S.H. DRUGS AND SOLUTIONS.
Philadelphia: Saunders, 1965.
Kitzinger, A., and Hill, P.J. DRUG ABUSE: a source book
and guide for teachers. Sacramento: California State

Department of Education, 1957.
Krimm, Irwin F. NARCOTICS AND HAPPINESS. New York: Vintage Press, 1962.
Land, H.W. WHAT YOU CAN DO ABOUT DRUGS AND YOUR CHILD. New York: Hart Publishing Company, 1969.
Laurie, Peter. DRUGS: MEDICAL, PSYCHOLOGICAL AND SOCIAL FACTS. Baltimore: Penguin Books, 1967.
Leech, K., and Jordan, B. DRUGS FOR YOUNG PEOPLE: THEIR USE AND MISUSE. Oxford: The Religious Education Press, 1967.
Levi, Mario, et al. THE EFFECT OF DRUGS ON RESPONSES TO THE RORSCHACH AND BUSS-DURKEE TESTS. A paper given at the California State Psychological Convention, Los Angeles, Dec. 11, 1964.
Lewin, Louis. PHANTASTICA; narcotic and stimulating drugs, their use and abuse. New York: Dutton, 1964.
Lingeman, Richard R. DRUGS FROM A TO Z: A DICTIONARY. New York: McGraw-Hill, 1969.
Louria, D. NIGHTMARE DRUGS. New York: Pocket Books, 1966.
Malitz, Sidney, et al. "A comparison of drug induced hallucinations with those seen in spontaneously occurring psychoses," HALLUCINATIONS, by L. West. New York: Grune and Stratton, 1962, pp. 50-61.
Marin, Peter, et al. PARENT'S GUIDE TO DRUGS. New York: Harper, 1969.
Marrazzi, Amedeo S. "Pharmacodynamics of hallucinations," HALLUCINATIONS, by L. West. New York: Grune and Stratton, 1962, pp. 36-49.
Mason, P. "Drug dependence caused by non-narcotics," ANIMAL AND CLINICAL PHARMACOLOGIC TECHNIQUES IN DRUG EVALUATION, volume II. Chicago: Year Book Medical Publishers, 1967, pp. 383-388.
Maurer, David W., and Vogel, Victor H. NARCOTICS AND NARCOTIC ADDICTION, 3rd edition. Springfield, Illinois: C.C. Thomas, 1967.
Menconi, Leslie. THE NARCOTIC PROBLEM, revised edition. Sacramento: California Department of Justice, Bureau of Narcotic Enforcement, 1962.
Mayler, L., and Peck, Harold M. DRUG INDUCED DISEASES: a symposium organized by the Boerhaave courses for postgraduate medical education, State University, Leyden. Assen, Netherland: Thomas, 1962.
Michaux, Henry. LIGHT THROUGH DARKNESS. New York: Orion Press, 1963.
Mitchell, Alexander Ross Kerr. DRUGS; THE PARENTS' DILEMMA, ed C. Morris. Royston, England: Priory, 1969
Modell, Walter. DRUGS. New York: Time, Inc., 1967.
Moscow, Alvin. MERCHANTS OF HEROIN; an in-depth portrayal of business in the underworld. New York: Dial Press, 1968.
Murphy, J.S. IN QUEST OF ATARAXIA: a background note on the problem of narcotics. Washington: Department of Health, Education and Welfare, 1967.
"Narcotics and drug abuse," THE CHALLENGE OF CRIME IN A

FREE SOCIETY. Washington: Government Printing Office, 1967, pp. 211-231.
National Council for Civil Liberties (London). DRUGS AND CIVIL LIBERTIES. A report. London, 1967.
New Jersey. Committee on narcotic control. SEVENTH REPORT OF STUDY AND RECOMMENDATIONS. Trenton, 1962.
New York (State). Division of Health, Physical Education and Recreation. INSTRUCTION REGARDING NARCOTICS AND HABIT-FORMING DRUGS. Albany, 1960.
New York (State). Division of Parole. AN EXPERIMENT IN THE SUPERVISION OF PAROLED OFFENDERS ADDICTED TO NARCOTIC DRUGS. Final report of the special narcotic project. Albany, 1960.
Paribok, V.P. NARCOTICS AND CELL NARCOSIS IN CHEMOTHERAPY. New York: Consultants Bureau, 1962.
Parks, D.C. NARCOTICS AND NARCOTICS ADDICTION. New York: Carlton Press, 1969.
Polsky, N. HUSTLERS, BEATS AND OTHERS. Chicago: Aldine Publishing Company, 1967.
Popham, R.E., and Schmidt, W. A DECADE OF ALCOHOLISM RE-SEARCH; a review of the research activities of the Alcoholism and Drug Research Foundation of Ontario, 1951-1961. Toronto: University of Toronto Press, 1962.
Poser, M. INTERNATIONAL DICTIONARY OF DRUGS USED IN NEUROLOGY AND PSYCHIATRY. Springfield, Illinois: C.C. Thomas, 1962.
Rathbone, Josephine L. TOBACCO, ALCOHOL AND NARCOTICS. New York: Oxford Book Company, 1962.
Read, D. DRUGS AND PEOPLE. Boston: Allyn and Bacon, 1969.
Rodman, Morton J., and Smith, Dorothy W. "The narcotic analgesics," PHARMACOLOGY AND DRUG THERAPY IN NURSING. Philadelphia: Lippincott, 1968, pp. 146-217.
Schmidt, Jacob E. NARCOTICS, LINGO AND LORE. Springfield, Illinois: C.C. Thomas, 1960.
Schneider, Elisabeth. COLERIDGE, OPIUM AND KUBLA KHAN. New York: Octagon Press, 1966.
Sharoff, Robert L., et al. DOCTOR DISCUSSES NARCOTICS AND DRUG ADDICTION. Chicago: Budlong Press, 1969.
Shepherd, Michael, et al. CLINICAL PSYCHOPHARMACOLOGY. London: English Universities Press, 1968.
Shibutani, Tamotsu. "Society and personality," INTERAC-TIONIST APPROACH TO SOCIAL PSYCHOLOGY. Englewood Cliffs, New Jersey: Prentice-Hall, 1961, pp. 203-204 passim.
Smith, Kline and French Laboratories, Philadelphia. DRUG ABUSE: ESCAPE TO NOWHERE; a guide for educators. Philadelphia: Smith, Kline and French Laboratories in cooperation with the American Association for Health, Physical Education, and Recreation;[distributed by National Education Association, Washington], 1967.
Smith, Kline and French Laboratories, Philadelphia. TEN YEARS' EXPERIENCE WITH THORAZINE, 1954-1964; reference manual, 5th edition. Philadelphia, [c.1964].
Smith, Kline and French Laboratories, Philadelphia. THOR-AZINE R, BRAND OF CHLORPROMAZINE: tranquilizer, antieme-

tic, potentiator, a fundamental drug in both office and hospital practice; reference manual, 4th edition. [Philadelphia, c1961].
Suchman, E. SOCIOLOGY AND THE FIELD OF PUBLIC HEALTH. New York: Russell Sage Foundation, 1963
Surface, William. THE POISONED IVY. New York: Coward-McCann, 1968.
"Symposium on Evaluation of Drug Therapy in Neurologic and Sensory Diseases, University of Wisconsin, 1960," EVAL-UATION OF DRUG THERAPY, PROCEEDINGS, ed Francis M. Foster. Madison: University of Wisconsin Press, 1961.
Talalay, Paul, editor. DRUGS IN OUR SOCIETY. Baltimore: Johns Hopkins Press, 1964.
Taylor, C., editor. WIDENING HORIZONS IN CREATIVITY (5th Utah Creativity Research Conference Proceedings). New York: Wiley and Sons, 1964.
Taylor, Norman. NARCOTICS: NATURE'S DANGEROUS GIFT, revised edition. New York: Dell Publishing Company, 1966.
Time, Inc. THE DRUG TAKERS. New York: Time-Life Books, 1965.
Time, Inc. HOW TO IDENTIFY WHAT DRUGS A TEEN MAY BE TAKING. New York: Time-Life Books, 1966.
Trease, G., and Evans, W. A TEXTBOOK OF PHARMACOGNOSY. London: Bailliere, Tindall and Cassell, 1966.
Turkel, Peter. THE CHEMICAL RELIGION; facts about drugs and teens. Glen Rock, New Jersey: Paulist Press, 1969.
Uhr, L., and Miller, J.G. DRUGS AND BEHAVIOR. New York: John Wiley and Sons, Inc., 1960.
United Nations. ESTIMATED WORLD REQUIREMENTS OF NARCOTIC DRUGS IN 1962. Statement issued by the Supervisory Body under article 5 of the Convention of 13 July 1931 for limiting the manufacture and regulating the distribution of narcotic drugs. New York, 1961.
United Nations. NARCOTIC DRUGS UNDER INTERNATIONAL CONTROL. New York, 1963.
United Nations. Commission on Narcotic Drugs. REPORT OF THE FOURTEENTH SESSION, 27 April-15 May 1959, Economic and Social Council, official records, twenty-eighth session, supplement no. 9. New York, 1961.
United Nations. Commission on Narcotic Drugs. REPORT OF THE SIXTEENTH SESSION, 24 April-10 May 1961, Economic and Social Council, official records, thirty-second session, supplement no. 9. New York, 1961.
United Nations. Commission on Narcotic Drugs. REPORT OF THE EIGHTEENTH SESSION, 29 April-17 May 1963. New York, 1964.
United Nations. Commission on Narcotic Drugs. SUMMARY OF ANNUAL REPORTS OF GOVERNMENTS RELATING TO OPIUM AND OTHER NARCOTIC DRUGS 1959. This summary covers annual reports submitted by governments in accordance with the treaties dealing with the international control of narcotic drugs. New York, 1961.
United Nations. Permanent Central Opium Board. REPORT TO THE ECONOMIC AND SOCIAL COUNCIL ON THE WORK OF THE BOARD

IN 1959. New York, 1960.
--REPORT TO THE ECONOMIC AND SOCIAL COUNCIL ON THE WORK
OF THE BOARD IN 1961. New York, 1961.
United Nations. WORLD HEALTH ORGANIZATION EVALUATION OF
DEPENDENCE-PRODUCING DRUGS: report of a WHO Scientific
Group. New York: WHO Technical Report Series 287:1-25,
1964.
United Nations. World Health Organization Expert Committee
on addiction-producing drugs. ELEVENTH REPORT. New
York: WHO Technical Report Series 211:1-16, 1961.
--TWELFTH REPORT. New York: WHO Technical Report Series
229:1-12, 1962.
--THIRTEENTH REPORT. New York: WHO Technical Report Ser-
ies 273:1-20, 1964.
United States. Congress. Appropriations Subcommittee.
90th Congress. HEARINGS ON THE TREASURY DEPARTMENT,
FEDERAL BUREAU OF NARCOTICS. Washington: Government
Printing Office, 1967.
United States. Congress. Committee on Labor and Public
Welfare. CONTROL OF PSYCHOTOXIC DRUGS. Hearing before
the Subcommittee on Health of the Committee on Labor
and Public Welfare, U.S. Senate. 88th Congress, 2d session, on S. 2628, a bill to protect the public health
by amending the Federal food, drug, and cosmetic act to
regulate the manufacture, compounding, processing, distribution, delivery, and possession of psychotoxic drugs,
Aug. 3, 1964. Washington: Government Printing Office,
1964.
--PSYCHOTOXIC DRUG CONTROL ACT OF 1964: report to accompany S. 2628. WASHINGTON: Government Printing Office,
1964.
United States. Department of Health, Education and Welfare. Food and Drug Administration. THE USE AND MIS-
USE OF DRUGS. Washington: Government Printing Office,
1968.
United States. Department of Health, Education and Wel-
fare. National Institute of Mental Health. HOOKED.
PHS, no. 1610. Washington: Government Printing Office,
1967.
--LSD: SOME QUESTIONS AND ANSWERS. PHS, no. 1828. Wash-
ington: Government Printing Office, 1968.
--MARIHUANA: SOME QUESTIONS AND ANSWERS. PHS, no. 1829.
Washington: Government Printing Office, 1968.
--THE UP AND DOWN DRUGS: AMPHETAMINES AND BARBITURATES.
PHS, no. 1830. Washington: Government Printing Office,
1968.
United States. Interdepartmental Committee on Narcotics.
REPORT TO THE PRESIDENT OF THE UNITED STATES. Washing-
ton: Government Printing Office, 1961.
United States. President's advisory Committee on Narcotic
and Drug Abuse. FINAL REPORT. Washington: Government
Printing Office, 1963.
United States. Treasury Department. Federal Bureau of
Narcotics. ACTIVE NARCOTIC ADDICTS AS OF DEC. 31, 1963.

Annual Tabulation. Washington: Government Printing Office, 1964.
Usdin, Earl, and Efron, Daniel H. PSYCHOTROPIC DRUGS AND RELATED COMPOUNDS. Washington: Public Health Service, United States Department of Health, Education and Welfare; Government Printing Office, 1967.
Vogel, Victor H., and Vogel, Virginia E. FACTS ABOUT NARCOTICS AND OTHER DANGEROUS DRUGS. Chicago: Science Research Associates, 1967.
Waife, Sholom O., and Shapiro, Alvin P. CLINICAL END OF NEW DRUGS. New York: Harper, 1960.
Watt, J., and Breyer-Brandwijk, M. THE MEDICINAL AND POISONOUS PLANTS OF SOUTHERN AND EASTERN AFRICA, second edition. Edinburgh: E & S Livingstone, 1962.
Weinswig, M.H., et al. DRUG ABUSE: A COURSE FOR EDUCATORS. Indianapolis: Butler University Press, 1968.
Welsh, Ashton L. FIXED ERUPTION, A POSSIBLE HAZARD OF MODERN DRUG THERAPY. Springfield, Illinois: C.C. Thomas, 1961.
West, Louis Jolyon, editor. HALLUCINATIONS. New York: Grune and Stratton, 1962.
White House Conference on Narcotic and Drug Abuse. PROCEEDINGS, Sept. 27-28, 1962. Washington: Government Printing Office, 1962.
Williams, J. B. NARCOTICS AND HALLUCINOGENICS: A HANDBOOK, revised edition. New York: Glencoe Press, 1967.
Williams, John B., editor. NARCOTICS. Dubuque, Iowa: William C. Brown, 1963.
Wilner, D.M. and Kassebaum, G., editors. NARCOTICS. New York: McGraw-Hill, 1965.
Wilson, Charles O., and Jones, Tony E. AMERICAN DRUG INDEX. Philadelphia: Lippincott, 1965.
Wisconsin. Division for Children and Youth. NARCOTICS AND YOUTH, by Harvey W. Rowe [revised edition]. Madison, 1961.
Wittenborn, J.R., et al, editors. DRUGS AND YOUTH: PROCEEDING OF THE RUTGERS SYMPOSIUM ON DRUG ABUSE. Springfield, Illinois: C.C. Thomas, 1969.
Wolfe, Tom. ELECTRIC KOOL-AID ACID TEST. New York: Farrar, Straus, 1968.
Yolles, Stanley F. RECENT RESEARCH ON LSD, MARIHUANA, AND OTHER DANGEROUS DRUGS. Statement before the subcommittee on juvenile delinquency of the Committee on the Judiciary, United States Senate, March 6, 1968. Washington: Department of Health, Education and Welfare, 1968.

NARCOTICS: Doctoral Dissertations

Fangman, John Joseph. "The effects of morphine on two forms of experimental pain" (Thesis, unpublished, Fordham University). DISSERTATION ABSTRACTS. 24(2):846-847, 1963.

Harpel, Howard S., Jr. "Fetal malformations induced by
high subcutaneous doses of morphine sulfate in CF-1
mice" (Thesis, unpublished, Temple University). DIS-
SERTATION ABSTRACTS. 28(10-B):4222, 1968.
Luther, Baldev R. "A comparative study of some arousal-
related measures in psychiatric patients and surgical
patients" (Thesis, unpublished, University of Minnesota).
DISSERTATION ABSTRACTS. 27(6-B):2140, 1966.

NARCOTICS: Periodical Literature

General Publications

"Absorption of morphine from opium by porous earthen pots,"
by Ramanathan, V.S., et al. BULLETIN ON NARCOTICS. 17
(4):21-25, Oct.-Dec., 1965.
"Addicting and nonaddicting drugs," by Flick, A.L. JOURNAL
OF THE AMERICAN MEDICAL ASSOCIATION. 194(8):937, 1965.
"Addicting drugs: narcotics and non-narcotics," by Mason,
P. JOURNAL OF THE MOUNT SINAI HOSPITAL, New York. 33:
28-31, Jan.-Feb., 1966.
"The addiction liability of codeine," by Brown, C.T. MIL-
ITARY MEDICINE. 129:1077-1080, 1964.
"Adolescence and drugs," by Feldbeg, M. SCIENCE. 162:307,
Oct. 18, 1968.
"Adverse drug effects available to all." SCIENCE NEWS LET-
TER. 88:326, Nov. 20, 1965.
"Advice on drugs and alcohol." TIMES (London) EDUCATIONAL
SUPPLEMENT. 2673:326, Aug. 12, 1966.
"Alcohol, drugs, and the adolescent," by Glatt, M.M. PUB-
LIC HEALTH. 80:284-294, Sept., 1966.
"Alcohol - narcotics - poison," by Dattoli, J.A. PENNSYL-
VANIA MEDICAL JOURNAL. 68:41-43, 1965.
"America's pill horror," by Roper, W.L. LISTEN. 16(2):
9-10, 1963.
"Anatomy of a project: 'The prohibited plant'." TECHNICAL
ASSISTANCE NEWSLETTER. 2:1-8, May-June, 1963.
"Anti-depressant drugs," by Feldstein, A. THE AMERICAN
BIOLOGY TEACHER. 24:434, Oct., 1962.
"Anti-narcotic testing: a physician's point of view," by
Hurley, C.T. FEDERAL PROBATION. 27(2):32-41, June, 1963.
"Antitussive drugs," by Chappel, C.I., and Von Seemann, C.
PROGRESS IN MEDICAL CHEMISTRY. 3:89-145, 1963.
"Appetite suppressants." BULLETIN ON NARCOTICS. 21(1):
45, Jan.-Mar., 1969.
"Before your kid tries drugs," by Yolles, S.F. NEW YORK
TIMES MAGAZINE. pp. 124 ff, Nov. 17, 1968.
"Begin in kindergarten; teaching respect for drugs." MICH-
IGAN EDUCATION JOURNAL. 46:35, Feb., 1969.

"Botanical sources of the new world narcotics," by Schulters, R.E. PSYCHEDELIC REVIEW. no. 1:157, Feb., 1963.
"The Bureau of Narcotics and American Pharmacy," by Giordano, H.L. MILITARY MEDICINE. 130:763-767, 1965.
"Capsules." RN. 24:24-26, Aug., 1961.
"Carl Koller and cocaine," by Becker, H.K. PSYCHOANALYTIC QUARTERLY. 32:309-373, 1963.
"Carl Koller and cocaine," by Crohn, B.B. JOURNAL OF THE MOUNT SINAI HOSPITAL, New York. 31:430-432, 1964.
"A case of chloral hydrate addiction," by Robinson, J.T. INTERNATIONAL JOURNAL OF SOCIAL PSYCHIATRY. 12:66-71, 1966.
"Central nervous system stimulants in drug abuse," by Knotts, G.R. JOURNAL OF SCHOOL HEALTH. 39:353-356, June, 1969.
"Changing attitudes about drug use and cigarette smoking," by Middendorf, J.L. AUDIOVISUAL INSTRUCTION. 14:55-56, June, 1969.
"Chemical mind-changers," by Coughlan, R. LIFE. 54:81-82+, Mar. 15, 1963.
"Chemical psychoses," by Hollister, L. ANNUAL REVUE OF MEDICINE. 15:203-214, 1964.
"Child on drugs," by Wyden, B.W. NEW YORK TIMES MAGAZINE. p. 63 passim, Aug. 20, 1967.
"The choice of analgesics in general practice," by Craddock, D. PRACTITIONER. 189:192-200, 1962.
"Class A narcotic drugs." JOURNAL OF THE INDIANA STATE MEDICAL ASSOCIATION. 57:688-689, 1964.
"Coca paste. Residues from the industrial extraction of cocaine. Ecgonine and anhydroecgonine," by Toffoli, Francesco, and Avico, Ulstik. BULLETIN ON NARCOTICS. 17(4):27-36, Oct.-Dec., 1965.
"Cocaine tachyphylaxis," by Teeters, W.R., et al. LIFE SCIENCES. 7:509-518, 1963.
"Codeine addiction with death possible due to abrupt withdrawal," by Margolis, J. JOURNAL OF THE AMERICAN GERIATRICS SOCIETY. 15(10):951-953, 1967.
"Codeine to morphine ratio of illicit heroin hydrolysates," by Nakamura, Georges R., and Ukita, Tyunosin. BULLETIN ON NARCOTICS. 15(1):43-44, Jan.-Mar., 1963.
"College guidance on drugs; Columbia University." SCHOOL AND SOCIETY. 95:139, Mar. 4, 1967.
"Conference on narcotics studies liaison of medicine, law." JOURNAL OF THE MEDICAL ASSOCIATION OF THE STATE OF ALABAMA. 36:1156-1157, 1967.
"Consultative group on coca leaf problems," by Avalos Jibaja, Carlos. BULLETIN ON NARCOTICS. 16:25-37, July-Sept., 1964.
"Content and method in controversial areas," by Shimmel, G.M. JOURNAL OF SCHOOL HEALTH. 31:230-235, Sept., 1961.
"Cool talk about hot drugs; misconceptions about heroin, LSD, and marijuana," by Louria, D.B. NEW YORK TIMES MAGAZINE. pp. 12-13 passim, Aug. 6, 1967.
"The cough syrup quagmire," by Taylor, W.J.R. APPLIED THERAPEUTICS. 6:197-206, 1964.

"Counterfeit drug dangers." SCIENCE NEWS LETTER. 78:324, Nov. 12, 1960.
"The criminogenic action of cannabis (marihuana) and narcotics," by Moraes Andrade, Oswald. BULLETIN ON NARCOTICS. 16:23-28, Oct.-Dec., 1964.
"Cultivation of the opium poppy and opium production in Yugoslavia," by Kusevic, V. BULLETIN ON NARCOTICS. 12(2):5-13, Apr.-June, 1960.
"Cyclazocine curbs craving for heroin." AMERICAN DRUGGIST. 156:38, Dec. 4, 1967.
"Dangerous drugs?" NEWSWEEK. 41:74, Jan. 12, 1965.
"Dangerous drugs." SAFETY EDUCATION. 42:14, Jan, 1963.
"The dangerous drug problem." NEW YORK MEDICINE. 22:14, July 20, 1966.
"Deaths from narcotism in New York City. Incidence, circumstances, and postmortem findings," by Helpern, M., and Rho, Y.M. NEW YORK STATE JOURNAL OF MEDICINE. 66: 2391-2408, 1966.
"The development of non-narcotic analgesics," by Cass, L.J., and Frederik, W.S. JOURNAL OF ORAL THERAPEUTICS AND PHARMACOLOGY. 2:107-109, 1965.
"Diagnosis and management of depressant drug dependence," by Ewing, J.A., et al. AMERICAN JOURNAL OF PSYCHIATRY. 123:909-917, Feb., 1967.
"The diagnosis of death from intravenous narcotism. With emphasis on the pathologic aspects," by Siegel, H., et al. JOURNAL OF FORENSIC SCIENCES. 11:1-16, 1966.
"Disciplining drug users; drugs on campus." SCHOOL AND SOCIETY. 95:381, Oct. 28, 1967.
"Dissident youth," by Unwin, J.R. CANADA'S MENTAL HEALTH. 17:4-10, Mar.-Apr., 1969.
"Do nurses spend too much time counting narcotics?" by McKillop, A.R. HOSPITALS. 37:138 passim, 1963.
"Don't dodge the drug questions; stimulants," by Hawkins, M.E. SCIENCE TEACHER. 33:33-34, Nov., 1966.
"Dream drugs: questions and answers." SOCIAL HEALTH NEWS. 38(9):2, 1963.
"A drug abuse project," by Jordan, C. JOURNAL OF SCHOOL HEALTH. 38:692-695, 1968.
"Drug dangers attacked." SCIENCE NEWS LETTER. 86:6, July 3, 1965.
"Drug notes," by McClure, M. EVERGREEN REVIEW. 6:103-117, July-Aug., 1962.
"Drug use in a normal population of young negro men," by Robins, L., and Murphy, G. AMERICAN JOURNAL OF PUBLIC HEALTH. 57:1580-1596, Sept., 1967.
"Drug use on high school and college campuses," by Cwalina, G.E. JOURNAL OF SCHOOL HEALTH. 38:638-646, Dec., 1968.
"Drug use: symptom, disease, of adolescent experimentation - the task of therapy,: by Liebert, R.S. JOURNAL OF THE AMERICAN COLLEGE HEALTH ASSOCIATION. pp. 25-29, Oct., 1967.
"Drugs." SCHOOL MANAGEMENT. pp. 95-107, June, 1966.
"Drugs." TIMES (London) EDUCATIONAL SUPPLEMENT. 2720:33,

July 7, 1967.
"Drugs: a student report," by Lake, Alice. SEVENTEEN. 25:
170-171 passim, Sept., 1966.
"Drugs: a tool for research in psychiatry," by Saunders,
J.C. JOURNAL OF MENTAL SCIENCE. 107:31-39, 1961.
"Drugs and children," by Costello, J.M., et al. NEW ZEALAND
MEDICAL JOURNAL. 67:402-405, Mar., 1968.
"Drugs and delinquency," by Stewart, H., et al. MEDICO-
LEGAL JOURNAL. 33(2):56-71, 1965.
"Drugs and doctors. Problem in the production of certain
behavioral disorders," by Hagedorn, A.B., et al. MINNE-
SOTA MEDICINE. 50:1187-1189, Aug., 1967.
"Drugs and drug addiction: opinions on the taking of 'soft'
drugs." MEDICINE, SCIENCE AND THE LAW. 6:167-168, 1966.
"Drugs and drug addiction: unjust operation of the danger-
ous drugs act." MEDICINE, SCIENCE AND THE LAW. 6:168,
1966.
"Drugs and jazz." TIME. 75:67, May 2, 1960.
"Drugs and mysticism," by Pahnke, W.N. INTERNATIONAL JOUR-
NAL OF PARAPSYCHOLOGY. 8(2):295-314, 1966.
"Drugs and obesity." JOURNAL OF THE AMERICAN MEDICAL ASSOC-
IATION. 204:328-329, Apr. 22, 1968.
"Drugs and pain," by Smith, S.E. NURSING TIMES. 59:1607-
1608, 1963.
"Drugs and people," by Wheeler, R.B. ILLINOIS MEDICAL JOUR-
NAL. 130:512-516, Oct., 1966.
"Drugs and psychiatry." MEDICAL WORLD (London). 93(8):
135-137, 1960.
"Drugs and public opinion: New York State residents speak
out on drug abuse." THE ATTACK ON NARCOTIC ADDICTION
AND DRUG ABUSE. 3(4):3-5, Fall, 1969.
"Drugs and schools: monkey on the backs of educators," by
Weissman, R. MINNESOTA JOURNAL OF EDUCATION. 49:10-
13, Mar., 1969.
"Drugs and the educational process," by Ungerleider, J.T.
THE AMERICAN BIOLOGY TEACHER. 30:625-628, Oct., 1968.
"Drugs and the mind," by Weil, A. HARVARD REVIEW. 1:3-5,
1963.
"Drugs and the young law-breaker," by Gibbens, T.C. MENTAL
HEALTH. 25(3):36-37, 1966.
"Drugs and their abuse," by Barber, G.O. JOURNAL OF THE
ROYAL INSTITUTE OF PUBLIC HEALTH AND HYGIENE. 28:16-
20, 1965
"Drugs and tobacco; films," by Falconer, V. SENIOR SCHOL-
ASTIC. 91(suppl.):15-16, Nov. 16, 1967.
"Drugs and youth." SENIOR SCHOLASTIC. 88:4-7, Apr. 29,
1966.
"Drugs, behavior, and crime," by Blum, R.H. ANNALS OF THE
AMERICAN ACADEMY OF POLITICAL AND SOCIAL SCIENCE. 374:
135-146, Nov., 1967.
"Drugs: caution." NEWSWEEK. 58:75, Aug. 7, 1961.
"Drugs for addicts." NEWSWEEK. 67:75, Oct. 12, 1961.
"Drugs hook 11 percent of narcotics victims," by Frazer,
H.F. OIL, PAINT AND DRUG REPORT. 186:4, July 6, 1964.

"Drugs left at home by psychiatric inpatients," by Robin, A.A., et al. BRITISH MEDICAL JOURNAL. 2:424-425, Aug. 17, 1968.

"Drugs, narcotics, and the flight from reality; with interview and press comments." SENIOR SCHOLASTIC. 90:4-12, Feb. 10, 1967.

"Drugs of abuse," by Long, R.E., et al. JOURNAL OF THE AMERICAN PHARMACEUTICAL ASSOCIATION. 8:12-14 passim, Jan., 1968.

"Drugs of confusion." PUBLIC HEALTH. 81:265-266, Sept., 1967.

"Drugs of dependence," by Wilson, C.W. PRACTITIONER. 200:102-112, Jan., 1968.

"Drugs on campus: turned on and tuned out," by Freedman, M.B., and Powelson, H. NATION. 202:125-127, Jan. 31, 1966.

"Drugs on the market; steps to remove ineffective remedies from the market." NEWSWEEK. 71:56-57, Feb. 5, 1968.

"Drugs that even scare hippies," by Rosenfeld, A. LIFE. 63:81-82, Oct. 27, 1967.

"Drugs; the mounting menace of abuse," by Berg, Roland H. LOOK. pp. 11-28, Sept. 8, 1967.

"Drugs you use." TODAY'S HEALTH. 43:38-39, Mar., 1965.

"Effects of drugs on conditioned 'anxiety'," by Blackman, D. NATURE. 217(5130):769-770, 1968.

"Effects of drugs on handwriting," by Purtell, D.J. JOURNAL OF FORENSIC SCIENCES. 10:335-346, 1965.

"Enlightened attitude toward narcotics urged," by Lewis, D.C. CURRENT MEDICAL PRACTICE. 1(5):2-7, 1964.

"Excessive consumption of drugs," by Segal, M. BRITISH MEDICAL JOURNAL. 5414:942-943, 1964.

"Explanatory trials of new drugs in man," by Pfeiffer, C. CLINICAL PHARMACOLOGY AND THERAPEUTICS. 3:397-399, 1962.

"Exploratory study of drugs and interaction," by Cheek. F. ARCHIVES OF GENERAL PSYCHIATRY. 9:566-574, 1963.

"The Fifteenth Session of the Commission on Narcotic Drugs and the Thirtieth Session of the Economic and Social Council." BULLETIN ON NARCOTICS. 12(4):43-46, Oct.-Dec., 1960.

"18th Session of the Commission on Narcotic Drugs and 36th Session of the Economic and Social Council." BULLETIN ON NARCOTICS. 15(3-4):39-42, July-Dec., 1963.

"The fight against narcotics," by Mabileau, J.F. UNITED NATIONS REVIEW. 11:29-34, Feb., 1964.

"First facts about drugs," by Kelsey, F.O. JOURNAL OF HEALTH, PHYSICAL EDUCATION AND RECREATION. 36:26-27, Feb., 1965.

"Great narcotics muddle," by DeMott, B. HARPERS. 224:46-50+, Mar., 1962.

"Heads and seekers: drugs on campus, counter-cultures and American society," by Keniston, K. AMERICAN SCHOLAR. 38:97-112, Winter, 1968/69.

"Heroin." THE ATTACK ON NARCOTIC ADDICTION AND DRUG ABUSE. 3:3, Spring, 1969.

"Heroin and the new prescribers." BRITISH MEDICAL JOURNAL.
1:719-720, Mar. 23, 1968.
"Heroin (diamorphine)." DRUG AND THERAPEUTICS BULLETIN.
5:11-12, 1967.
"Heroin in the provinces." CANADIAN MEDICAL ASSOCIATION
JOURNAL. 99(6):286, 1968.
"Heroin trap." THE ATTACK ON NARCOTIC ADDICTION AND DRUG
ABUSE. 3:10, Summer, 1969.
"The hill tribes of northern Thailand and the opium pro-
blem," by Saihoo, Patya. BULLETIN ON NARCOTICS. 15:
35-45, Apr.-June, 1963.
"The hill tribes of Thailand and the place of opium in
their socio-economic setting." BULLETIN ON NARCOTICS.
20(3):7-17, July-Sept., 1968.
"History, culture and subjective experience: an exploration
of the social bases of drug-induced experiences," by
Becker, H. JOURNAL OF HEALTH AND SOCIAL BEHAVIOR. 8:
163-176, Sept., 1967.
"History of the opium and narcotic drug legislation, Canada," by Trasov, G.E. CRIMINAL LAW QUARTERLY. 4:274,
1962.
"The history of the poppy and of opium and their expansion
in antiquity in the eastern Mediterranean area," by Krit-
ikos, P.G., and Papadaki, S.P, pt. I. BULLETIN ON NAR-
COTICS. 19(3):17-38, July-Sept., 1967.
--pt. II. BULLETIN ON NARCOTICS. 19(4):5-10, Oct.-Dec.,
1967.
"Hong Kong: its many splendored face," by Boal, S. DINERS'
CLUB MAGAZINE. 14:28-35, Oct., 1963.
"The horrors of heroin," by Severo, R. READER'S DIGEST.
96(573):72-75, Jan., 1970.
"How drugs act--second series. II. Drugs and addiction,"
by Smith, S.E. NURSING TIMES. 63:388-389, Mar. 24, 1967.
"How opiates change behavior," by Nichols, J.R. SCIENTIFIC
AMERICAN. 212(2):80-88, 1965.
"How to teach about drugs and sex," by Fort, J. CTA JOUR-
NAL. 65:22-24, Jan., 1969.
"Influence of drugs on driving," by Neil, W.H. TEXAS STATE
JOURNAL OF MEDICINE. 58(2):92-97, 1962.
"Inhalation psychosis and related states. A review," by
Glaser, F.B. ARCHIVES OF GENERAL PSYCHIATRY. 14(3):315-
32, 1966.
"Inter-American Consultative group on coca leaf problems,
Lima, 14-21 Dec., 1964." BULLETIN ON NARCOTICS. 17(4):
37-41, Oct.-Dec., 1965.
"Laboratory testing of new drugs for morphine-like drug de-
pendence," by Buckett, W.R. BRITISH JOURNAL OF ADDIC-
TION. 62:387-390, Dec., 1967.
"A land of lotus-eaters?" by Carstairs, G.M. AMERICAN JOUR-
NAL OF PSYCHIATRY. 125:1576-1580, May, 1969.
"Latin America; dog days for cocaine men." ECONOMIST.
223:785-786, May 20, 1967.
"Limitation and control of natural narcotics raw materials:
schemes of the League of Nations and United Nations,"

by Renborg, B. BULLETIN ON NARCOTICS. 15(2):13-26, Apr.-June, 1963.
"Little idea of dangers of drugs," by Binyon, M. TIMES (London) EDUCATIONAL SUPPLEMENT. 2785:686, Oct. 4, 1968.
"Mass drug catastrophies and the roles of science and technology," by Modell, W. SCIENCE. 156:346-351, 1967.
"The major medical complications of heroin addiction," by Louria, D.B., et al. ANNALS OF INTERNAL MEDICINE. 67: 1-22, July, 1967.
"Manufacture of alkaloids from the poppy plant in Hungary," by Bayer, I. BULLETIN ON NARCOTICS. 13(1):21-28, Jan.-Mar., 1961.
"Marcus Aurelius and mandragora," by Witke, E.C. CLASSICAL PHILOLOGY. 60:23-24, Jan., 1965.
"The meeting of the Inter-American Consultative Group on Narcotics Control. Rio de Janeiro, 27 November - 7 December 1961," by Parreiras, D. BULLETIN ON NARCOTICS. 15(2): 47-53, Apr.-June, 1963.
"Methadone blocks craving for heroin." AMERICAN DRUGGIST. 154:41, Sept. 26, 1966.
"Methods and limitations of narcotic use testing with nalorphine in California, minutes of the 24th meeting of the Committee on Drug Addiction and Narcotics," by Terry, J.G. APPENDIX 5, NATIONAL ACADEMY OF SCIENCE AND NATIONAL RESEARCH COUNCIL. pp. 12756ff, Jan. 29, 1962.
"The Middle East narcotics survey mission of the United Nations (Sept.-Oct., 1959)," by United Nations Department of Social Affairs. BULLETIN ON NARCOTICS. 12(4):37-42, 1960.
"Mind, drugs and behavior," by McGeer, P.L. AMERICAN SCIENTIST. 50:322-338, 1962.
"Misapprehensions about drug addiction - some origins and repercussions," by Brill, H. COMPREHENSIVE PSYCHIATRY. 4(3):150-159, 1963.
"Mischievous drugs," by Rossi, G. AMERICAN JOURNAL OF PHARMACY. 140:38-43, 1968.
"Misuse of dristan inhaler," by Greenberg, H.R., and Lustig, N. NEW YORK STATE JOURNAL OF MEDICINE. 66:613-617, 1966.
"The most commonly used drugs," by Higgins, L. LISTEN. 13: 17-22, Jan.-Feb., 1960.
"Multilingual list of narcotic drugs under international control." BULLETIN ON NARCOTICS. 21(3):47, July-Sept., 1969.
"Narcotic and narcotic antagonist analgesics," by Fraser, H.F., and Harris, L.S. ANNUAL REVIEW OF PHARMACOLOGY. 7:277-300, 1967.
"Narcotic antagonists " LANCET. 1:1310, 1967.
"Narcotic antagonist activity of naloxone," by Blumberg, H., et al. FEDERATION PROCEEDINGS. 24(2, pt.1):676, 1965.
"Narcotic antagonists and analgesics," by Archer, S. SCIENCE. 137:541-542, Aug., 1962.
"Narcotic antagonists as analgesics. Laboratory aspects," by Archer, S., et al. ADVANCES IN CHEMISTRY SERIES. 45:162-169, 1964.

"Narcotic blockade," by Dole, V.P., et al. ARCHIVES IN IN-
TERNAL MEDICINE. 118:304-309, 1966.
"Narcotic drugs commission; twenty-second session. UN MONTH-
LY CHRONICLE. 5:41-44, Feb., 1968.
"The narcotic problem," by Schwartz, G. WESTERN MEDICINE.
6:335-338, 1965.
"Narcotics and crime: why our cities are taking a new look."
SENIOR SCHOLASTIC. 81:16-19, Nov. 14, 1962.
"Narcotics and drug abuse: the federal response," by Walsh,
J. SCIENCE. 162:1254 passim, Dec. 13, 1968.
"Narcotics and medical practice. Medical use of morphine
and morphine-like drugs and management of persons depen-
dent on them." JOURNAL OF THE AMERICAN MEDICAL ASSOCIA-
TION. 202:209-212, Oct. 16, 1967.
"Narcotics and medical practice. The use of narcotic drugs
in medical practice and the medical management of narcot-
ic addicts." JOURNAL OF THE AMERICAN MEDICAL ASSOCIATION.
185(12):976-982, 1963.
"Narcotics and nalline: six years of testing," by Brown, T.
FEDERAL PROBATION. 27(2):27-32, June, 1963.
"Narcotics and related bases," by Farmilo, C.G., and Genest,
K. PROGRESS IN CHEMICAL TOXICOLOGY. 1:199-295, 1963.
"Narcotics and the premature infant." BULLETIN ON NARCOTICS.
20(4):7, Oct.-Dec., 1968.
"Narcotics and their regulation - lawyer's view," by Ache-
son, D.C. ILLINOIS MEDICAL JOURNAL. 130:432-436, 1966.
"Narcotics dilemma: crime or disease?" by Kobler, J. SAT-
URDAY EVENING POST. 235:64-66, 1962.
"Narcotics in Delaware." DELAWARE PHARMACIST. 17(11):4,
1963.
"Narcotics, negroes, and the South," by Bates, W.M. SOCIAL
FORCES. 45(1):61-67, Sept., 1966.
"Narcotics on campus," by Beall, L.L. JOURNAL OF SECONDARY
EDUCATION. 43:233-235, May, 1968.
"Narcotics policing; President asking for lots more of it."
OIL, PAINT AND DRUG REPORT. 191:7, Feb. 13, 1967.
"The narcotics problem." NEW ORLEANS STATE AND ITEMS. Oct.
26, 1965.
"The narcotics racket. How the pipeline works," by Scaduto,
A. NEW YORK POST. Nov. 10, 1965.
"Narcotics: the international picture," by Fort, J. CALI-
FORNIA YOUTH AUTHORITY QUARTERLY. 14:3-17, Summer, 1961.
"Narcotics: United States Government. Dangerous drugs unit."
SCIENCE. 161(3840):447, 1968.
"Narcotics use and abuse," by Trellis, E.S. PENNSYLVANIA
MEDICINE. 69:50-52, 1966.
"Narcotine in Indian opium," by Ramanathan, V.S., et al.
BULLETIN ON NARCOTICS. 18(4):25-29, Oct.-Dec., 1966.
"Nature of the mind and the effect of drugs upon it," by
Wilms, J.H. NATIONAL ASSOCIATION OF WOMEN DEANS AND
COUNSELORS JOURNAL. 31:24-30, Fall, 1967.
"A new antitussive agent of the thiaxanthene group." BUL-
LETIN ON NARCOTICS. 20(2):44, Apr.-June, 1968.
"New drugs of addiction," by Bachrich, P.R. BRITISH MEDICAL

JOURNAL. 5386:834-835, 1964.
"New Names." JOURNAL OF THE AMERICAN MEDICAL ASSOCIATION.
185(12):958-959, 1963.
"New opium alkaloid," by Brochmann-Hanssen, E., and Furuya,
T. JOURNAL OF PHARMACEUTICAL SCIENCES. 53(5):575, 1964.
"A new phenothiazine derivative with analgesic properties,"
by Lasagna, L., and DeKornfeld, T.J. JOURNAL OF THE AMER-
ICAN MEDICAL ASSOCIATION. 178:887-890, 1961.
"A non-narcotic analgesic: darvon. BULLETIN ON NARCOTICS.
20(4):14, Oct.-Dec., 1968.
"Non-narcotic analgesics. MEDICAL LETTER ON DRUGS AND THER-
APEUTICS. 8:7-8, 1966.
"Non professionals deliver narcotics in this new system,"
by Brown, W.S., and Leydon, J.J. MODERN HOSPITAL. 104:
136-137, 1965.
"Not for money: stewardess Simonne Christmann. NEWSWEEK.
57:33, June 5, 1961.
"Notes on the use of drugs to facilitate group psychother-
apy," by Eisner, B.G. PSYCHIATRIC QUARTERLY. 38(2):310-
328, 1964.
"Nutmeg as a narcotic," by Weil, A.T. ECONOMIC BOTANY.
19(3):194-217, 1965.
"One hundred years of progress in the drug treatment of di-
sease," by Keele, C.A. ROYAL SOCIETY OF HEALTH JOURNAL.
83:325-330, 1963.
"Opium as a tranquilizer," by Carlson, E.T., and Simpson,
M.M. AMERICAN JOURNAL OF PSYCHIATRY. 120, 1963.
"The opium-producing hill tribes of northern Thailand -
recommendations made by the UN Survey Team." BULLETIN
ON NARCOTICS. 21(1):1-29, Jan.-Mar., 1969.
"Our far-flung correspondents; few puffs on Mr. Su's pipe,"
by Busch, N.F. NEW YORKER. 35:162-164+, Nov. 28, 1959.
"An overview of the problem of drug abuse: as a clinical
entity," by Cameron, D.C. JOURNAL OF THE HILLSIDE HOS-
PITAL. 16(2):120-127, 1967.
"Pain: one mystery solved," by Beecher, H.K. SCIENCE.
151:840-841, 1966.
"Pain relieving drugs: the new versus the old," by Adriana,
J., and Robinson, D.W. JOURNAL OF THE LOUISIANA STATE
MEDICAL SOCIETY. 116:385-390, 1964.
"The pain-relieving properties of pentazocine, a new non-
narcotic analgesic," by Ende, M. JOURNAL OF THE AMER-
ICAN GERIATRICS SOCIETY. 13(8):775-778, 1965.
"Pennsylvania Department of Health notes dangers of con-
junctive use of alcohol and drugs." MARYLAND STATE
MEDICAL JOURNAL. 16:134-136, May, 1967.
"Pentazocine, a new attempt to separate analgesia from lia-
bility to dependence." DRUG AND THERAPEUTICS BULLETIN.
5:33-34, 1967.
"Pentazocine: a potent nonaddicting analgesic," by Henshaw,
J.R., et al. AMERICAN JOURNAL OF THE MEDICAL SCIENCES.
251(1):57-62, 1966.
"Pentazocine and its relation to addiction," by Eddy, N.B.
JOURNAL OF THE AMERICAN MEDICAL ASSOCIATION. 195(5):

322-323, 1966.
"Pentazocine as an analgesic. Clinical evaluation," by Cass, L.H., et al. JOURNAL OF THE AMERICAN MEDICAL ASSOCIATION. 188(2):112-115, 1964.
"Pentazocine for the relief of pain following urological procedures," by Wilkey, J.L., et al. JOURNAL OF UROLOGY. 97(3):550-551, 1967.
"Personality structure as the main determinant of drug induced (model) psychoses," by Fischer, R., et al. NATURE. 218(5138):296-298, 1968.
"Pharmacy in 1967." PHARMACEUTICAL JOURNAL. 199:649-650, 1967.
"Pills--the new menace," by Lefkowitz, B. NEW YORK POST. June 1, 1965.
"Poppy cultivation in Bulgaria and the production of opium," by Dalev, D., et al. BULLETIN ON NARCOTICS. 12(1): 25-36, Jan.-Mar., 1960.
"The position of the Bureau of Narcotics," by Gaffnery, G.H. ILLINOIS MEDICAL JOURNAL. 130:516-520, 1966.
"Possibility of crop substitution for the coca bush in Bolivia," by Rodriguez, A.A. BULLETIN ON NARCOTICS. 17: 13-23, 1965.
"Primitive but effective herb medicines of the Amazon Jungle," by Saul, F.W. JOURNAL OF THE KANSAS MEDICAL SOCIETY. 65:458-464, 1964.
"The problem of narcotic drugs," by Khalifa, A.M. INTERNATIONAL ANNALS OF CRIMINOLOGY. 1:108-116, 1964.
"Problems related to teaching about drugs," by Bland, H.B. JOURNAL OF SCHOOL HEALTH. 39:117-119, Feb., 1969.
"Progress in the production of opium and opium-alkaloids in India," by Ramanathan, V.S. SCIENCE AND CULTURE. 32(1):3-8, 1966.
"Psychoactive drug action and group interaction process," by Lennard, H.L., et al. JOURNAL OF NERVOUS AND MENTAL DISEASE. 145(1):69-78, 1967.
"Psycho-active drugs, exploratory activity and fear," by Kumar, R. NATURE. 218(5141):587-588, 1968.
"Psychometabolism," by Huxley, J. JOURNAL OF NEUROPSYCHIATRY. 3(suppl. 1), 1962.
"Psychopharmacological revolution," by Jarvik, M.E. PSYCHOLOGY TODAY. 1(1):51-59, May, 1967.
"Psychopharmacology and psychiatry: towards a classification of psychotropic drugs," by Delay, J. BULLETIN ON NARCOTICS. 19(1):1-5, 1967.
"Psychotherapeutic drugs: a guide for social workers," by Garetz, F.K., and Janecek, J. SOCIAL CASEWORK. 44(4): 206-209, 1963.
"Psychotoxic drugs (barbiturates, amphetamines and hallucinogenic drugs)," by Shaffer, H.B. EDITORIAL RESEARCH REPORTS. pp. 64-80, Jan. 27, 1965.
"Recent changes in the incidence in all types of drug dependence in Great Britain," by Bewley, T. PROCEEDINGS OF THE ROYAL SOCIETY OF MEDICINE. 61:175-177, 1968.
"Recreational drugs." JOURNAL OF HEALTH AND SOCIAL BEHAV-

IOR. 9(2), June, 1968 [whole issue on drugs].

"Relief without risk? New analgesics promise fast pain-killing with little danger of addiction: narcotic antagonists." CHEMICAL WEEK. 94:55-56, May 23, 1964.

"Requirement and evaluations of narcotics tests," by Mannering, G.J. PSYCHOPHARMACOLOGY BULLETIN; NATIONAL CLEARINGHOUSE FOR MENTAL HEALTH INFORMATION. 3:27-29, Dec., 1966.

"Responsibility of the physician in the prescription of drugs, etc., in the symptoms of toxicomania," by Varenne, G. BELGISCH TIJDSCHRIFT VOOR GENEESKUNDIGE DOCUMENTATIE. 19:830-840, 1963.

"A review of narcotic and non-narcotic analgesics," by De-Kornfeld, T.J. MICHIGAN MEDICINE. 65:359-361, 1966.

"Review of the 22nd session of the Commission on Narcotic Drugs and the 44th session of the Economic and Social Council." BULLETIN ON NARCOTICS. 20(2):37-41, Apr.-June, 1968.

"Schoolman's guide to illicit drugs." SCHOOL MANAGEMENT. 12:57-59, Feb., 1968.

"Self image and attitudes toward drugs," by Brehm, M.L., and Back, K.W. JOURNAL OF PERSONALITY. 36:299-314, June, 1968.

"Shortening of coma duration in narcotic poisoning," by Myschetzky, A. INTERNATIONAL ANESTHESIOLOGY CLINICS. 4:351-358, 1966.

"6-methyl-codeine. A new opium alkaloid," by Brochmann-Hanssen, E., and Nielsen, B. JOURNAL OF PHARMACEUTICAL SCIENCES. 54(9):1393, 1965.

"The sixteenth session of the Commission on Narcotic Drugs and the thirty-second session of the Economic and Social Council." BULLETIN ON NARCOTICS. 13(4):39-41, Oct.-Dec., 1961.

"The single convention on narcotic drugs, 1961," by Lande, A. INTERNATIONAL ORGANIZATION. 16:776-797, Autumn, 1962.

"Slang terms associated with drugs in the United Kingdom," by Bewley, T. BULLETIN ON NARCOTICS. 18(4):10-13, 1966.

"Solvent sniffing: physiologic effects and community control measures for intoxication from the intentional inhalation of organis solvents," by Press, E., and Done, A.K. PEDIATRICS. 39:451, Mar., 1967; 611, Apr., 1967.

"Some actions of morphine on the circulation," by Flacke, W. FEDERATION PROCEEDINGS. 24(2, pt.I):613, 1965.

"Some derivatives of metamorphinan," by Gates, M., and Klein, D.A. JOURNAL OF MEDICINAL CHEMISTRY. 10(3): 380-383, 1967.

"Some narcotic antagonists in the benzomorphan series," by Harris, L.S., and Pierson, A.K. JOURNAL OF PHARMACOLOGY AND EXPERIMENTAL THERAPEUTICS. 143:141-148, 1964.

"Some problems in prescribing narcotic drugs: the doctor-patient relationship," by Zinberg, N.E., and Lewis, D.C. BULLETIN ON NARCOTICS. 19(1):333-335, Jan.-Mar., 1967.

"Some statistical aspects of pyrolysis-GLC in the identification of alkaloids," by Kingston, C.R., and Kirk, P.L.

BULLETIN ON NARCOTICS. 17(2):19-25, Apr.-June, 1965.
"Spon cases: a quick method of identifying heroin," by King,
W. POLICE. 5(1):73, Sept.-Oct., 1960.
"Stimulants and tranquilizers: their use and abuse," by
Braceland, F.J. BULLETIN OF THE NEW YORK ACADEMY OF
MEDICINE. 39:649-665, 1963.
"Straight talk about the drug problem." SCHOOL MANAGEMENT.
12:52-56 passim, Feb., 1968.
"Stramonium poisoning in 'Teeny-Boppers'," by Teitelbaum,
D.T. ANNALS OF INTERNAL MEDICINE. 68:174, 1968.
"Symposium on side effects and drug toxicity," by Schiele,
B.C. PSYCHOPHARMACOLOGY BULLETIN; NATIONAL CLEARING-
HOUSE FOR MENTAL HEALTH INFORMATION. 4(1):56-61, 1967.
"Technical questions - narcotic drugs." INTERNATIONAL
CRIMINAL POLICE REVIEW. 203:290-296, 1966.
"Test your drug I.Q." FEDERAL PROBATION. 32:15-17, Sept.,
1968.
"Those wonderful pills," by Clark, S.E. LISTEN. 14:7-8,
May-June, 1961.
"Today's drugs: drugs of addiction." BRITISH MEDICAL JOUR-
NAL. 2(5417):1119-1120, 1964.
"To label or not to label," by Council on Drugs. JOURNAL
OF THE AMERICN MEDICAL ASSOCIATION. 194(12):1311, 1965.
"Toward the year 2000." DAEDALUS. Summer, 1967.
"The toxicity of some of the newer narcotic analgesics,"
by Lister, R.E. JOURNAL OF PHARMACY AND PHARMACOLOGY.
18(6):374-383, 1966.
"United Nations Consultative Group on Narcotics Problems in
Asia and the Far East." BULLETIN ON NARCOTICS. 17(2):
3946, Apr.-June, 1965.
"Use and abuse of drugs," by Rapp, M.S. CANADIAN MEDICAL
ASSOCIATION JOURNAL. 98:922, 1968.
"The use of hyoscyamine as a hallucinogen and intoxicant,"
by Keeler, M.H., and Kane, F.J., Jr. AMERICAN JOURNAL
OF PSYCHIATRY. 124(6):852-854, 1967.
"The use of nutmeg as a psychotropic agent," by Weil, A.T.
BULLETIN ON NARCOTICS. 18(4):15, 1966.
"What are narcotic drugs?" TODAY'S EDUCATION. 58:48-50,
Mar., 1969.
"What to tell young people about alcohol and narcotics,"
by Northup, D.W. WEST VIRGINIA MEDICAL JOURNAL. 59:
374-377, 1963.
"Why drugs?" by Trocchi, A. NEW SOCIETY. 5(138):9-10,
1965.
"World Health Organization Expert Committee on Addiction-
producing Drugs: tenth report." BULLETIN ON NARCOTICS.
12(2):47-49, Apr.-June, 1960.
--Thirteenth report. BULLETIN ON NARCOTICS. 16:53-55,
Apr.-June, 1964.
--Fourteenth report. BULLETIN ON NARCOTICS. 17(4):43-
46, Oct.-Dec., 1965.
--Fifteenth report. BULLETIN ON NARCOTICS. 19(1):29-32,
Jan.-Mar., 1967.
--Sixteenth report. TECHNICAL REPORT SERIES no. 407, 1969.

"Zu Gottfried Benns drogenlyrik: interpretation der gedichte
Betaubung und Entwurzelungen," by Rothmann, K. MODERN
LANGUAGE NOTES. 82:454-461, Oct., 1967.

NARCOTICS: Periodical Literature

Scientific Publications

"Absence of trans-n-methylation of morphine in the rat,"
by Mule, S.J., and Mannering, G.J. BULLETIN ON NARCOTICS.
17(2):27-28, Apr.-June, 1965.
"Abuse liability and narcotic antagonism of pentazocine: re-
port on two cases," by Keup, W. DISEASES OF THE NERVOUS
SYSTEM. 29(9):599-602, 1968.
"Accelerated painless labor," by Louros, N.C., et al. AMER-
ICAN JOURNAL OF OBSTETRICS AND GYNECOLOGY. 98:555-561,
1967.
"The action of drugs on the circular muscle strip from the
guinea-pig isolated ileum," by Harry, J. BRITISH JOURNAL
OF PHARMACOLOGY. 20:399-417, 1963.
"The action of some CNS and local anesthetic drugs on the
stimulated glycolysis of frog sartorius muscle," by Smith,
C., and Abood, L. INTERNATIONAL JOURNAL OF NEUROPHARMA
COLOGY. 5:255-261, 1966.
"Actions and interactions of norepinephrine. Tyramine and
cocaine on aortic strips of rabbit and left atria of gui-
nea pig and cat," by Furchgott, R.F., et al. JOURNAL OF
PHARMACOLOGY AND EXPERIMENTAL THERAPEUTICS. 142(1):39,
1963.
"Actions of tyramine and cocaine on catecholamine levels
in subcellular fractions of the isolated cat heart," by
Campos, H.A., et al. JOURNAL OF PHARMACOLOGY AND EXPER-
IMENTAL THERAPEUTICS. 141(3):290-300, 1963.
"Acute poisoning," by Jacobson, T., and Kahanpaa, A. NORD-
ISK MEDICIN. 69:698-700, 1963.
"Acute tolerance to morphine following systemic and intra-
cerebral injection in the rat," by Lotti, V.J., et al.
INTERNATIONAL JOURNAL OF NEUROPHARMACOLOGY. 5(1):35-42,
1966.
"The addiction cycle to narcotics in the rat and its rela-
tion to catecholamines," by Akera, T., et al. BIOCHEMI-
CAL PHARMACOLOGY. 17:675-688, May, 1968.
"Addiction liability of I-C-26 (dextro-3-dimethylamino-1,
1-diphenylbutyl ethyl sulfone hydrochloride), and I-D-20
(ethyl 1-carbamethyl)-4-phenylpiperidine-4-carboxylate
hydrochloride)," by Wolbach, A.B., Jr., and Fraser, H.F.
BULLETIN ON NARCOTICS. 15(1):25-28, Jan.-Mar., 1963.
"The addiction potential of oxycodone (pereodan)." CALI-
FORNIA MEDICINE. 99:127-130, Aug., 1963.
"Addiction Research Center Inventory (ARCI): development

of a general drug estimation scale," by Haertzen, C.A.
JOURNAL OF NERVOUS AND MENTAL DISEASE. 141:300-307,
1965.
"The Addiction Research Center Inventory: appendix. I.
Items comprising empirical scales for seven drugs. II.
Items which do not differentiate placebo from any drug
condition,: by Hill, H.E., et al. PSYCHOPHARMACOLOGIA.
4(3):167-183, 1963.
"Addictiveness of 1,2-dimethyl, 3-phenyl, 3-propionoxy pyr-
rolidine hydrochloride (ARC 1-0-1)," by Fraser, H.F.
BULLETIN ON NARCOTICS. 16:37-43, Jan.-Mar., 1964.
"Adjunctive use of prozine in somatic illness. A controlled
study," by Bradley, W.F. OHIO MEDICAL JOURNAL. 58:765-
768, 1962.
"Advances in pharmacology related to anesthesia and surgery,"
by Collins, V.J. INDUSTRIAL MEDICINE AND SURGERY. 35
(6):465-471, 1966.
"Alcoholism and reliance upon drugs as depressive equiva-
lents," by Fox, R.P. AMERICAN JOURNAL OF PSYCHOTHERAPY.
21:585-596, 1967.
"Alkaloid biosynthesis. I. The biosynthesis of papaverine,"
by Battersby, A.R., and Harper, B.J.T. JOURNAL OF THE
CHEMICAL SOCIETY (London). pp. 3526-3533, Sept., 1962.
"Alkaloid biosynthesis. II. The biosynthesis of morphine,"
by Battersby, A.R., et al. JOURNAL OF THE CHEMICAL SOC-
IETY (London). pp. 3534-3544, Sept., 1962.
"Alkaloid biosynthesis. VIII. Use of ootically active pre-
cursors for investigations on the biosynthesis of mor-
phine alkaloids," by Battersby, A.R., and Foulkes, D.M.
JOURNAL OF THE CHEMICAL SOCIETY (London). pp. 3323-3332,
May, 1965.
"The alkaloids of papaver somniferum L. I. Evidence for
a rapid turnover of the major alkaloids," by Fairbairn,
J.W., and Wassel, G. PHYTOCHEMISTRY. 3(2):253-258,
1964.
"The alkaloids of papaver somniferum L. V. Fate of the
'end-product' alkaloid morphine," by Fairbairn, J.W.,
and El-Masry, S. PHYTOCHEMISTRY. 6(4):499-504, 1967.
"Alterations in response to somatic pain associated with
anaesthesia. XII. Further studies with atropine," by
Moore, J., and Dundee, J.W. BRITISH JOURNAL OF ANAES-
THESIA. 34:712-716, 1962.
"Alterations in response to somatic pain associated with
anaesthesia. XIII. The 'lytic cocktail'," by Nicholl,
R,M,m et al. BRITISH JOURNAL OF ANAESTHESIA. 34(10):
717-720, 1962.
"American College of Neuropsychopharmacology: fifth annual
meeting," by Cole, J., and Davis, J. PSYCHOPHARMACOLOGY
BULLETIN; NATIONAL CLEARINGHOUSE FOR MENTAL HEALTH IN-
FORMATION. 4(1):28-31, 1967.
"Amiphenazole in the treatment of morphine and opium addic-
tion," by Bruce, D.W. LANCET. 7341:1010-1012, 1964.
"Analgesia for postpartum pain," by Headley, C.R. BULLETIN
OF THE GEISINGER MEDICAL CENTER. 15:75-79, 1963.

"Analgesia in myocardial infraction: double blind compari-
son of piminodine and morphine," by Hoff, H.R., et al.
AMERICAN JOURNAL OF THE MEDICAL SCIENCES. 249(5):495-
498, 1965.
"Analgesia in obstetrics. The effect of analgesia on uter-
ine contractility and fetal heart rate," by Filler, W.W.,
Jr., et al. AMERICAN JOURNAL OF OBSTETRICS AND GYNECOL-
OGY. 98:832-846, 1967.
"Analgesic abuse and renal disease in north-east Scotland,"
by Prescott, L.F. LANCET. 2:1143-1145, 1966.
"Analgesic effect of florinal with codeine," by Madore, P.,
and Chiricosta, A. ANESTHESIA AND ANALGESIS: CURRENT
RESEARCHES. 46(4):405-409, 1967.
"Analgesic effect of methotrimeprazine and meperidine in
postoperative patients. Double-blind study in 24 cases,"
by Bronwell, A.W., et al. AMERICAN SURGEON. 32:641-644,
1966
"Analgesic effect of methotrimeprazine and morphine. A
clinical comparison," by Montilla, E., et al. ARCHIVES
OF INTERNAL MEDICINE. 11:725-728, 1963.
"The analgesic effect of opiate-opiate antagonist combinations in the rat," by Grumbach, L., and Chernov, H.I.
JOURNAL OF PHARMACOLOGY AND EXPERIMENTAL THERAPEUTICS.
149(3):385-396, 1965.
"Analgesic effects in monkeys of morphine, nalorphine, and
a benzomorphan narcotic antagonist," by Weis, B., and
Laties, V.G. JOURNAL OF PHARMACOLOGY AND EXPERIMENTAL
THERAPEUTICS. 143(2):169-173, 1964.
"The analgesic efficacy and respiratory effects in man of
benzomorphan 'narcotic antagonist'," by Lasagna, L., et
al. JOURNAL OF PHARMACOLOGY AND EXPERIMENTAL THERAPEU-
TICS. 144(1):12-16, 1964.
"Analysis of terpin hydrate and codeine elixir for codeine
content." AMERICAN JOURNAL OF HOSPITAL PHARMACY. 24
(10):585-586, 1967.
"An analysis of the direct and indirect actions of drugs
on the isolated guinea-pig ileum," by Day, M., and Vane,
J.R. BRITISH JOURNAL OF PHARMACOLOGY AND CHEMOTHERAPY.
20:150-170, 1963.
"Anesthesia for voiding cytography in children," by McDon-
ald, J.L., and Good, H.D. ANESTHESIA AND ANALGESIA:
CURRENT RESEARCHES. 45:450-452, 1966.
"Anesthesia in toxicomania," by Gualandi, W. MINERVA AN-
ESTESIOLOGICA (Torino). 30:273-278, 1964.
"Antagonism by caffeine of the respiratory effects of co-
deine and morphine," by Bellville, J.W., et al. JOURNAL
OF PHARMACOLOGY AND EXPERIMENTAL THERAPEUTICS. 136:38-
42, 1962.
"Antagonism by nalorphine of the hypothermic effect of mor-
phine in the rat," by Lotti, V.J. FEDERATION PROCEEDINGS.
24(2, pt.I):548, 1965.
"Antagonism of convulsive and lethal effects induced by pro-
poxyphene," by Fiut, R.E., et al. JOURNAL OF THE PHAR-
MACEUTICAL SCIENCES. 55(10):1085-1087, 1966.

"Antagonism of guanethidine and bretylium by various agents,"
by Day, M.D., and Rand, M.J. LANCET. 2:1282-1283, 1962.
"Antagonism of morphine and of reserpine by the levorotatory
and dextrorotatory isomers of 2,2-diphenyl 4(2-piperidyl-
1,3-dioxolane HCl," by Hidalgo, J., and Thompson, C.R.
PROCEEDINGS OF THE SOCIETY FOR EXPERIMENTAL BIOLOGY AND
MEDICINE. 114(1):92, 1963.
"Antagonism of the analgesic effect of morphine and other
drugs by p-chlorophenylamine, a serotonin derivative,"
by Tenen, S.S. PSYCHOPHARMACOLOGIA. 12(4):278-285, 1968.
"Antibiotic activity of various types of cannabis resin,"
by Radosevič, A., et al. NATURE. 195(4845):1007-1009,
1962; also UN DOCUMENT ST-SOA-SER. S-6, 1962.
"Anticholinergic hallucinosis: effect of atropine and JB-
329 on 'caudate spindle' phenomena and electrical activity of cat hippocampus," by Spradlin, W., et al. RECENT
ADVANCES IN BIOLOGICAL PSYCHIATRY. 8:175-185, 1966.
"Antidepressants. II. Derivatives of polynuclear indoles,"
by Freed, M.E., et al. JOURNAL OF MEDICINAL CHEMISTRY.
7(5):628-632, 1964.
"Antidiuretic effects of oxytocin, morphine and pethidine
in pregnancy and labour. AUSTRALIAN AND NEW ZEALAND
JOURNAL OF OBSTETRICS AND GYNAECOLOGY. 3:81-83, 1963.
"Antidiuretic effects of subnarcotic doses of phenazocine,"
by Calesnick, B., and Milligan, D. ANESTHESIOLOGY. 23:
81-85, 1962.
"Anti-epileptic drugs and the foetus, by Lawrence, A. BRI-
TISH MEDICAL JOURNAL. 5367:1267, 1963.
"Antitussive activity of narcotine derivatives," by Ota, Y.,
et al. CHEMICAL AND PHARMACEUTICAL BULLETIN. 12(5):
569-578, 1964.
"Antitussives," by Bickerman, H.A. AMERICAN JOURNAL OF NURS-
ING. 63:61-64, 1963.
"Apomorphine and levallorphan tartrate in acute poisonings.
A preliminary report," by Berry, R.A., and Lambdin, M.A.
AMERICAN JOURNAL OF DISEASES OF CHILDREN. 105(2):160-
163, 1963.
"Apomorphine induces reinforcement," by Robinson, Paul, et
al. PSYCHONOMIC SCIENCE. 7(3):117-118, 1967.
"Apparent concentration quenching of morphine fluorescence,"
by Brandt, R., et al. SCIENCE. 139(3559):1063-1064,
1963.
"Apparent lack of interaction between dimenthyl sulfoxide
(DMSO) and a variety of drugs," by Dixon, R.L., et al.
PROCEEDINGS OF THE SOCIETY FOR EXPERIMENTAL BIOLOGY AND
MEDICINE. 118:756-759, 1965.
"Application of activation analysis to forensic science.
II. Drugs," by Bate, L.C., and Pro, M.J. INTERNATIONAL
JOURNAL OF APPLIED RADIATION. 15:111-114, 1964.
"Application of e-analysis to pharmaceuticals. II. De-
termination of morphine," by Casimelli, J.L., and Sis-
heimer, J.E. JOURNAL OF PHARMACEUTICAL SCIENCES. 51:
336-338, 1962.
"Application of paper chromatography to the investigation

217

of opium and opiun alkaloids," by Buchi, J., et al. BUL-
LETIN ON NARCOTICS. 12(2):25-45, Apr.-June, 1960.
"Application of the Ariens theory of drug action to narcotic
antagonist interactions on serum esterase activity," by
Ettinger, M.J., and Gero, A. FEDERATION PROCEEDINGS.
24(2, pt.I):549, 1965.
"Are postoperative narcotics necessary?" by Roe, B.B. AR-
CHIVES OF SURGERY. 87:912-915, 1963.
"Assessing subjective effects of drugs: an index of careless-
ness and confusion for use with the Addiction Research
Center Inventory (ARCI)," by Haertzen, C.A., and Hill,
H.E. JOURNAL OF CLINICAL PSYCHOLOGY. 19:407-412, 1963.
"An assessment of inhalation as a mode of administration of
heroin by addicts," by Pui-nin Mo, B., and Way, E.L.
JOURNAL OF PHARMACOLOGY AND EXPERIMENTAL THERAPEUTICS.
154(1):142-151, 1966.
"Assessment of the dependence-producing properties of dihydrocodeinone and codoxime," by Jasinski, D.R., and Martin, W.R. CLINICAL PHARMACOLOGY AND THERAPEUTICS. 8:
266-270, 1967.
"Atropine sulfate premedication and fractional pneumography:
effect on electrocardiographic changes," by Davie, J.C.,
and Baldwin, M. ARCHIVES OF NEUROLOGY. 2:258-264, 1963.
"Basal narcosis or sedation for cardiac catheterization,"
by Norris, W. BRITISH JOURNAL OF ANAESTHESIA. 35:358-
367, 1963.
"Behavior effects of caffeine, methamphetamine, and methylphenidate in the rat," by Mechner, F., and Latranyi, M.
JOURNAL OF THE EXPERIMENTAL ANALYSIS OF BEHAVIOR. 6(3):
331-342, 1963.
"A behavioral method for the study of pain perception in
the monkey. The effects of some pharmacological agents,"
by Weitzman, E.D., and Ross, G.S. NEUROLOGY. 12(4):
264-272, 1962.
"The biochemical transformation of the morphothebaine to
the morphine ring system," by Gross, S., and Dawson, R.F.
BIOCHEMISTRY. 2(1):186-188, 1963.
"The biological disposition of morphine and its surrogates,"
by Way, E.L., and Adler, T.K. BULLETIN OF THE WORLD
HEALTH ORGANIZATION. 27:359-394, 1962.
--2. BULLETIN OF THE WORLD HEALTH ORGANIZATION. 26:51-
66, 1962.
--3. BULLETIN OF THE WORLD HEALTH ORGANIZATION. 26:261-
284, 1962.
"The biological fabric of time (part 1): 1. The history of
the concepts of time. 2. Biological unity of time. 3.
Psychotomimetic varieties of time contraction," by Fischer, R. ANNALS OF THE NEW YORK ACADEMY OF SCIENCE.
138:440-488, 1967.
"Biosynthesis of alkaloids. On the occurence of keot acids
of papaver somniferum L. plants," by Jindra, A., et al.
EXPERIENTIA. 20(7):371-372, 1964.
"Blocking effect of puromycin, ethanol, and chloroform on
the development of tolerance to an opiate," by Smith,

A.A., et al. BIOCHEMICAL PHARMACOLOGY. 15(11):1877-1879, 1966.
"Blood glucose and brain catecholamine levels in the cat following the injection of morphine into the cerebrospinal fluid," by Moore, K.E., et al. JOURNAL OF PHARMACOLOGY AND EXPERIMENTAL THERAPEUTICS. 148(2):169-175, 1965.
"Bromism induced by 'safe' medications, old and new: some psychological considerations," by Martin, I. MEDICAL JOURNAL OF AUSTRALIA. 1:95-98, Jan. 21, 1967.
"Cardiovascular actions of narcotic analgesics," by Elliott, H.W., and Abdel-Rahman, M.A. AMERICAN HEART JOURNAL. 69:567-568, 1965.
"Catecholamine metabolism amd morphine abstinence," by Gunne, L.M. ANNALS OF THE NEW YORK ACADEMY OF SCIENCES. 96: 205-210, 1962.
"Catecholamine metabolism in morphine withdrawal in the dog," by Gunne, L.M. NATURE. 195(4843):815-816, 1962.
"Centrally mediated inhibition of gastrointestinal propulsive motility by morphine over a non-neural pathway," by Margolin, S. PROCEEDINGS OF THE SOCIETY FOR EXPERIMENTAL BIOLOGY AND MEDICINE. 112(2):311-315, 1963.
"Certain aspects of the effects of levorphanol on water metoabolism in rats," by Newsome, H.H., et al. JOURNAL OF PHARMACOLOGY AND EXPERIMENTAL THERAPEUTICS. 139(3): 368-376, 1963.
"Characteristics and sequelae of paregoric abuse," by Lerner, A.M., et al. ANNALS OF INTERNAL MEDICINE. 65: 1019-1030, Nov., 1966.
"Chemical constituents of the alkaloid-free fraction from opium," by Matsui, K., et al. CHEMICAL AND PHARMACEUTICAL BULLETIN. 10:872-875, 1962.
"Children, drugs, and local anesthesia," by Tarsitano, J.J. JOURNAL OF THE AMERICAN DENTAL ASSOCIATION. 70:1153-1158, 1965.
"Chlorphentermine," by Craig, D.D. BRITISH MEDICAL JOURNAL. 5367:1269, 1963.
"Chromatographic separation of rauwolfia serpentina and opium alkaloids on thin layers of alumina," by Ikram, M., et al. JOURNAL OF CHROMATOGRAPHY. 11:260-263, 1963.
"Cinegastroscopic observations on the effect of anticholinergic and related drugs on gastric and pyrolic motor activity," by Barowsky, H., et al. AMERICAN JOURNAL OF DIGESTIVE DISEASES. 10(6):506-513, 1965.
"Circulatory effects of heroin in patients with myocardial infraction," by MacDonald, H.R., et al. LANCET. 1:1070-1073, 1967.
"Circulatory response to tilting following methotrimeprazine and morphine in man," by Helrich, M., and Gold, M.I. ANESTHESIOLOGY. 25:662-667, 1964.
"Classical conditioning of a morphine abstinence phenomenon, reinforcement of opoid-drinking behavior and 'relapse' in morphine-addicted rats," by Wikler, A., and Pescor, F.T. PSYCHOPHARMACOLOGIA. 10(3):255-284, 1967.

"Clinical appraisal of analgesic agents," by Batterman,
R.C. CURRENT THERAPEUTIC RESEARCH. 4:75-80, 1962.
"Clinical assessnebt of analgesic drugs. I. Initial trial,"
by Masson, A.H. ANAESTHESIA. 17:373-378, 1962.
--2. Observer trial. Anaesthesia. 17:411-418, 1962.
--Spirometry trial. ANESTHESIA AND ANALGESIA; CURRENT RE-
SEARCHES. 41:615-622, 1962.
"A clinical comparison of the analgesic and side effects of
lethotrimeprazine and morphine," by Wallenstein, S.L.,
et al. FEDERATION PROCEEDINGS. 24(2, pt.I):548, 1965.
"A clinical determination of pain relief in office patients.
A controlled comparative study," by Koldony, A.L. PSY-
CHOSOMATICS. 7:11-13, 1966.
"The clinical effect of drugs and their influence on animal
behavior," by Jacobsen, E. REVUE DE PSYCHOLOGIE APPLI-
QUEE. 11:421-432, 1961.
"Clinical effectiveness of drugs used for tropical anes-
thesia," by Adriana, J., and Zepernick, R. JOURNAL OF
THE AMERICAN MEDICAL ASSOCIATION. 188(8):711-716, 1964.
"The clinical evaluation of morphine and its substitutes
as analgesics," by Lasagna, L. PHARMACOLOGICAL REVIEWS.
16(1):47-83, 1964.
"Clinical experience with promethazine and meperidine in
relief of pain," by Hashkes, H.R. CLINICAL MEDICINE.
69:1587-1590, 1962.
"Clinical investigation of antitussive properties of phoco-
dine," by Mulinos, M.G., et al. NEW YORK STATE JOURNAL
OF MEDICINE. 62:2373-2377, 1962.
"Clinical pharmacology of antitussive agents," by Bickerman,
H.A. CLINICAL PHARMACOLOGY AND THERAPEUTICS. 3(3):353
368, 1962.
"Clinical pharmacology of potent analgesics," by Murphree,
H.B. CLINICAL PHARMACOLOGY AND THERAPEUTICS. 3(4):473-
504, 1962.
"Clinical pharmacology of the narcotic analgesics," by Vandam, L.D. CLINICAL PHARMACOLOGY AND THERAPEUTICS. 3:
827-838, 1962.
"Clinical studies of induction agents. VI. Miscellaneous
observations with G.29.505," by Riding, J.E., et al.
BRITISH JOURNAL OF ANAESTHESIA. 35:480-483, 1963.
"Clinical syndromes and biochemical alterations following
mescaline, lysergic acid diethylamide, psilocybin and a
combination of the three psychotomimetic drugs," by Hol-
lister, L.E., and Sjoberg, B.M. COMPREHENSIVE PSYCHIATRY
5(3):170-178, 1964.
"Clinical trial of a new antitussive agent," by Thalberg,
R.E. WESTERN MEDICINE. 3:473-474, 1962.
"Clinical use of analgesics: some basic pharmacologic prin-
ciples," by Calesnick, B. CLINICAL PEDIATRICS. 2:9-12,
1963.
"Cocaine tachyphylaxis," by Teeters, W.R., et al. LIFE
SCIENCES. 7:509-518, 1963.
"Codeine vs. caramiphen in cough control," by Glick, J.
DELAWARE MEDICAL JOURNAL. 35:180, 1963.

"Codeinone as the intermediate in the biosynthetic conversion of thebaine to codeine," by Blaschke, G., et al. JOURNAL OF THE AMERICAN CHEMICAL SOCIETY. 89(6):1540-1541, 1967.

"Collaborative study of the determination of morphine in paregoric," by Smith, E. JOURNAL OF THE ASSOCIATION OF OFFICIAL AGRICULTURAL CHEMISTS. 51(6):1315-1318, Nov., 1968.

"Comparative analgesic potency of heroin and morphine in postoperative patients," by Reichle, C.W., et al. JOURNAL OF PHARMACOLOGY AND EXPERIMENTAL THERAPEUTICS. 136 (1):43-46, 1962.

"A comparative clinical test of pholcodine with codeine as control," by Kelly, D.F. NORTHWEST MEDICINE. 62:871-874, 1963.

"Comparative effects of age, sex, and drugs upon two tasks of auditory vigilance," by Neal, G.L., and Pearson, R.G. PERCEPTUAL AND MOTOR SKILLS. 23(3, pt.1):967-974, 1966.

"Comparative effects of codeine and morphine in man," by Kay, D.C., et al. JOURNAL OF PHARMACOLOGY AND EXPERIMENTAL THERAPEUTICS. 156(1):101-106, 1967.

"The comparative enhancement of the depressant action of alcohol by eight representative ataractic and analgesic drugs," by Forney, R.B., et al. EXPERIENTIA. 18:468-470, 1962.

"Comparative evaluation of analgesic agents in post-partum patients: oral dextropropoxyphene, codeine, and meperidine," by Gruber, C.M., Jr., et al. ANESTHESIA AND ANALGESIA; CURRENT RESEARCHES. 41:538-544, 1962.

"Comparative pharmacological reactions of certain wild and domestic mammals to thebaine derivatives in the M-series of compounds," by Harthoorn, A.M. FEDERATION PROCEEDINGS. 26(4):1251-1261, 1967.

"Comparative pharmacology of drugs affecting behavior," by Weiss, B., and Laties, V.G. FEDERATION PROCEEDINGS. 26(4):1146-1156, 1967.

"The comparative potencies of codeine and its demethylated metabolites after intraventricular injection in the mouse," by Adler, T.K. JOURNAL OF PHARMACOLOGY AND EXPERIMENTAL THERAPEUTICS. 140(2):155-161, 1963.

"The comparative potency and effectiveness of topical anesthetics in man," by Adriana, J., et al. CLINICAL PHARMACOLOGY AND THERAPEUTICS. 5(1):49-62, 1964.

"A comparative study of four premedications," by Feldman, S.A. ANAESTHESIA. 18:169-184, 1963.

"Comparative study of physiological and subjective effects of heroin and morphine administered intravenously in post-addicts," by Martin, W.R., and Fraser, H.F. JOURNAL OF PHARMACOLOGY AND EXPERIMENTAL THERAPEUTICS. 133:388-399, 1961.

"A comparative study of the effects of listica and meprobamate upon motor functioning," by Lawton, M.P., and Cahn, B. JOURNAL OF PSYCHOLOGY. 54(1):131-137, 1962.

"Comparative toxicity of heroin, morphine and methadone.

BULLETIN ON NARCOTICS. 21(1):40, Jan.-Mar., 1969.
"A comparison between acute and chronic physical dependence
in the chronic slinal dog," by Martin, W.R., and Eades,
C.G. JOURNAL OF PHARMACOLOGY AND EXPERIMENTAL THERAPEU-
TICS. 146(3):385-394, 1964.
"Comparison of analgesic and side effects of parenteral d-
propowyphene and meperidine," by Stoelting, V.K., et al.
ANESTHESIOLOGY. 23:21-26, 1962.
"Comparison of chemical tests with the pupillary method for
the diagnosis of narcotic use," by Way, E.L., et al.
BULLETIN ON NARCOTICS. 15(1):29-33, Jan.-Mar., 1963.
"Comparison of drug effects on approach avoidance and es-
cape motivation," by Barry, H., and Miller, N.E. JOURNAL
OF COMPARATIVE AND PHYSIOLOGICAL PSYCHOLOGY. 59(1):18-
24, 1965.
"A comparison of fentanyl, droperidol, and morphine," by
Gorodetsky, G.W., and Martin, W.R. CLINICAL PHARMACOLOGY
AND THERAPEUTICS. 6(6):731-739, 1965.
"Comparison of phenobarbital and pentobarbital actions upon
water ingestion," by Schmidt, H., and Dry, L. JOURNAL OF
COMPARATIVE AND PHYSIOLOGICAL PSYCHOLOGY. 56(1):179-182,
1963.
"Comparison of phenyramidol and placebo in musculo-skeletal
pain syndrome," by Bodi, T., et al. CURRENT THERAPEUTIC
RESEARCH. 4:135-145, 1962.
"Comparison of potency of injectable meperidine and prometh-
azine-meperidine capsules in postoperative pain," by Man-
narelli, A.A. JOURNAL OF THE AMERICAN OSTEOPATHIC ASSOC-
IATION. 63:1034-1037, 1964.
"A comparison of the analgesic effects of pentazocine and
morphine in patients with cancer," by Beaver, W.T., et
al. CLINICAL PHARMACOLOGY AND THERAPEUTICS. 7:740-751,
1966.
"A comparison of the analgesic effects of pentazocine and
pethidine in post-operative pain," by Erb, H. GYNAECO-
LOGIA. 162(4):275-282, 1967.
"A comparison of the analgesic potencies of morphine, pentazocine, and a mixture of methamphetamine and pentazocine
in the rat," by Evans, W.O., and Bergner, D.P. JOURNAL
OF NEW DRUGS. 4(2):82-85, 1964; also United States Army,
MEDICAL RESEARCH LABORATORY. no. 602:1-7, Feb., 1964.
"A comparison of the analgetic potency of some analgesics as
measured by the 'flinch-jump' procedure," by Evans, W.O.
PSYCHOPHARMACOLOGIA. 3(1):51-54, 1962.
"Comparison of the effects of single doses of morphine and
thebaine on body temperature, activity, and brain and
heart levels of catecholamines and serotonin," by Sloan,
J.W., et al. PSYCHOPHARMACOLOGIA. 3(4):291-301, 1962.
"A comparison of the intellectual performance of the juven-
ile addict with standardization norms," by Laskowitz.
JOURNAL OF CORRECTIONAL EDUCATION. 14(2):31-32, 1962.
"Comparison of the nalorphine test and urinary analysis in
the detection of narcotic use," by Elliott, H.W., et al.
CLINICAL PHARMACOLOGY AND THERAPEUTICS. 5:405-413, 1964.

"A comparison of the pharmacologic effects of morphine and
N-methyl morphine," by Foster, R.S., et al. JOURNAL OF
PHARMACOLOGY AND EXPERIMENTAL THERAPEUTICS. 157(1):185-
195, 1967.
"Comparison of two drugs with psychotomimetic effects (LSD
and ditran)," by Wilson, R.E., and Shagass, C. JOURNAL
OF NERVOUS AND MENTAL DISEASE. 138:277-286, 1964.
"A comparison of two narcotics. Numorphan and demeral, in
obstetrics, by double-blind technique," by Sherline, D.M.,
and Roddick, J.W., Jr. QUARTERLY BULLETIN OF NORTHWEST-
ERN UNIVERSITY MEDICAL SCHOOL. 36:54-56, 1962.
"Compendium of neuropsychopharmacology. Analgesics," by La-
Verne, A.A. JOURNAL OF NEUROPSYCHIATRY. 5:201-211, 1964.
"Compounds possessing morphine-antagonizing or powerful an-
algesic properties," by Bentley, K.W., et al. NATURE.
206(4979):102-103, 1965.
"Conditioned suppression in rats and the effect of pharmaco-
logical agents thereon," by Lauener, H. PSYCHOPHARMACO-
LOGIA. 4:311-325, 1963.
"Conduction block by cocaine in sodium-depleted nerves with
activity maintained by lithium, hydrazinium or guandium
ions," by Condouris, G.A. JOURNAL OF PHARMACOLOGY AND
EXPERIMENTAL THERAPEUTICS. 141(2):253-259, 1963.
"Configuration of reticuline in the opium poppy," by Batters-
by, A.R., et al. TETRAHEDRON LETTERS. 18:1275-1278,
1965.
"Consistency of psilocybin induced changes in the Minnesota
Multiphasic Personality Inventory," by Keeler, M.H., and
Doehne, E.F. JOURNAL OF CLINICAL PSYCHOLOGY. 21(3):284,
1965.
"The control of severe pain with oral oxymorphone hydro-
chloride," by Cass, L.J., and Frederik, W.S. CURRENT
THERAPEUTIC RESEARCH. 5:579-586, 1963.
"Controlled clinical trials of antitussive agents: an ex-
perimental evaluation of different methods," by Nicolis,
F.B., and Pasquariello, G. JOURNAL OF PHARMACOLOGY AND
EXPERIMENTAL THERAPEUTICS. 136(2):183-189, 1962.
"A controlled evaluation of deanol and benactyzine-mepro-
bamate," by Loranger, A.W., and Prout, C.T. NEW ENGLAND
JOURNAL OF MEDICINE. 266(21):1073-1078, 1962.
"Cough control of chronic coughs with an antitussive aon-
taining two cough suppressants," by Chesrow, E.J., et al.
CLINICAL MEDICINE. 73(10):47-49, 1966.
"Counteraction of narcotic antagonist analgesics by the nar-
cotic antagonist naloxone," by Blumberg, H., et al. PRO-
CEEDINGS OF THE SOCIETY FOR EXPERIMENTAL BIOLOGY AND MED-
ICINE. 123:755-758, 1966.
"Cross-cellular adaptation to methadone and meperidine in
cerebral cortical slices from morphinized rats," by Take-
mori, A.E. JOURNAL OF PHARMACOLOGY AND EXPERIMENTAL
THERAPEUTICS. 135:252-255, 1962.
"A critical appraisal of chlordiazepoxide," by Ayd, F.J.,
Jr. JOURNAL OF NEUROPSYCHIATRY. 3:177-180, 1962.
"Cyclazocine, a long acting narcotic antagonist; its vol-

untary acceptance as a treatment modality by narcotic
abusers," by Jaffe, J.H., and Brill, L. INTERNATIONAL
JOURNAL OF THE ADDICTIONS. 1(1):99-123, 1966.
"Cyclazocine and methadone in narcotic addiction," by Freed-
man, A., et al. JOURNAL OF THE AMERICAN MEDICAL ASSOCIA-
TION. 202:191-194, 1967.
"Demonstration of tolerance to and physical dependence of
N-allylnormorphine (nalorphine)," by Martin, W.R., et al.
JOURNAL OF PHARMACOLOGY AND EXPERIMENTAL THERAPEUTICS.
150:437-442, Dec., 1965.
"Dependence on dextromoramide," by Cormack, J. BRITISH MED-
ICAL JOURNAL. 1:362, Feb. 11, 1967.
"Dependence on dextromoramide (pt.1)," by Seymour-Shove, R.,
et al. BRITISH MEDICAL JOURNAL. 1:88-90, Jan. 14, 1967.
--pt.2. BRITISH MEDICAL JOURNAL. 1:568-569, Mar. 4, 1967.
"Detection and determination of various organic poisons in
biological fluids," by Bourdoin, R., et al. ANNALES DE
BIOLOGIE CLINIQUE. 21:187-218, 1963.
"Detection and estimation of cocaine by gas chromatography,"
by Scaringelli, F.P. JOURNAL OF THE ASSOCIATION OF OFFI-
CIAL AGRICULTURAL CHEMISTS. 46(4):643-645, 1963.
"Detection of narcotic drugs, tranquilizers, amphetamines,
and barbiturates in urine," by Dole, V.P., et al. JOUR-
NAL OF THE AMERICAN MEDICAL ASSOCIATION. 198:349-352,
1966.
"Detection of narcotic usage by the pupillary method," by
Way, E.L. PSYCHOPHARMACOLOGY BULLETIN; NATIONAL CLEAR-
INGHOUSE FOR MENTAL HEALTH INFORMATION. 3:61-63, Dec.,
1966.
"Detection of narcotic use. Comparison of the nalorphine
(pupil) test with chemical tests," by Elliott, H.W., et
al. CALIFORNIA MEDICINE. 109:121-125, Aug., 1968.
"Determination of codeine in terpin hydrate and codeine
elixir," by Blake, M.I., and Carlstedt, B. JOURNAL OF
PHARMACEUTICAL SCIENCES. 55(12):1462, 1966.
"The determination of morphine in opium," by Avico, U.
BULLETIN ON NARCOTICS. 19(4):1-3, Oct.-Dec., 1967.
"Development of the Addiction Research Center Inventory
(ARCI): selection of items that are sensitive to the
effects of various drugs," by Haertzen, C.A., et al.
PSYCHOPHARMACOLOGIA. 4:155-166, 1963.
"Determination of narcotic analgesics in human biological
materials. Application of thin layer chromatography,"
by Mule, S.J. PSYCHOPHARMACOLOGY BULLETIN; NATIONAL
CLEARINGHOUSE FOR MENTAL HEALTH INFORMATION. 3:37-39,
Dec., 1966; also ANALYTICAL CHEMISTRY. 36:1907-1914,
1964.
"Development and loss of tolerance to morphine in the rat
after single and multiple injections," by Cochin, J.,
and Kornetsky, C. JOURNAL OF PHARMACOLOGY AND EXPERI-
MENTAL THERAPEUTICS. 145(1):1-10, 1964.
"Development of scales based on patterns of drug effects,
using the Addiction Research Center Inventory (ARCI),"
by Haertzen, C.A. PSYCHOLOGICAL REPORTS. 18:163-194,

1966.
"Dextromethorphan in antitussive mixtures. I. Combined
with an antihistamine." PRACTITIONER. 190:657-659, 1963.
"Diethylpropion: the risk of dependence." DRUG AND THER-
APEUTICS BULLETIN. 6:12, Feb. 2, 1968.
"Diffuse systems of the brain: physiological and pharmaco-
logical mechanisms," by Bradley, P.B. DEVELOPMENTAL MED-
ICINE AND CHILD NEUROLOGY. 4(1):49-54, 1962.
"Dihydrocodeine as a cough suppressant." PRACTITIONER.
193:86-88, 1964.
"Dilaudid in acute cardiac emergencies," by Goodman, R.D.
ACADEMY OF MEDICINE OF NEW JERSEY BULLETIN. 9:11-19,
1963.
"A direct titrimetic method for the determination of some
organic bases in pharmaceutical preparations," by John-
son, C.A., and Ring, R.E. JOURNAL OF PHARMACEUTICAL
PHARMACOLOGY. 15:584-588, 1963.
"Distribution of N-C-14-methyl labeled morphine. I. In
central nervous system of nontolerant and tolerant dogs,"
by Mule, S.J., and Woods, L.A. JOURNAL OF PHARMACOLOGY
AND EXPERIMENTAL THERAPEUTICS. 136:232-241, 1962.
--II. Effect of nalorphine in the central nervous system
of nontolerant dogs and observations on metabolism," by
Mule, S.J., et al. JOURNAL OF PHARMACOLOGY AND EXPERI-
MENTAL THERAPEUTICS. 136(2):242-249, 1962.
--III. Effect of nalorphine in the central nervous system
and other tissues of tolerant dogs," by Mule, S.J. JOUR-
NAL OF PHARMACOLOGY AND EXPERIMENTAL THERAPEUTICS. 148
(3):393-398, 1965.
"Dolorimetry and its value as a method of evaluating anal-
gesic agents," by Sweeney, D.R. DISSERTATION ABSTRACTS.
23(9):3506, 1963.
"Double blind evaluation of analgesic agents in the post-
partum patient," by Benson, R.C. WESTERN JOURNAL OF SUR-
GERY. 71:167-169, 1963.
"Double-blind evaluation of two analgesic combinations for
pain after minor oral surgical procedures," by Koslin,
A.J. JOURNAL OF ORAL SURGERY, ANESTHESIA, AND HOSPITAL
DENTAL SERVICE. 21:414-419, 1963.
"A double blind study of a new analgesic combination," by
Uhland, H. NORTHWEST MEDICINE. 61:843-845, 1962.
"Double-blind study of methotrimeprazine, morphine, and meperidine for preanesthetic medication," by Dobkin, A.B.,
et al. ANESTHESIA AND ANALGESIA; CURRENT RESEARCHES.
44(5):510-516, 1965.
"Double blind trial of dextromoramide, methadone and pethidine in the treatment of severe pain," by Matts, S.G.F.,
et al. POSTGRADUATE MEDICAL JOURNAL. 40(460):103-105,
1964.
"Drug administration to cerebral cortex of freely moving
dogs," by Kobayashi, T. SCIENCE. 135(3509):1126-1127,
1962.
"Drug and placebo responses in chronic alcoholics," by Kissin, B., et al. PSYCHIATRIC RESEARCH REPORTS. 24:44-
60, 1968.

"Drug and strain effects on performance and reversal of a head-position habit," by Coppock, H.W., et al. JOURNAL OF COMPARATIVE AND PHYSIOLOGICAL PSYCHOLOGY. 56:551-557, 1963.
"Drug dangers to the fetus from maternal medications," by Arena, J.M. CLINICAL PEDIATRICS. 3:450-465, 1964.
"Drug effects on the behavior of animals," by Cook, L., and Kelleher, R.T. ANNALS OF THE NEW YORK ACADEMY OF SCIENCES. 96:315-335, 1962.
"Drug effects on motor coordination," by Watzman, N., and Barry, H. PSYCHOPHARMACOLOGIA. 12(5):414-423, 1968.
"Drug-induced modifications of discriminated avoidance behavior in rats," by Morpurgi, C. PSYCHOPHARMACOLOGIA. 8:91-99, 1965.
"Drug-induced respiratory depression in man. A method of assessment," by Campbell, D., et al. CLINICAL PHARMACOLOGY AND THERAPEUTICS. 5(2):193-200, 1964.
"Drug-induced skin eruptions treated at the Helsinki University dermatological clinic 1956-1960," by Kauppinen, K. DUODECIM. 79:269-272, 1963.
"Drug interaction in the field of analgesic drugs," by Lasagna, L. PROCEEDINGS OF THE ROYAL SOCIETY OF MEDICINE. 58(11, pt.2):978-983, 1965.
"Drug metabolism and forensic toxicology," by Smith, R.L. JOURNAL OF THE FORENSIC SCIENCE SOCIETY. 7(2):71-85, Apr., 1967.
"Drug therapy," by Cole, J., et al. PROGRESS IN NEUROLOGY AND PSYCHIATRY. 15:540-576, 1960.
"Drug withdrawal and fighting in rats," by Florea, J., and Thor, D.H. PSYCHONOMIC SCIENCE. 12(1):33, 1968.
"Drug withdrawal with promazine hydrochloride," by Rolo, A. NEW YORK STATE JOURNAL OF MEDICINE. 62:1429-1431, 1962.
"Drugs and alcohol as toxicological problems," by Kácl, K. CASOPIS LEKARU CESKYCH. 104:884-888, 1965.
"Drugs and judgement: effects of amphetamine and secobarbital on self-evaluation," by Smith, G., and Beecher, H. JOURNAL OF PSYCHOLOGY. 58:397-405, 1964.
"Drugs and placebos: a model design," by Ross, S., et al. PSYCHOLOGICAL REPORTS. 10(2):383-392, 1962.
"Drugs and the driver," by Jolles, K.E. MEDICAL WORLD. 97:338-342, 1962.
"Drugs that modify actions of pharmacologically active polypeptides," by Walaszek, E.J., et al. ANNALS OF THE NEW YORK ACADEMY OF SCIENCES. 104:281-289, 1963.
"Duquenois-Levine test modification," by Butler, W. JOURNAL OF THE ASSOCIATION OF OFFICIAL AGRICULTURAL CHEMISTS. 45:597, 1962.
"Effect of a potent non-narcotic analgesic agent (pentazocine) on uterine contractility and fetal heart rate," by Filler, W.W., and Filler, N.W. OBSTETRICS AND GYNECOLOGY. 28:224-232, 1966.
"Effect of actinomycin D on morphine tolerance," by Cohen, M., et al. PROCEEDINGS OF THE SOCIETY OF EXPERIMENTAL BIOLOGY AND MEDICINE. 119(2):381-384, 1965.

"The effect of addiction to and abstinence from morphine on rat tissue catecholamine and serotonin level," by Sloan, J.W., et al. PSYCHOPHARMACOLOGIA. 4(4):261-270, 1963.

"The effect of altering liver microsomal N-demethylase activity on the development of tolerance to morphine in rats," by Clouet, D.H., and Ratner, M. JOURNAL OF PHARMACOLOGY AND EXPERIMENTAL THERAPEUTICS. 144(3):362-372, 1964.

"Effect of an hallucinogenic agent on verbal behavior," by Honigfeld, G. PSYCHOLOGICAL REPORTS. 13(2):383-385, 1963.

"Effect of cocaine, desipramine, amd angiotensin on uptake of noradrenaline in tissues of pithed rats," by Pals, D.T., amd Masucci, F.D. NATURE. 217(5130):772-773, 1968.

"Effect of cocaine, phenoxybenzamine and phentolamine on the catecholamine output from spleen and adrenal medulla," by Kirpekar, S.M., and Cervoni, P. JOURNAL OF PHARMACOLOGY AND EXPERIMENTAL THERAPEUTICS. 142(1):59-70, 1963.

"Effect of drugs on survival time from scorpion envenomation," by Greenberg, L., and Ingalis, J.W. JOURNAL OF PHARMACEUTICAL SCIENCES. 52:159-161, 1963.

"Effect of common drugs on urinary excretion of gonadotropins," by Ciprut, S., et al. JOURNAL OF CLINICAL ENDOCRINOLOGY AND METABOLISM. 22(5):535-536, 1962.

"Effect of drugs on coronary circulating during experimental spasm of the cardiac vessels," by Kareva, G.F. FEDERATION PROCEEDINGS; TRANSLATION SUPPLEMENT. 22:866-868, 1963.

"Effect of local anesthetics on the cardiovascular system of the dog," by Stewart, D.M., et al. ANESTHESIOLOGY. 24(5):620-624, 1963.

"Effect of meperidine in uterine contractility during pregnancy and prelabor," by Sica-Blanco, Y., et al. AMERICAN JOURNAL OF OBSTETRICS AND GYNECOLOGY. 97(8):1096-1100, 1967.

"The effect of morphine on diverticulosis of the colon," by Painter, N.S. PROCEEDINGS OF THE ROYAL SOCIETY OF MEDICINE. 56(9):800, 1963.

"The effect of morphine, meperidine, and thiopental in hypovolemic shock," by Chasnow, E.A., et al. SURGERY. 55(4):567-573, 1964.

"Effect of morphine on breathing pattern. A possible factor in atelectasis," by Egbert, L.D., and Bendixen, H.H. JOURNAL OF THE AMERICAN MEDICAL ASSOCIATION. 188(6):485-488, 1964.

"Effect of morphine on diverticula of the colon," by Painter, N.S. DISEASES OF THE COLON AND RECTUM. 8:40-41, 1965.

"Effect of morphine on rats bearing Walker carcinosarcoma 256," by Sobel, H., and Bonorris, G. NATURE. 196(4857):896-897, 1962.

"The effect of morphine on the discharge of muscle spindles with intact motor innervation." INTERNATIONAL JOURNAL OF NEUROPHARMACOLOGY. 4(3):177-183, 1965.

"Effect of morphine on the morphological alterations of the endocrine glands induced by castration and oestrogen hormone administration," by David, M.A., and Kovacs, K. ACTA ANATOMICA. 50:90-102, 1962.

"Effect of morphine sulfate on spontaneous activity level of the albino rat," by Collins, L.G. PSYCHOLOGICAL REPORTS. 16:694-696, 1965.

"Effect of morphine upon uterine contraction in late pregnancy," by Eskes, T.K.A.B. AMERICAN JOURNAL OF OBSTETRICS AND GYNECOLOGY. 84(3):281-289, 1962.

"Effect of nitrous oxide and morphine on the minimum anesthetic concentration of fluroxene," by Munson, E.S., et al. ANESTHESIOLOGY. 26(2):134-139, 1965.

"The effect of preanesthetic and anesthetic agents on the respiration-heart rate response of dogs," by McCrady, J.D., et al. AMERICAN JOURNAL OF VETERINARY RESEARCH. 26:710-716, 1965.

"Effect of psychotogens on approach and avoidance behavior," by Ray, O.S. INTERNATIONAL JOURNAL OF NEUROPSYCHIATRY. 1:98, 1965.

"The effect of psychotropic drugs on food reinforced behaviour and on food consumption," by Bainbridge, J.G. PSYCHOPHARMACOLOGIA. 12(3):204-213, 1968.

"Effect of reserpine and alpha-methyl-tyrosine on morphine analgesia," by Verri, R.A., et al. INTERNATIONAL JOURNAL OF NEUROPHARMACOLOGY. 7(3):283-292, 1968.

"The effect of reserpine on animal behavior and bioelectric activity of the brain," by Damlycek, V.P. PHARMACEUTICAL-MEDICAL JOURNAL. 1:4-8, 1965.

"The effect of sleep plus morphine on the respiratory response to carbon dioxide," by Forrest, W.H., Jr., and Bellville, J.W. ANESTHESIOLOGY. 25:137-141, 1964.

"Effect of some blocking drugs on the pressor response to physostigmine in the rat," by Gokhale, S.D., et al. BRITISH JOURNAL OF PHARMACOLOGY AND CHEMOTHERAPY. 21(2):273-284, 1963.

"The effect of some centrally-acting drugs on disjunctive reaction time," by Evans, W.O., and Jewett, A. PSYCHOPHARMACOLOGIA. 3(2):124-127, 1962.

"Effect of some drugs upon rat brain histamine content," by Green, H., and Erickson, R.W. INTERNATIONAL JOURNAL PF NEUROPHARMACOLOGY. 3:315-320, 1964.

"The effect of stimulant and depressant drugs on the latency of auptokinetic illusion," by Singh, S.D., and Singh, V. ACTA PSYCHOLOGICA (Amsterdam). 18(5):354-359, 1961.

"Effect of the morphine-group analgesics on the central inhibitory machanisms," by Kruglov, N.A. INTERNATIONAL JOURNAL OF NEUROPHARMACOLOGY. 3(2):197-203, 1964.

"Effect of the narcotic kat (catha edulis) on certain functions of the human body," by Galkin, V.A., and Mironychev, A.V. FEDERATION PROCEEDINGS. 23(4):T.741-T.742, 1964.

"The effect of various environmental factors on cocaine and ephedrine toxicity," by Peterson, D.I., et al. JOURNAL

OF PHARMACY AND PHARMACOLOGY. 19(12):810-814, 1967.
"Effect of various pharmacologic agents on cerebral arteries," by Karlsberg, P., et al. NEUROLOGY. 13(9):772-778, 1963.
"The effect of y-phenyl-propylcarbamate compared with meprobamate and placebo," by Idestrom, C.M. PSYCHOPHARMACOLOGIA. 3(1):15-22, 1962.
"The effectiveness of dextro-propoxyphene hydrochloride in the control of pain after periodontal surgery," by Berdon, J.K., et al. JOURNAL OF PERIODONTOLOGY. 35:106-111, 1964.
"Effects of a bacterial polysaccharide (piromen) on the pituitary-adrenal axis: modification of ACTH release by morphine and salicylate," by Wexler, B.C. METABOLISM. 12:49-56, 1963.
"Effects of addiction to intravenous heroin on patterns of physical activity in man," by Fraser, H.F., et al. CLINICAL PHARMACOLOGY AND THERAPEUTICS. 4(2):188-196, 1963.
"The effects of aggregation, electric shock, and adrenergic blocking drugs on inhibition of the 'writhing syndrome'," by Okun, R., et al. JOURNAL OF PHARMACOLOGY AND EXPERIMENTAL THERAPEUTICS. 139:107-109, 1963.
"The effects of anesthetics upon the ear. V. Cochlear potentials and behavioral thresholds," by Strotcher, W.F., et al. ANNALS OF OTOLOGY, RHINOLOGY AND LARYNGOLOGY. 73:141-152, 1964.
"Effects of atropine, morphine, and epinephrine on electrically stimulated contractions of isolated intestines of several species," by Goldenberg, M.M. FEDERATION PROCEEDINGS. 24(2, pt.1):710, 1965.
"Effects of certain drugs on perfused human placenta. I. Narcotic analgesics, serotonin and relaxin," by Gautieri, R.F., and Ciuchta, H.P. JOURNAL OF PHARMACEUTICAL SCIENCES. 51(1):55-58, 1962.
--II. Vasodilators, by Ciuchta, H.P., and Gautieri, R.F. JOURNAL OF PHARMACEUTICAL SCIENCES. 52(10):974-978, 1963.
"The effects of bretylium and cocaine on noradrenaline depletion," by Callingham, B.A., and Cass, R. JOURNAL OF PHARMACY AND PHARMACOLOGY. 14:385-389, 1962.
"Effects of cocaine administered on brain, adrenal and urinary adrenaline and noradrenaline in rats," by Gunne, L.M., and Jonsson, J. PSYCHOPHARMACOLOGIA. 6(2):125-129, 1964.
"Effects of drugs on the electric knife fish, eigenmannia virescens," by Krivoy, W.A., et al. PROCEEDINGS OF THE SOCIETY FOR EXPERIMENTAL BIOLOGY AND MEDICINE. 114(3):640-644, 1963.
"The effects of drugs on uptake and exit of cerebral amino acids," by Lajtha, A., and Toth, J. BIOCHEMICAL PHARMACOLOGY. 14:729-738, 1965.
"Effects of drugs used in pregnancy on availability of fetal cerebral oxygen," by Mairahy, G.A., et al. ANESTHESIOLOGY. 24(2):198-202, 1963.
"Effects of levorphanol and levallorphan on osmolality of

serum from water loaded rats," by Fujimoto, J.M., et al. PROCEEDINGS OF THE SOCIETY FOR EXPERIMENTAL BIOLOGY AND MEDICINE. 114(1):193, 1963.

"Effects of ligation and morphine on electric and motor activity of dog duodenum," by Bass, P., and Wiley, J.N. AMERICAN JOURNAL OF PHYSIOLOGY. 208:908-913, 1965.

"Effects of magnesium pemoline and dextroamphetamine on human learning," by Burns, John T., et al. SCIENCE. 155 (3764):849-851, 1967.

"Effects of meperidine hydrochloride and morphine sulfate on the lung capacity of intact dogs," by Shemano, I., and Wendel, H. JOURNAL OF PHARMACOLOGY AND EXPERIMENTAL THERAPEUTICS. 149(3):379-384, 1965.

"Effects of meperidine on the newborn infant," by Shnider, S.M. AMERICAN JOURNAL OF OBSTETRICS AND GYNECOLOGY. 89(8):1009-1015, 1964.

"The effects of morphine and pethidine on somatic evoked responses in the midbrain of the cat, and their relevance to analgesia," by McKenzie, J.S., and Beechey, N.R. ELECTROENCEPHALOGRAPHY AND CLINICAL NEUROPHYSIOLOGY. 14: 501-519, 1962.

"Effects of morphine and trofanil on the incorporation of phosphate into phospholopids of rat brain slices," by Brossard, M., and Quastel, J.H. BIOCHEMICAL PHARMACOLOGY. 12(7):766-768, 1963.

"Effects of morphine, levallorphan and respiratory gases on increased intracranial pressure," by Weitzner, S.W., et al. ANESTHESIOLOGY. 24:291-298, 1963.

"Effects of morphine, nalorphine, cyclazocine and naloxone on the flexor reflex," by McClane, T.K., and Martin, W.R. INTERNATIONAL JOURNAL OF NEUROPHARMACOLOGY. 6(2):89-98, 1967.

"Effects of morphine on the hormonal control of metabolism. I. In vitro effects of morphine and hydrocortisone on utilization of glucose by muscle of normal and chronically morphinized rats," by Lee Peng, C.H., and Walsh, E. BIOCHEMICAL PHARMACOLOGY. 12(9):921, 1963.

--II. Invitro effects of adrenaline and hydrocortisone on utilization of glucose by muscle of normal and chronically morphinized rats," by Walsh, E. BIOCHEMICAL PHARMACOLOGY. 14(6):1003-1009, 1965.

"Effects of morphine on the operant behaviour in rats," by Molinengo, L. PSYCHOPHARMACOLOGIA. 6(5):347-367, 1964.

"Effects of morphine on uptake of glucose and synthesis of glycogen in muscle of normal and chronically morphinized rats," by Lee Peng, C.H., and Walsh, E.O.F. NATURE. 196(4850):171, 1962.

"Effects of morphine on ventricular performance," by Vasko, J.S., et al. SURGICAL FORUM; CLINICAL CONGRESS OF THE AMERICAN COLLEGE OF SURGEONS. 16:162-165, 1965.

"The effects of morphine, pentobarbital, pentazocine and nalorphine on bioelectrical potentials evoked in the brain stem of the cat by electrical stimulation of the tooth pulp," by Straw, R.N., and Mitchell, C.L. JOURNAL OF

PHARMACOLOGY AND EXPERIMENTAL THERAPEUTICS. 146:7-15, 1964.

"The effects of preanesthetic, anesthetic, and postoperative drugs on renal function," by Papper, S., and Papper, E.M. CLINICAL PHARMACOLOGY AND THERAPEUTICS. 5(2):205-215, 1964.

"Effects of premedicant drugs on respiration and gas exchange in man," by Smith, T.C., et al. ANESTHESIOLOGY. 28(5):883-890, 1967.

"The effects of psychotomimetic drugs on primary suggestibility," by Sjoberg, B.M, Jr., and Hollister, L.E. PSYCHOPHARMACOLOGIA. 8(4):251-262, 1965.

"Effects of reserpine and morphine on behavior suppressed by punishment," by Geller, I., et al. LIFE SCIENCES. 4:226-231, 1963.

"The effects of SKF 525-A on hepatic glycogen and rate of hepatic drug metabolism," by Rogers, L.A., et al. BIOCHEMICAL PHARMACOLOGY. 12:341-348, 1963.

"Effects of shock intensity, deprivation, and morphine in a simple approach-avoidance conflict situation," by Lead, R.C., and Muller, S.A. PSYCHOLOGICAL REPORTS. 17:819-823, 1965.

"The effects of smooth muscle stimulants on the movement of calcium-47 in the guinea-pig ileum in vitro," by Banerjee, A.K., and Lewis, J.J. JOURNAL OF PHARMACY AND PHARMACOLOGY. 15:409-410, 1963.

"Effects of sodium pentobarbital and d-amphetamine on latency of the escape response in the rat," by Mize, D., and Isaac, W. PSYCHOLOGICAL REPORTS. 10:643-645, 1962.

"Effects of stimulant and depressant drugs on physical persistence," by Singh, S.D. PERCEPTUAL AND MOTOR SKILLS. 14:270, 1962.

"Effects of time and 8-azaguanine on the development of morphine tolerance," by Spoerlein, M.T., and Scrafani, J. LIFE SCIENCES. 6(14, pt.2):1549-1564, 1967.

"Effects of various drugs on a conditioned avoidance response in dogs resistant to extinction," by Domino, E.F., et al. JOURNAL OF PHARMACOLOGY AND EXPERIMENTAL THERAPEUTICS. 141:92-99, 1963.

"The effects of two phenylacetic acid derivatives on the analgesic action of morphine in mice," by Madakovic, M., and Banic, B. JOURNAL OF PHARMACY AND PHARMACOLOGY. 15(10):660-665, 1963.

"The efficacy of placebo on pain perception threshold," by Blair, A.E. ORAL SURGERY, ORAL MEDICINE AND ORAL PATHOLOGY. 20(3):384-391, 1965.

"Elevation of plasma histamine levels in the dog following administration of muscle relaxants, opiates and macromolecular polymers," by Thompson, W.L., and Walton, R.P. JOURNAL OF PHARMACOLOGY AND EXPERIMENTAL THERAPEUTICS. 143(1):131-136, 1964.

"Emergence delirium," by Bastron, R., and Moyers, J. JOURNAL OF THE AMERICAN MEDICAL ASSOCIATION. 200(10):179, 1967.

"Energy metabolism in dogs during anesthesia, curarization, or acute arterial hypotension," by Galvao, P.E., et al. AMERICAN JOURNAL OF PHYSIOLOGY. 204:337-342, 1963.
"Environmental temperature effects on the thermoregulatory response to systemic and hypothalamic administration of morphine," by Paolino, R.M., and Pernard, B.K. LIFE SCIENCES. 7(15):857-863, 1968.
"Enzymatic formation of morphine and nicotine in a mammal," by Azelrod, J. LIFE SCIENCES. 1:29-30, 1962.
"Establishing the presence of cocaine in novocaine mixtures - qualitative aspect." BULLETIN ON NARCOTICS. 20(3):40, July-Sept., 1968.
"Estimating the acceptibility of morphine and noracymethadol in postpartum patients," by Gruber, C.M., and Baptisti, A. CLINICAL PHARMACOLOGY AND THERAPEUTICS. 4(2):172-181, 1963.
"Estimation of codeine in pharmaceutical preparations," by Bose, P.C., et al. JOURNAL OF SCIENTIFIC AND INDUSTRIAL RESEARCH (India), SECTION D. 21(10):386-387, 1962.
"The estimation of morphine, codeine and thebaine in opium and in poppy latex by paper chromatography," by Fairbairn, J.W., and Wassel, G. JOURNAL OF PHARMACY AND PHARMACOLOGY. 15(suppl.):216T-221T, 1963.
"Evaluation of analgesics by the rating of patient behavior," by Steinhaus, J.E., et al. ANESTHESIOLOGY. 25(1):64-70, 1964.
"Evaluation of carisoprodol and phenyramidol for addictiveness," by Fraser, H.F., et al. BULLETIN ON NARCOTICS. 13(4):1-6, Oct.-Dec., 1961.
"Evaluation of ethchlorvynol in the preoperative medication of mentally ill and mentally retarded patients," by Kralemann, H., and Tyce, F.A. ANESTHESIA AND ANALGESIA: CURRENT RESEARCHES. 44(2):180-185, 1965.
"Evaluation of opiates for pain and premedication," by Steinhaus, J.E., and Lee, W.J. JOURNAL OF THE MEDICAL ASSOCIATION OF GEORGIA. 52:396-398, 1963.
"An evalutaion of oxymorphone in labor," by Sentor, M.H., et al. AMERICAN JOURNAL OF OBSTETRICS AND GYNECOLOGY. 84:956-961, 1962.
"Evaluation of phenazocine with meperidine as an analgesic agent during labor, by the double blind method," by Olson, R.O., and Riva, H.L. AMERICAN JOURNAL OF OBSTETRICS AND GYNECOLOGY. 88(5):601-605, 1964.
"Evalutaion of psychotherapeutic drugs on general practice," by Wheatley, C. PSYCHOPHARMACOLOGY SERVICE CENTER BULLETIN. 2:25-31, 1962.
"Evaluation of the nalorphine pupil diagnostic test for narcotic usage in longterm heroin and opium addicts," by Way, E.L., et al. CLINICAL PHARMACOLOGY AND THERAPEUTICS. 7(3):300-311, May-June, 1966.
"Evaluation of two screening procedures for detecting the use of opiates," by Mason, C.C., and Shepherd, H.G. AMERICAN JOURNAL OF CLINICAL PATHOLOGY. 37:176-181, 1962.
"Evaluation of tranquilizing drugs in the management of

acute mental disturbance," by Abse, D.W., et al. AMER-
ICAN JOURNAL OF PSYCHIATRY. 116:973-980, 1960.
"An evaluation of the efficacy of methopholine for the re-
lief of postoperative pain," by Moore, J., et al. AMER-
ICAN JOURNAL OF THE MEDICAL SCIENCES. 244(3):337-343,
1962.
"The excretion of pethidine and its derivatives," by Asa-
toor, A.M., et al. BRITISH JOURNAL OF PHARMACOLOGY AND
CHEMOTHERAPY. 20(2):285-298, 1963.
"Experience with a new cough preparation: report of 203
cases," by Phillips, F.J., et al. CURRENT THERAPEUTIC
RESEARCH. 5:17-23, 1963.
"Experience with intravenous demerol with lorfan for anal-
gesia and anesthesia in obstetrics," by Rowe, D.H., and
Fealy, J. JOURNAL OF THE FLORIDA MEDICAL ASSOCIATION.
48:635-639, 1962.
"Experimental and clinical toxicology of chlordiazepoxide
(librium R)," by Zbinden, G., et al. TOXICOLOGY AND AP-
PLIED PHARMACOLOGY. 3:619-637, 1961.
"An experimental pain method sensitive to morphine in man,
the submaximum effort tourniquet technique," by Smith,
G.M., et al. JOURNAL OF PHARMACOLOGY AND EXPERIMENTAL
THERAPEUTICS. 154(2):324-332, 1966.
"Experimental production of human 'blue velvet' and 'red
devil' lesions," by Puro, H.E., et al. JOURNAL OF THE
AMERICAN MEDICAL ASSOCIATION. 197:1100-1102, 1966.
"Experimental use of morphine in mine accidents." PROCEED-
INGS OF THE MINE MEDICAL OFFICERS' ASSOCIATION. 43:81-
88, 1964.
"Experiments in relief of clinical pain with N-(2,3-xylyl)-
anthranilic acid (CI-473;mefenramic acid)," by Cass, L.J.,
and Frederik, W.S. JOURNAL OF PHARMACOLOGY AND EXPERI-
MENTAL THERAPEUTICS. 139(2):172-176, 1963.
"Factors modifying chlorpromazine hyperthermia in young al-
bino mice," by Bagdon, W.J., and Mann, D.E. JOURNAL OF
PHARMACEUTICAL SCIENCES. 54:240-246, 1965.
"Factors regulating oral consumption of an opioid (etonita-
zene) by Morphine-addicted rats," by Wikler, A., et al.
PSYCHPHARMACOLOGIA. 5:55-76, 1963.
"Fetal response to maternal medication," by Kovar, W.R.
NEBRASKA STATE MEDICAL JOURNAL. 49:540-546, 1964.
"Fighting narcotic bondage and other forms of narcotic dis-
orders," by Rado, S. COMPREHENSIVE PSYCHIATRY. 4:160-
167, 1963.
"Fluorometric identification of submicrogram amounts of mor-
phine and related compounds on thin-layer chromatographs,"
by Jupferberg, H.J., et al. JOURNAL OF CHROMATOGRAPHY.
16(3):558-559, 1964.
"Focal convulsions during barbiturate abstinence in dogs
with cerebrocortical lesions," by Essig, C.F. PSYCHO-
PHARMACOLOGIA. 3:432-437, 1962.
"Foetal death after pethidine and promazine," by Amias,
A.G., and Fairbairn, D. BRITISH MEDICAL JOURNAL. 5354:
432-433, 1963.

"Foetal death after pethidine and promazine," by Macvicar,
J. BRITISH MEDICAL JOURNAL. 5363:999, 1963.
"Further study of performance errors on Ravens Progressive
Matrices (1938)," by Sheppard, C., et al. JOURNAL OF PSY-
CHOLOGY. 71(1):127-132, 1969.
"Gas chromatography of the morphine alkaloids and the re-
lated compounds," by Yamaguchi, S., et al. CHEMICAL AND
PHARMACEUTICAL BULLETIN. 10(8):755-757, 1963.
"Gas-liquid chromatography of aporphine alkaloids," by Arndt,
R.R., and Baarschers, W.H. CHEMISTRY AND INDUSTRY. 28:
1163-1165, 1963.
"The general outlook in toxicology," by Eichholtz, F.
DEUTSCHE MEDIZINISCHE WOCHENSCHRIFT. 16:29-35, 1965.
"Glutamic acid metabolism in vivo: the effects of pretreat-
ment with morphine sulphate," by Maynard, L.S., and
Schenker, V.J. BIOCHEMICAL PHARMACOLOGY. 13(11):1507-
1511, 1964.
"H-allylnoroxymorphone: a new potent narcotic antagonist,"
by Foldes, F.F., et al. AMERICAN JOURNAL OF THE MEDICAL
SCIENCES. 245(1):25-30, 1963.
"Hazards to health. Chronic-meprobamate intoxication," by
Johnson, A.M. NEW ENGLAND JOURNAL OF MEDICINE. 267(3):
145, 1962.
"Hemodynamics studies of dogs under pentobarbital and mor-
phine chloralose anesthesia," by Shabetal, R., et al.
JOURNAL OF SURGICAL RESEARCH. 3:263-267, 1963.
"Hemolytic anemias caused by drugs," by Frick, P.G. SCHWIE-
ZERISCHE MEDIZINISCHE WOCHENSCHRIFT. 94:531-533, 1964.
"Histamine-induced hypotension due to morphine and arfonad
in the dog," by Morris, K.J., and Zeppa, R. JOURNAL OF
SURGICAL RESEARCH. 3:313-317, 1963.
"Histamine liberation by codeine and polymysin B in urti-
caria pigmentosa," by Sutter, M.C., et al. ARCHIVES OF
DERMATOLOGY. 86:217-221, 1962.
"Human pharmacology and addiction-liabilities of phenazocine
and levophenacylmorphan," by Fraser, H.F., and Isbell, H.
BULLETIN ON NARCOTICS. 12(2):15-23, Apr.-June, 1960.
"The human pharmacology and abuse potential of N-allylnoro-
xymorphone (naloxone)," by Jasinski, D.R., et al. JOUR-
NAL OF PHARMACOLOGY AND EXPERIMENTAL THERAPEUTICS. 157:
420-426, 1967.
"Human pharmacology and addictiveness of ethyl 1-(3-cyano-3,
3-phenylpropyl) 4-phenyl-4-piperidine carboxylate hydro-
chloride (R-1132, diphenoxylate)," by Fraser, H.F., and
Isbell, H. BULLETIN ON NARCOTICS. 13(1):29-43, Jan.-
Mar., 1961.
"The human pharmacology and clinical use of narcotic antag-
onists," by Foldes, F.F. MEDICAL CLINICS OF NORTH AMER-
ICA. 48(2):421-443, 1964.
"Hydroxyzine-meperidine analgesia and neonatal response,"
by Benson, C., and Benson, R.C. AMERICAN JOURNAL OF OB-
STETRICS AND GYNECOLOGY. 84(1):37-43, 1962.
"Hyperventilation studies during nitrous oxide-narcotic-re-
laxant anaesthesia," by Markello, R., et al. ANAESTHES-

IOLOGY. 24:225-230, 1963.
"The identification and determination of morphine," by Ehr-
lich-Rogozinsky, S., and Cheronis, N.D. MICROCHEMICAL
JOURNAL. 7(3):336, 1963.
"The identification of drugs of addiction and habituation,"
by Cann, F.L. JOURNAL OF THE FORENSIC SCIENCE SOCIETY.
3(1):33-36, 1962.
"Identification of morphine and codeine in the urine by
thin-layer chromatography and ultraviolet spectrophoto-
metry," by Harms, D.R. AMERICAN JOURNAL OF MEDICAL TECH-
NOLOGY. 31(1):1-8, 1965.
"Identification of nasal inhaler by gas chromatography," by
Cromp, C.C. JOURNAL OF FORENSIC SCIENCES. 8:477-480,
1963.
"Identification of the opium poppy," by Thornton, J.I., and
Dillon, D.J. JOURNAL OF THE FORENSIC SCIENCE SOCIETY.
6:42-43, 1966.
"Identifying the names and dosage of drugs," by Poulton,
E.C. JOURNAL OF PHARMACY AND PHARMACOLOGY. 16:213-219,
1964.
"Ill-advised medication with drugs leading to habituation
and addiction," by Blair, D. BRITISH JOURNAL OF ADDIC-
TION. 59(2):3-11, 1963.
"Importance of mood amelioration in relief of pain. A con-
trolled comparative study of three analgesic agents," by
Kolodny, A.L. PSYCHOSOMATICS. 4:230-233, 1963.
"Indigenous drug research," by Shama-Rau, T., and Mukerji,
G. PROBE. 1:205-210, 1962.
"Induced hypersensitivity to barbital in the female rat,"
by Aston, R., and Hibbeln, P. SCIENCE. 157:1463-1464,
Sept. 22, 1967.
"Influence of (-) 3-hydroxy-N-propargyl-morphinan on the
respiratory depressant action of codeine," by Rao, D.A.,
and Hofmann, H. EXPERIENTIA. 18:7-8, 1962.
"The influence of drugs on bioelectrical responses evoked
by interacting light flash and tooth pulp simuli," by
Mitchell, S.L., and Killam, K.F. INTERNATIONAL JOURNAL
OF NEUROPHARMACOLOGY. 3:383-396, 1964.
"The influence of morphine and pethidine on somatic evoked
responses in the hippocampal formation of the cat," by
McKenzie, J.S. ELECTROENCEPHALOGRAPHY AND CLINICAL NEURO-
PHYSIOLOGY. 17(4):428-431, 1964.
"Influence of morphine-antagonists on the respiratory de-
pressant action of ethylmorphine and Vo,021," by Anand,
R.D. INDIAN JOURNAL OF PHARMACY. 27(5):143-145, 1965.
"The influence of morphine on glucose utilization in cere-
bral preparations of rats," by Takemori, A.E. JOURNAL OF
PHARMACOLOGY AND EXPERIMENTAL THERAPEUTICS. 145(1):20-26,
1964.
"The influence of narcotics on some age-associated changes
in aerobacter aerogenes," by Blankenship, L.C., and
Doetsch, R.N. JOURNAL OF GERONTOLOGY. 19:39-44, 1964.
"The influence of phenothiazine premedication on methohexi-
tone dosage," by Dundee, J.W., et al. ANAESTHESIA. 18:
41-45, 1963.

"Infra-red spectral analysis of Soviet opium: simultaneous
determination of narcotine, thebaine and papaverine," by
Merlis, V.M., et al. BULLETIN ON NARCOTICS. 20(2):5-8,
Apr.-June, 1968.
"The inhibition of autonomic neuro-effector on transmission
by morphine-like drugs and its use as a screening test
for narcotic analgesic drugs," by Gyang, E.A., et al.
ARCHIV FUR EXPERIMENTELLE PATHOLOGIE UND PHARMAKOLOGIE.
248:231-246, 1964.
"Inhibition of bacterial growth by drugs of the morphine
series," by Simon, E.J. SCIENCE. 144(3618):543-544,
1964.
"Inhibition of evoked potentials by caudate stimulation and
its antagonism by centrally acting drugs," by Collins,
R.J., and Simonton, V.R. INTERNATIONAL JOURNAL OF NEURO-
PHARMACOLOGY. 6(5):349-356, 1967.
"Inhibition of hexobarbital metabolism by ethylmorphine and
codeine in the intact rat," by Rubin, A., et al. BIO-
CHEMICAL PHARMACOLOGY. 13(7):1053-1057, 1964.
"Inhibition of phenylquinone-induced writhing by narcotic
antagonists," by Taber, R.I., et al. NATURE. 204(4954):
189-190, 1964.
"Inhibition of synthesis of RNA in E. coli by narcotic drug
laeverphanel," by Simon, E.J. NATURE. 198(4882):794-
795, 1963.
"The inhibition of the liver microsomal N-demethylation of
morphine by N-allylnornorphine and its pharmacological
implications," by Leadbeater, L., and Davies, D.R. BIO-
CHEMICAL PHARMACOLOGY. 13(12):1569-1576, 1964.
"Inhibition of writhing by narcotic antagonists," by Pearl,
J., and Harris, L.S. JOURNAL OF PHARMACOLOGY AND EXPER-
IMENTAL THERAPEUTICS. 154(2):319-323, 1966.
"Interaction of asarone with mescaline, amphetamine and tre-
morine," by Dandiya, P.C., and Menon, M.K. LIFE SCIENCES.
4(17):1635-1641, 1965.
"Interaction of caffeine and morphine on respiration," by
Bellville, J.W. JOURNAL OF PHARMACOLOGY AND EXPERIMENTAL
THERAPEUTICS. 143(2):165-168, 1964.
"Interaction of cocaine and G-strophanthin on the membrane
potential of frog sartorius muscle fibers," by Draper,
M.H. MEDICINA EXPERIMENTALIS. 8:242-250, 1963.
"Interaction of cocaine and tyramine on the isolated mammal-
ian heart," by Farmer, J.B., and Petch, B. JOURNAL OF
PHARMACY AND PHARMACOLOGY. 15(10):939-943, 1963.
"The interaction of morphine and d-tubocurarine on respira-
tion and grip strength in man," by Bellville, J.W., et
al. CLINICAL PHARMACOLOGY AND THERAPEUTICS. 5(1):35-
43, 1964.
"Interaction of pharmaceuticals with Schardinger dextrains.
II. Interaction with selected compounds," by Lach, J.L.,
and Cohen, J. JOURNAL OF PHARMACEUTICAL SCIENCES. 52:
137-142, 1963.
"Interaction of the analgesic effects of morphine and codeine in rats. NATURE. 205(4973):811-812, 1965.

"Interactions between cocaine, tyramine and noradrenaline at the noradrenaline store," by Farrant, J. BRITISH JOURNAL OF PHARMACOLOGY AND CHEMOTHERAPY. 20(3):540-549, 1963.
"Interactions between nalorphine and morphine in the decerebrate cat," by Martin, W.R., and Eiseman, A.J. JOURNAL OF PHARMACOLOGY AND EXPERIMENTAL THERAPEUTICS. 138(1): 113-119, 1962.
"Intravenous nisentil and lorfan in dental anaesthesia: a report on 2,000 cases," by Burbank, P.M. ANESTHESIA AND ANALGESIA; CURRENT RESEARCHES. 42:275-282, 1963.
"The intravenous use of a new analgesic agent, piminodine, in office urologic operative procedures," by Howard, A.H., et al. ANESTHESIA AND ANALGESIA; CURRENT RESEARCHES. 41(3):471-474, 1962.
"Investigations on the biosynthesis of morphine alkaloids," by Barton, D.H.R., et al. JOURNAL OF THE AMERICAN CHEMICAL SOCIETY. 2423-2438, Apr., 1965.
"Irreversible effects of glutethimide addiction," by Lingl, F.A. AMERICAN JOURNAL OF PSYCHIATRY. 123:349-351, Sept., 1966.
"Laboratory and clinical experience with phenazocine during anaesthesia," by Stephen, C.R., and Macmillan, R.W. CANADIAN ANAESTHETIST'S SOCIETY JOURNAL. 10(3):217-227, 1963.
"Laboratory evaluation of analgetic effectiveness in human subjects," by Sherman, H., et al. EXPERIMENTAL NEUROLOGY. 7:435-456, 1963.
"Laboratory investigation of drug addiction," by Marks, V. BRITISH JOURNAL OF ADDICTION. 61:291-294, Aug., 1966.
"Lack of addiction from high doses of tybamate," by Feldman, H.S., et al. JOURNAL OF NEW DRUGS. 6:354-360, Nov.-Dec., 1966.
"Lack of dependence and withdrawal symptoms in healthy volunteers given high doses of tybamate," by Colmore, J.P., and Moore, J.D. JOURNAL OF CLINICAL PHARMACOLOGY AND JOURNAL OF NEW DRUGS. 7(6):319-323, 1967.
"Lack of effect of dexoxadrol in self-maintained morphine dependence in rats," by Collins, R.J., and Weeks, J.R. PSYCHOPHARMACOLOGIA. 11(4):287-292, 1967.
"Lethal effects of aggregation and electric shock in mice treated with cocaine," by Lal, H., and Chessick, R.D. NATURE. 208:295-296, 1965.
"Liberation of antidiuretic hormone: pharmacologic blockade of ascending pathways," by Mills, E., and Wang, S.C. AMERICAN JOURNAL OF PHYSIOLOGY. 207(6): 1405-1410, 1964.
"Liver function tests in morphine-addicted and in nonaddicted rhesus monkeys," by Brooks, F.P., et al. GASTROENTEROLOGY. 44(3):287-290, 1963.
"The local effect of glyceryl trinitate, nitrite, papaverine, and atropine upon coronary vascular resistance," by Frohlich, E.D., and Scott, J.B. AMERICAN HEART JOURNAL. 63 (3):362-366, 1962.
"A long-acting antitussive preparation," by Ellison, S.E., et al. PRACTITIONER. 188:249-252, 1962.

"Loss of biological activity of apomorphine from auto-oxi-
dation," by Burkman, A.M. JOURNAL OF PHARMACY AND PHAR-
MACOLOGY. 15(7):461-465, 1963.
"The management of intractable pain due to advanced malig-
nant disease," by Hay, R.K. WINNIPEG CLINIC QUARTERLY.
16:24-32, 1963.
"Management of postoperative pain," by Silk, R.E. MEDICAL
TIMES. 91:187-190, 1963.
"Mania associated with the use of I.N.H. and cocaine," by
Kane, F.J., and Taylor, T.W. AMERICAN JOURNAL OF PSY-
CHIATRY. 119:1098-1099, 1963.
"Manual for the determination of narcotics and dangerous
drugs in the urine," by Parker, K.D., et al. PSYCHO-
PHARMACOLOGY BULLETIN; NATIONAL CLEARINGHOUSE FOR MENTAL
HEALTH INFORMATION. 3:18-42, July, 1966; also BULLETIN
ON NARCOTICS. 19(2):51-57, Apr.-June, 1967.
"Mass spectrometry of the morphine alkaloids," by Audier, H.,
et al. TETRAHEDRON LETTERS. 1:13-22, 1965.
"Mass spectrometry of morphine alkaloids. I. Fragmentation
of morphinan and related compounds," by Nakata, H., et al.
TETRAHEDRON LETTERS. 13:829-836, 1965.
"Maternal-fetal effects of propiomazine-meperidine analges-
ia," by Ellery, J.C., and Bair, J.R. AMERICAN JOURNAL OF
OBSTETRICS AND GYNECOLOGY. 84:1051-1056, 1962.
"Measurement of narcotic potency using houseflies," by Brad-
bury, E.R., and O'Carroll, F.M. ANNALS OF APPLIED BIO-
LOGY. 57(1):15-31, 1966.
"The measurement of pain: a new approach to an old problem,"
by Kast, E.C. JOURNAL OF NEW DRUGS. 2:344-351, 1962.
"Mechanism of action of cocaine and amphetamine in the brain,"
by Van Rossum, J.M., et al. EXPERIENTIA. 18(5):229-231,
1962.
"The mechanism of meperidine action on the pancreas," by
Byrne, J.J., and Toutounghi, F.M. AMERICAN JOURNAL OF
DIGESTIVE DISEASES. 8:411-418, 1963.
"The mechanism of shock following suicidal doses of barbit-
urates, narcotics and tranquilizer drugs, with observa-
tions on the effects of treatment," by Shubin, H., et al.
AMERICAN JOURNAL OF MEDICINE. 38:853-863, 1965.
"Mechanisms of action of morphine in the treatment of exper-
imental pulmonary edema," by Vasko, J.S., et al. AMERI-
CAN JOURNAL OF CARDIOLOGY. 18(6):876-883, 1966.
"Membrane potentials in isolted and electrically stimulated
mammalian cerebral cortex. Effects of chlorpromazine,
cocaine, phenobarbitone and protamine on the tissue's
electrical and chemical responses to stimulation," by
Hillman, H.H., et al. JOURNAL OF NEUROCHEMISTRY. 10:
325-339, 1963.
"Meperidine in cataract surgery," by Fishof, F.E. AMERICAN
JOURNAL OF OPHTHALMOLOGY. 53:672-676, 1962.
"Metabolism of cocaine," by Montesinos, F. BULLETIN ON NAR-
COTICS. 17(2):11-17, Apr.-June, 1965.
"Metabolism of codeine: urinary excretion rate of codeine
and morphine," by Redmond, N., and Parker, J.M. CANADIAN

JOURNAL OF BIOCHEMISTRY AND PHYSIOLOGY. 41(4):243-245, 1963.

"The metabolism of drugs by liver microsomes from alloxyn-diabetic rats: long term diabetes," by Dixon, R.L., et al. JOURNAL OF PHARMACOLOGY AND EXPERIMENTAL THERAPEU-TICS. 142(3):312-317, 1963.

"Metabolism of heroin and its pharmacologic implications," by Way, L.E., et al. BULLETIN ON NARCOTICS. 17(1):25-33, Jan.-Mar., 1965.

"Methadone poisoning in a child," by Ratcliffe, S.G. BRI-TISH MEDICAL JOURNAL. 5337:1069-1070, 1963.

"Method for evaluating diphenoxylate hydrochloride. Compar-ison of its antidiarrheal effect with that of camphor-ated tincture of opium," by Barowsky, J., and Schwartz, S.A. JOURNAL OF THE AMERICAN MEDICAL ASSOCIATION. 180:1058-1061, 1962.

"A method for the thin-layer chromatography of analgesic drugs and related compounds in non-aqueous systems," by Emmerson, J.L., and Anderson, R.C. JOURNAL OF CHROMA-TOGRAPHY. 17:495-500, 1965.

"A method of isolating porphyroxine from opium," by Szen-drei, K. BULLETIN ON NARCOTICS. 20(1):51-54, Jan.-Mar., 1968.

"A method of maximally assisted ventilation," by Elam, J.O. INTERNATIONAL ANESTHESIOLOGY CLINICS. 3:297-314, 1965.

"A method utilizing morphine as an indicator of an altera-tion in the blood-brain barrier," by Koestner, A. COR-NELL VETERINARIAN. 52:191-199, 1962.

"Methodological models for the study of drugs in the treat-ment of alcoholism," by Sherman, L.J., and Rothstein, E. PSYCHOSOMATIC MEDICINE, PART 2. 28(4):627-635, 1966.

"Methods and problems of measuring drug-induced changes in emotions and personality," by Steinberg, H. REVUE DE PSYCHOLOGIE APPLIQUEE. 11:361-372, 1961.

"Methods for studying mood changes produced by drugs," by Nowlis, V. REVUE DE PSYCHOLOGIE APPLIQUEE. 11:373-386, 1961.

"Methopholine, a new analgesic agent," by Cass, L.J., and Frederik, W.S. AMERICAN JOURNAL OF THE MEDICAL SCIENCES. 246(5):550-557, 1963.

"The methylation of normorphine in rat brain and liver," by Clouet, D.H. LIFE SCIENCES. 1:31-34, 1962.

"Microchemical identification of modern analgesic drugs - part II," by Clarke, E.G.C. BULLETIN ON NARCOTICS. 13(4):17-20, Oct.-Dec., 1961.

"Microcrystal tests for O^3-monoacetylmorphine in comparison with O^6-monoacetylmorphine, diacetylmorphine, morphine, and codeine," by Fulton, C.C. MICROCHEMICAL JOURNAL. 6(1):51-65, 1962.

"Mode of action of apomorphine and dexa-amphetamine on gnaw-ing compulsion in rats," by Ernst, A.M. PSYCHOPHARMACO-LOGIA. 10(4):316 passim, 1967.

"Modern analgesia in obstetrics," by Black, E.F.E. APPLIED THERAPEUTICS. 6:653-656, 1964.

"Modification of affect, social behavior and preformance by
sleep deprivation and drugs," by Latis, V.G. JOURNAL OF
PSYCHIATRIC RESEARCH. 1(1):12-24, 1961.
"Modification of physical properties of certain antitussive
and antihistiminic agents by formation of N-cyclohexyl-
sulfamate salts," by Campbell, J.A., and Slater, J.G.
JOURNAL OF PHARMACEUTICAL SCIENCES. 51(10):931-934, 1962.
"Morphine antagonistic actions of N-propargyl-14-hydroxydi-
hydronormorphinine hydrochloride and related compounds,"
by Minakami, H., et al. LIFE SCIENCES. 10:503-507, 1962.
"Morphine-induced hyperglycemia in the cat," by Borison,
H.L., et al. JOURNAL OF PHARMACOLOGY AND EXPERIMENTAL
THERAPEUTICS. 138:229-235, 1962.
"Morphine inhibition of drug metabolism in the rat," by
Bousquet, W.F., et al. BIOCHEMICAL PHARMACOLOGY. 13(1):
123-125, 1964.
"Morphine manufacture from poppy straw and its concentrate."
BULLETIN ON NARCOTICS. 20(2):50, Apr.-June, 1968.
"Morphine self-administration, food-reinforced, and avoid-
ance behaviors in rhesus monkeys," by Thompson, T., and
Schuster, C.R. PSYCHOPHARMACOLOGIA. 5(2):87-94, 1964.
"Morphine: single dose tolerance," by Kornetsky, C., and
Bain, G. SCIENCE. 162:1011-1012, Nov. 29, 1968.
"Morphine tolerance, physical dependence and synthesis of
brain 5-hydroxytryptamine," by Way, E.L., et al. SCIENCE.
162:1290-1292, Dec. 13, 1968.
"N-allylnorapomorphine," by Hensiak, J.F., and Cannon, J.G.
JOURNAL OF MEDICINAL CHEMISTRY. 8(5):557-559, 1965.
"N- and O-demethylation of some narcotic analgesics by brain
slices from male and female Long-Evans rats," by Elison,
C., and Elliott, H.W. BIOCHEMICAL PHARMACOLOGY. 12(12):
1363-1366, 1963.
"N-dealkylation of morphine and nalorphine in the brain of
living rats," by Milthers, K. NATURE. 195(4841):607,
1962.
"N-methylation of normorphine by rat tissues in vitro," by
Clouet, D.H., et al. BIOCHEMICAL PHARMACOLOGY. 12(9):
957-966, 1963.
"Nalorphine antagonism to the narcotic action of chlorpro-
mazine, meprobamate and metaminodiazeposide (librium),"
by von Ledebur, I., et al. MEDICINA EXPERIMENTALIS.
7:177-179, 1962.
"Narcotic analgesics in heart disease," by Modell, W. AMER-
ICAN HEART JOURNAL. 65(5):709-711, 1963.
"Narcotic and methamphetamine use during pregnancy. Effect
on newborn infants," by Sussman, S. AMERICAN JOURNAL OF
DISEASES OF CHILDREN. 106(3):325-330, 1963.
"Narcotic antagonists as analgesics," by Archer, S., et al.
SCIENCE. 137(3529):541-543, 1962.
"Narcotic drugs in the postanesthetic recovery room," by
Ditzler, J.W., et al. HENRY FORD HOSPITAL MEDICAL BUL-
LETIN. 10:339-346, 1962.
"Narcotic usage. I. A spectrum of a difficult medical pro-
blem," by Zinberg, N.E., and Lewis, D.C. NEW ENGLAND

JOURNAL OF MEDICINE. 270:989-993, 1964.
--II. A historical perspective on a difficult medical pro-
blem," by Lewis, D.C., and Zinberg, N.E. NEW ENGLAND
JOURNAL OF MEDICINE. 270:1045-1050, 1964.
"Narcotic withdrawal syndrome in newborns," by Dikshit,
S.K. INDIAN JOURNAL OF PSYCHIATRY. 28:11-15, 1961.
"Narcotic withdrawal syndrome: suppression of, by means of
electric compulsine therapy," by Kelman, H. MINNESOTA
MEDICINE. 47:525-527, 1964.
"Narcotics analysis - a simple approach," by Lerner, M., et
al. JOURNAL OF FORENSIC SCIENCES. 8:126-131, 1963.
"Narcotics and medical practice. The use of narcotic drugs
in medical practice and the medical managemant of nar-
cotic addicts." JOURNAL OF THE AMERICAN MEDICAL ASSOC-
IATION. 185:976-982, 1963.
"Narcotics control in the hospital. A re-examination of
ASHP's 'suggested regulation'," by Trygstad, V.O. HOS-
PITALS. 37:88 passim, 1963.
"Narcotics in the post-operative period - a reappraisal,"
by Ulert, I.A. SOUTHERN MEDICAL JOURNAL. 60:1289-1292,
1967.
"Near fatal poisoning due to accidental ingestion of an over-
dose of dextro propoxyphene hydrochloride by a two-year
old child," by Hyatt, H.W., Sr. NEW ENGLAND JOURNAL OF
MEDICINE. 267:710, 1962.
"New benzomorphan analgesics," by Gordon, M., et al. JOUR-
NAL OF MEDICINAL AND PHARMACEUTICAL CHEMISTRY. 5(3):633-
635, 1963.
"A new concept of the mode of interaction of narcotic anal-
gesics with receptors," by Portoghese, P.S. JOURNAL OF
MEDICINAL CHAMISTRY. 8:609-616, 1965.
"New drugs and developments in therapeutics." JOURNAL OF
THE AMERICAN MEDICAL ASSOCIATION. 184:709-710, 1963.
"New drugs and developments in therapeutics by the Council
on Drugs." JOURNAL OF THE AMERICAN MEDICAL ASSOCIATION.
183:469-470, 1963.
"A new nonaddicting analgesic. A double-blind evaluation in
postoperative pain," by Sadove, M.S., and Balagot, R.C.
JOURNAL OF THE AMERICAN MEDICAL ASSOCIATION. 193(11):
887-892, 1965.
"A new noscapine formulation for the relief of symptoms as-
sociated with respiratory tract disorders," by Rohr, J.H.
CURRENT THERAPEUTIC RESEARCH. 4:21-23, 1962.
"New potent analgesics in the morphine series," by Bentley,
K.W., and Hardy, D.G. PROCEEDINGS OF THE AMERICAN CHEMI-
CAL SOCIETY. p. 220, July, 1963.
"A new synthetic method of codeine from thebaine," by Ya-
mada, M. CHEMICAL AND PHARMACEUTICAL BULLETIN. 10:871-
872, 1962.
"A new test for morphine-like physical dependence (addiction
liability) in rats," by Buckett, W.R. PSYCHOPHARMACO-
LOGIA. 6(6):410-416, 1964.
"Newborn attention as affected by medication during labor,"
by Stechler, G. SCIENCE. 144:315-317, 1964.

"Nitrous oxide inhalation as a fad. Dangers in uncontrolled sniffing for psychedelic effects," by Dillon, J.B. CALIFORNIA MEDICINE. 106(6):444-446, 1967.

"A note on the identification of dimenoxadol," by Clarke, A.G.C. BULLETIN ON NARCOTICS. 12(1):41, Jan.-Mar., 1960.

"A note on the paper chromatographic separation of codeine, morphine, and nalorphine," by Street, H.V. JOURNAL OF PHARMACY AND PHARMACOLOGY. 14(1):56-57, 1962.

"Objective assessment of antitussive agents in patients with chronic cough," by Sevelius, H., et al. JOURNAL OF CLINICAL PHARMACOLOGY AND THE JOURNAL OF NEW DRUGS. 6:216-223, 1966.

"Objective evidence of mental effects of heroin, morphine and placebo in normal subjects," by Smith, G.M., et al. JOURNAL OF PHARMACOLOGY AND EXPERIMENTAL THERAPEUTICS. 136 (1):53-58, 1962.

"Objective measurements of the effects of drugs on driver behavior," by Miller, J.G. JOURNAL OF THE AMERICAN MEDICAL ASSOCIATION. 179(12):940-943, 1962.

"On carbohydrate metabolism in the rat under brevin and urethane narcosis," by Rausch, J., and Ankermann, H. ARCHIVES INTERNATIONALES DE PHARMACODYNAMIE ET DE THERAPIE. 138:591-596, 1962.

"On the biosynthesis of isothebaine," by Battersby, A.R., et al. CHEMICAL COMMUNICATIONS. 11:230-232, 1965.

"On the detection of various habit-forming drugs by round filter chromatography," by Paulus, W., et al. ARZNEIMITTEL FORSCHUNG. 12:1086-1087, 1962.

"On the mechanism of spasmolytic effect of papaverine and certain derivatives," by Santi, R., et al. BIOCHEMICAL PHARMACOLOGY. 13(1):153-158, 1964.

"One year follow-up of depressed patients treated in a multi-hospital drug study. I. Social worker's evaluation," by Honigfeld, G., and Lasky, J.J. DISEASES OF THE NERVOUS SYSTEM. 23:555-562, 1962.

"An operant reinforcement paradigm in the study of drug effects," by Brady, J.P., et al. DISEASES OF THE NERVOUS SYSTEM. 23(9):497-502, 1962.

"Opiate antagonist drugs," by Gray, G.W. WISCONSIN MEDICAL JOURNAL. 61:533-535, 1962.

"Opium alkaloids. Separation and identification by gas, thin-layer, and paper chromatography," by Brochmann-Hanssen, E., and Furuya, T. JOURNAL OF PHARMACEUTICAL SCIENCES. 53(12):1549-1550, 1965.

--II. Isolation and characterization of codamine," by Brochmann-Hanssen, E., et al. JOURNAL OF PHARMACEUTICAL SCIENCES. 54(10):1531-1532, 1965.

"Opium as a tranquillizer," by Carlson, E.T., and Simpson, M.M. AMERICAN JOURNAL OF PSYCHIATRY. 120(2):112-117, 1963.

"Oral versus subcutaneous potency of codeine, morphine, levorphan and anileridine as measured by rabbit toothpulp changes," by Leaders, F.E., and Keasling, H.H. JOURNAL OF PHARMACEUTICAL SCIENCES. 51(1):46-49, 1962.

"The orienting response in chronic schizophrenics following morphine administration," by Collins, L.G., et al. BEHAVIORAL SCIENCE. 11:177-179, 1966.

"Oxycodone suppositories in the relief of intractible pain," by Stathers, D.N., and Hunnybun, J. PRACTITIONER. 190: 779-781, 1963.

"Oxymorphone, an effective analgesic in dogs and cats," by Palminteri, A. JOURNAL OF THE AMERICAN VETERINARY MEDICAL ASSOCIATION. 143(2):160-163, 1963.

"Pain and analgesia evaluated by the intraperitoneal bradykinin-evoked pain method in man," by Lin, R.K.S., et al. CLINICAL PHARMACOLOGY AND THERAPEUTICS. 8:521-542, 1967.

"Pain relieving drugs for advanced cancer," by Harrold, T. JOURNAL OF THE MEDICAL ASSOCIATION OF GEORGIA. 51:85, 1962.

"Papaverine hydrochloride as therapy for mentally confused geriatric patients," by LaBrecque, D.C. CURRENT THERAPEUTIC RESEARCH. 8:106-109, 1966.

"Papaverine-like pharmacological properties of rotenone," by Santi, R., et al. JOURNAL OF PHARMACY AND PHARMACOLOGY. 15(10):697-698, 1963.

"Paradoxical responses to chlorpromazine after LSD," by Schwarz, C.J. PSYCHOSOMATICS. 8(4, pt.1):210-211, 1967.

"Parenteral use of meperidine-promethazine as preanesthetic medication in ambulatory patients," by Catania, A.F., and Kringstein, G.J. JOURNAL OF ORAL SURGERY. 20:12-17, 1962.

"Parenteral use of promethazine-meperidine combination during labour," by Daro, A.F., et al. ILLINOIS MEDICAL JOURNAL. 12:53-56, 1962.

"Passage of drugs across the placenta," by Moya, F., and Thorndike, V. AMERICAN JOURNAL OF OBSTETRICS AND GYNECOLOGY. 84:1778-1798, 1962.

"Pentobarbital anaesthesia in the dog following preanesthetic administration of promazine and meperidine in clinical practice," by Clifford, D.H., and Kook, C.C. CORNELL VETERINARIAN. 53:199-212, 1963.

"Performance as a function of drug, dose, and level of training," by Ray, O.S., and Bivens, L.W. PSYCHOPHARMACOLOGIA. 101(2):103-109, 1966.

"A peri-surgical evaluation of oxymorphone," by Kane, A.A. WESTERN MEDICINE. 3:8-10, 1962.

"Permanent encephalopathy from toluene inhalation," by Knox, J.W., et al. NEW ENGLAND JOURNAL OF MEDICINE. 275:1494-1496, Dec. 29, 1966.

"Pharmacodynamics of human disease. I. Biochemical factors in the action of analgesic and narcotic drugs," by Axelrod, J. POSTGRADUATE MEDICINE. 34:328-333, 1963.

--II. Therapeutic application of opiates," by Dripps, R.D. POSTGRADUATE MEDICINE. 3:520-524, 1963.

"Pharmacologic basis for the increased sensitivity of the newborn rat to morphine," by Kupferberg, H.J., and Way, L.E. JOURNAL OF PHARMACOLOGY AND EXPERIMENTAL THERAPEUTICS. 141(1):105-112, 1963.

243

"Pharmacologic factors in relapse and the possible use of the narcotic antagonists in treatment," by Martin, W.R. ILLINOIS MEDICAL JOURNAL. 130:489-494, Oct., 1966.
"Pharmacological experiments on the release of the sympathetic transmitter," by Blackeley, A.G., et al. JOURNAL OF PHYSIOLOGY. 167:505-514, 1963.
"Pharmacological properties of morphine-potentiating serum obtained from morphine-tolerant dogs and men," by Kiplinger, G.F., and Clift, J.W. JOURNAL OF PHARMACOLOGY AND EXPERIMENTAL THERAPEUTICS. 146(2):139-146, 1964.
"Pharmacological studies of analgesics. VI. The administration of morphine and changes in acetylcholine metabolism mouse brain," by Hano, K., et al. BIOCHEMICAL PHARMACOLOGY. 13(3):441-447, 1964.
"Pharmacological studies of spinal cord adrenergic and cholinergic mechanisms and their relation to physical dependence on morphine," by Martin, W.R., and Eades, C.G. PSYCHOPHARMACOLOGIA. 11(3):195-223, 1967.
"Pharmacology and addiction-liability of dl- and d-propoxyphene," by Fraser, H.F., et al. BULLETIN ON NARCOTICS. 12(1):9-14, Jan.-Mar., 1960.
"The pharmacology and physiology of drug addiction," by Sherrod, T.M. ILLINOIS MEDICAL JOURNAL. 130:453-456, 1966.
"The pharmacology of pain control," by Mathewson, H.S. APPLIED THERAPEUTICS. 6:601-602, 1964.
"The pharmacology of the psychoactive drugs," by Cohen, S. NORTHWEST MEDICINE. 65:197-203, 1966.
"Phenazocine analgesia," by Brown, I.M., et al. PRACTITIONER. 188:365-367, 1962.
"Phenazocine (prinadol) in the treatment of psychotic patients," by Durland, A.A., and Gruenwald, F. DISEASES OF THE NERVOUS SYSTEM. 23:284-291, 1962.
"A phosphorimetric investigation of several representative alkaloids of the isoquinoline, morphine, and indole groups," by Hollifield, H.C., and Winefordner, J.D. TALANTA. 12(9):860-863, 1965.
"Physico-chemical methods for the identification of narcotics(cont.). Part Vb. Paper chromatographic data for narcotics and related compounds," by Genest, K., and Farmile, C.G. BULLETIN ON NARCOTICS. 12(1):15-24, Jan.-Mar., 1960.
--Part VI. Common physical constants, UV, IR and X-ray data for 12 narcotics and related compounds," by Martin, L., et al. BULLETIN ON NARCOTICS. 15(3-4):17-38, July-Dec., 1963.
"Physiochemical properties of drugs that control absorption rate after subcutaneous implantation," by Ballard, B.E., and Nelson, E. JOURNAL OF PHARMACOLOGY AND EXPERIMENTAL THERAPEUTICS. 135:120-127, 1962.
"Physiological and psychological functioning in chronic schizophrenics following a single dose of morphine sulfate," by Collins, L.G., et al. PSYCHOLOGICAL REPORTS. 16(3, pt.2):1303-1304, 1965.
"Piminodine as an adjunct to anesthesia," by Sadove, M.S.,

et al. ILLINOIS MEDICAL JOURNAL. 121:261-266, 1962.
"Piperidino groups in antitussive activity," by Kase, Y.,
et al. JOURNAL OF MEDICINAL AND PHARMACEUTICAL CHEMIS-
TRY. 6(2):118-122, 1963.
"Placebo reactor," by Parkhouse, J. NATURE. 199:308, 1963.
"Possibilities of crop substitution for the coca bush in
Bolivia," by Rodriguez, A.A. BULLETIN ON NARCOTICS.
17(3):13-23, July-Sept., 1965.
"A possible receptor role of the subformical organ in mor-
phine-induced hyperglycemia," by Borison, H.L., et al.
NEUROLOGY. 14(11):1049-1053, 1964.
"Post-operative analgesia in 200 podiatry patients. A stu-
dy of demerol apap and demerol compound tablets," by Har-
ris, M.D. JOURNAL OF THE AMERICAN PODIATRY ASSOCIATION.
53:820-822, 1963.
"Postoperative pain," by Cottingham, J.W. MEDICAL ANNALS
OF THE DISTRICT OF COLUMBIA. 33:495-498, 1964.
"Potential dangers of morphine in acute diverticulosis of
the colon," by Painter, N.S., and Truelove, S.C. BRI-
TISH MEDICAL JOURNAL. 5348:33-34, 1963.
"Potential reserpine analogues. Derivatives of reduced
isoquinolines and meconine," by Khan, N.H., and Sharp,
L.K. JOURNAL OF PHARMACY AND PHARMACOLOGY. 17:318-
322, 1965.
"Potentiation of actions of cathecholamines by a derivative
of hemicholinium," by Wong, S., and Long, J.P. JOURNAL
OF PHARMACOLOGY AND EXPERIMENTAL THERAPEUTICS. 156(3):
469-482, 1967.
"Potentiation of an effect of morphine in the rat by sera
from morphine-tolerant and abstinent dogs and monkeys,"
by Kornetsky, C., and Kiplinger, G.F. PSYCHOPHARMACO-
LOGIA. 4(1):66-71, 1963.
"Potentiation of ethanol-induced depression in dogs by re-
presentative ataractic and analgesic drugs," by Forney,
R.B., et al. QUARTERLY JOURNAL OF STUDIES ON ALCOHOL.
24:1-8, 1963.
"Potentiation of morphine by intraperitoneal injections of
iproniazid in rabbits," by Defalque, R.J. ANESTHESIA
AND ANALGESIA; CURRENT RESEARCHES. 44(2):190-193, 1965.
"The potentiation of opiate induced analgesia by stimulant
drugs: the effect of monoamine oxidase inhibitors and
caffeine," by Evans, W.O. UNITED STATES ARMY MEDICAL RE-
SEARCH LABORATORY REPORT. no. 519, 1961.
"Potentiation of some catechol amines by phenoxybenzamine,
guanethidine and cocaine," by Stafford, A. BRITISH JOUR-
NAL OF PHARMACOLOGY AND CHEMOTHERAPY. 21(2):361-367,
1963.
"Powerful analgesics. BRITISH MEDICAL JOURNAL. 5325:241-
242, 1963.
"A practical application of thin-layer chromatography in
the detection of narcotic drugs in the urine," by Kokoski,
R.J. PSYCHOPHARMACOLOGY BULLETIN; NATIONAL CLEARINGHOUSE
FOR MENTAL HEALTH INFORMATION. 3:34-36, Dec., 1966.
"Practice and pharmacy: list and classification of pharma-

ceutical specialities which may be offered for sale. INTERNATIONAL DIGEST OF HEALTH LEGISLATION. 15(1):118, 1964.
"Pre-anaesthetic medication. Phenazocine and levophenacyl-morphan compared with morphine, pethidine and a placebo," by Ciliberti, B.J., et al. BULLETIN ON NARCOTICS. 16: 41-51, Apr.-June, 1964.
"Preanesthetic medication with intramuscular administration of hydroxyzine hydrochloride: a parallel, double-blind study of hydroxyzine hydrochloride, meperidine hydrochloride, secobarbital sodium, and a placebo," by Bizzarri, D., et al. ANESTHESIA AND ANALGESIA; CURRENT RESEARCHES. 42:316-324, 1963.
"Preanesthetic medication without narcotics. A continuing analysis of 7,718 case studies from 15,000 patients treated," by Wallace, G., et al. JOURNAL OF THE INTERNATIONAL COLLEGE OF SURGEONS. 40:340-353, 1963.
"Preferences for punished and unpunished schedules of reinforcement under oxazepam, chlordiazepoxide, and amphetamine," by Margules, D.L., and Stein, L. PROCEEDINGS OF THE 74th ANNUAL CONVENTION OF THE AMERICAN PSYCHOLOGICAL ASSOCIATION. pp. 113-114, 1966.
"Premature labor and meperidine analgesia," by Kaltreider, D.F. AMERICAN JOURNAL OF OBSTETRICS AND GYNECOLOGY. 99:989-993, 1967.
"Premedication for children," by Corbett, M.C. JOURNAL OF DENTISTRY FOR CHILDREN. 33:125-127, 1966.
"Premedication for children undergoing anesthesia," by Seigne, T.D. CLINICAL PEDIATRICS. 5(9):549-553, 1966.
"Preoperative and postoperative use of pentazocine, a new nonnarcotic analgesic," by Gaines, H.R. ILLINOIS MEDICAL JOURNAL. 131:320-322, 1967.
"Preoperative medication in children," by Forster, K. SINAI HOSPITAL, DETROIT BULLETIN. 11:89-94, 1963.
"The preparation of O-methylporphyroxine and its detection in opium," by Hughes, D.W., and Farmilo, C.G. JOURNAL OF PHARMACY AND PHARMACOLOGY. 17(11):757-758, 1965.
"The preparation of porphyroxine from opium," by Genest, K., and Farmilo, C.G. JOURNAL OF PHARMACY AND PHARMACOLOGY. 15(3):197-201, 1963.
"The pressor response on the spinal cat to different groups of ganglion-stimulating agents," by Jones, A., et al. JOURNAL OF PHARMACOLOGY AND EXPERIMENTAL THERAPEUTICS. 139:312-320, 1963.
"A procedure which produces sustained opiate-directed behavior (morphine addiction) in the rat," by Nichols, J.R. PSYCHOLOGICAL REPORTS. 13(3):895-904, 1963.
"Procedures for assured identification of morphine, dihydromorphinone, codeine, norcodeine, methadone, quinine, methamphetamine, etc., in human urine," by Ono, M., et al. BULLETIN ON NARCOTICS. 21(2):31-40, Apr.-June, 1969.
"Propoxyphene hydrochloride, a drug of abuse," by Claghorn, J.L., et al. JOURNAL OF THE AMERICAN MEDICAL ASSOCIATION. 196:1089-1091, June 20, 1966.

"Provocation of serum enzyme activity in cholecystectomized patients given opiates," by Burckhardt, D., and Ladue, J.S. AMERICAN JOURNAL OF GASTROENTEROLOGY. 46:43-50, 1966.

"Prozine as an adjunct to psychotherapy with alcoholic outpatients in the withdrawal stage," by Haden, H.H., Jr., et al. QUARTERLY JOURNAL OF STUDIES ON ALCOHOL. 23(3): 442-448, 1962.

"Psychological and physiological functioning in chronic schizophrenics following a single dose of morphine sulfate," by Collins, L.G., et al. PSYCHOLOGICAL REPORTS. 16:1303-1304, 1965.

"The psychopharmacological profile: a systematic approach to the interaction of drug effects and personality traits," by Lehmann, H.E., and Knight, D.A. REVUE CANADIENNE DE BIOLOGIE. 20:631-641, 1961.

"The pupil test for diagnosing narcotic usage," by Way, E.L. TRIANGLE. 7:152 passim, 1965.

"Quantitative determination of morphine in opium by gas-liquid chromatography," by Brochmann-Hanssen, E., and Baerheim-Svendsen, A. JOURNAL OF PHARMACEUTICAL SCIENCES. 52(12):1134, 1963.

"Quantitative evaluation of surface anesthetics in albino mice," by Jones, W.R., and Weaver, L.C. JOURNAL OF PHARMACEUTICAL SCIENCES. 52:500-501, 1963.

"Rcn Tutor Section winter conference: drugs and addiction." NURSING TIMES. 63:161, Feb. 3, 1967.

"Rapid estimation of diacetylmorphine in the presence of acetylcodeine," by Nakamura, G.R. JOURNAL OF THE ASSOCIATION OF OFFICIAL AGRICULTURAL CHEMISTS. 46(4):769-770, 1963.

"Rapid identification of analgesic drugs in urine with thin-layer chromatography," by Cochin, H., and Daly, J.W. EXPERIENTIA. 18:294-295, 1962.

"A rapid screening test for potential addiction liability of new analgesic agents," by Shemano, I., and Wendel, H. TOXICOLOGY AND APPLIED PHARMACOLOGY. 6:334-339, 1964.

"Reaction time ('mental set') in control and chronic schizophrenic subjects and in postaddicts under placebo, LSD-25, morphine, pentobarbital and amphetamine," by Wikler, A., et al. PSYCHOPHARMACOLOGIA. 7(6):423-443, 1965.

"Recent advances in analgesic medications," by Cass, L.J., and Frederick, W.S. CURRENT THERAPEUTIC RESEARCH. 5: 81-86, 1963.

"Recent advances in the chemical research of cannabis," by Grlić, Ljubisa. BULLETIN ON NARCOTICS. 16:29-40, Oct.-Dec., 1964"Recent developments in the chemistry and biochemistry of narcotics," by Abood, L.G. ILLINOIS MEDICAL JOURNAL. 130:450-452, Oct., 1966.

"Reduction of dislocated shoulders using methocarbamol," by Tronzo, R.G. JOURNAL OF THE AMERICAN MEDICAL ASSOCIATION. 184:1044-1046, 1963.

"The relation between the levels of microsomal cytochromes and meperidine N-demethylase activity in rat liver," by

Clouet, D.H. LIFE SCIENCES. 4(3):365-371, 1965.
"The relationship between the analgesic effect of morphine and addiction liability in rats," by Nichols, J.R., and Evans, W.O. UNITED STATES ARMY MEDICAL RESEARCH LABORATORY REPORTS. 559:1-8, 1963.
"The relative analgesic and respiratory effects of phenazocine and morphine," by Houde, R.W., et al. JOURNAL OF PHARMACY AND EXPERIMENTAL THERAPEUTICS. 144(3):337-345, 1964.
"Relief of pain in labour," by Beazley, J.M., et al. LANCET. 1:1033-1035, 1967.
"The relief of pain - the search for the ideal analgesic," by Bentley, K.W. ENDEAVOUR. 23:97-101, 1964.
"Renal papillary mecrosis associated with analgesic abuse," by Plass, H.F. ANNALS OF INTERNAL MEDICINE. 60:111-114, 1964.
"Report from the Duke University Poison Control Center. Drug dangers (maternal medication) to the fetus," by Arena, J.M. NORTH CAROLINA MEDICAL JOURNAL. 25:210-211, 1964.
"Report on oxymorphone in obstetrics," by Snow, D.L., and Sattenspiel, E. AMERICAN JOURNAL OF OBSTETRICS AND GYNECOLOGY. 83:22-24, 1962.
"Report on vegetable drugs and their derivatives," by Levine, J. JOURNAL OF THE ASSOCIATION OF THE OFFICIAL AGRICULTURAL CHEMISTS. 47(1):55, 1964.
"Research on various kinds of fungi observed on Turkish opium and their removal with different sorts of fungicide," by Eltutar, H., and Igneciler, M. BULLETIN ON NARCOTICS. 12(3):25-34, July-Sept., 1960.
"The respiratory and subjective effects of pentazocine," by Bellville, J.W., and Green, J. CLINICAL PHARMACOLOGY AND THERAPEUTICS. 6(2):152-159, 1965.
"The respiratory effects of oxymorphone administered alone or in combination with levallorphan," by Foldes, F.F., et al. AMERICAN JOURNAL OF THE MEDICAL SCIENCES. 243:480-488, 1962.
"Respiratory sensitivity of the newborn infant to meperidine and morphine," by Way, W.L., et al. CLINICAL PHARMACOLOGY AND THERAPEUTICS. 6(4):454-461, 1965.
"Responses of adult heroin addicts to a total therapeutic program," by Freedman, A.M., et al. AMERICAN JOURNAL OF ORTHOPSYCHIATRY. 33(5):890-899, 1963.
"Response of experimental pain to analgesic drugs. I. Morphine, aspirin, and placebo," by Wolff, B.B., et al. CLINICAL PHARMACOLOGY AND THERAPEUTICS. 7(2):224-238, 1966
"The responses of the terminal bile duct to morphine and morphine-like drugs," by Crema, A., et al. JOURNAL OF PHARMACOLOGY AND EXPERIMENTAL THERAPEUTICS. 149(3):373-378, 1965.
"Reversal of hormonal effects as a result of chronic morphinization," by Walsh, E.O'F., et al. NATURE. 204 (4959):698, 1964

"The risk of dependence on chlormethiazole," by Lundquist, G. ACTA PSYCHIATRICA SCANDINAVICA. 42(suppl. 192):203+, 1966.
"The sedative central analgesic and anticonvulsant actions of local anesthetics," by Koppanyi, T. AMERICAN JOURNAL OF THE MEDICAL SCIENCES. 244(5):646-654, 1962.
"A selective method for the study of drug effects on behavior," by Milligan, M.M., and Kalman, G. PROCEEDINGS OF THE WESTERN PHARMACOLOGY SOCIETY. 6:7-8, 1963.
"Selective potentiation of the actions of catecholamines on rabbit auricles by phenoxybenzamines and cocaine." THE JOURNAL OF PHYSIOLOGY. 166(2):34, 1963.
"Selective quaternization in the morphine series," by Bognár, R., and Szabó, S. TETRAHEDRON LETTERS. 39:2867-2871, 1964.
"The separation and determination of morphine and thebaine," by Clair, E.G. ANALYST. 87(1035):499-500, 1962.
"Separation of acetylcodeine from illicit heroin by thin-layer chromatography," by Nakamura, G.R. JOURNAL OF THE ASSOCIATION OF OFFICIAL ANALYTICAL CHEMISTS. 49(5):1086-1090, 1966.
"Separation of tabletted mixtures of barbiturates, aspirine, phenacetin, caffeine, codeine, and quinine by ion-exchange paper chromatography," by Street, H.V., and Niyogi, S.K. JOURNAL OF PHARMACEUTICAL SCIENCES. 51:666-668, 1962.
"Serum enzyme activities following morphine. A study of transaminase and alkaline phosphates levels in normal persons and those with gallbladder disease," by Mossberg, S.M., et al. ARCHIVES OF INTERNAL MEDICINE. 109:429-437, 1962.
"Serum hepatitis and illicit drug use," by Johnson, J.S. ROCKY MOUNTAIN MEDICAL JOURNAL. 65:43-45, Feb., 1968.
"Serum transaminase activity following morphine, meperidine and codeine in normals," by Shuster, F., et al. AMERICAN JOURNAL OF THE MEDICAL SCIENCES. 246:714-716, 1963.
"Severe reaction to long-acting antitussive," by Gould, K.S. AMERICAN JOURNAL OF DISEASES OF CHILDREN. 105(5):497-498, 1963.
"A severe systemic reaction to demerol," by Johnson, K.J. ANNALS OF ALLERGY. 21(7):408, 1963.
"Side effects and double-blind studies: I. A clinical comparison between thioridazine hydrochloride and a combination of phenobarbital and atropine sulfate," by Grinspoon, L., et al. JOURNAL OF PSYCHIATRIC RESEARCH. 2(4):247-256, 1964.
"Side-effects of drugs. Drug metabolism and toxic side-effects," by Parke, D.V. ANGLO-GERMAN MEDICAL REVIEW. 1:460-472, 1962.
"A simple and rapid method for distinguishing opium of Mexican origin from other types of opium," by Grlic, L. JOURNAL OF CRIMINAL LAW, CRIMINOLOGY AND POLICE SCIENCE. 52:229-231, 1961.
"A simple method for producing tolerance to dihydromorphinone in mice," by Shuster, L., et al. JOURNAL OF PHARMA-

COLOGY AND EXPERIMENTAL THERAPEUTICS. 140(2):149-154, 1963.
"Simultaneous administration of narcotic and narcotic-antagonist drugs in the newborn rabbit," by Moore, W.M.O., and Davis, J.A. JOURNAL OF PEDIATRICS. 71(3):420-424, 1967.
"Simultaneous determination of morphine, codeine and prophyroxine in opium by infrared and visible spectometry," by Genest, K., and Farmilo, C.G. ANALYTICAL CHEMISTRY. 34 (11):1464-1468, 1962.
"Sir Walter Scott's laudanum?" by Wright, A.D. ANNALS OF THE ROYAL COLLEGE OF SURGEONS OF ENGLAND. 32:194-195, 1963.
"Site of synthesis of alkaloids in some plants," by Kapoor, L.D. CURRENT SCIENCES. 32(8):355-356, 1963.
"Sites of action of some central nervous system depressants," by Domino, E.F. ANNUAL REVIEW OF PHARMACOLOGY. 2:215-250, 1962.
"The social behaviour of laboratory rats and the action of chlorpromazine and other drugs," by Silverman, A.P. BEHAVIOUR. 27:1-38, 1966.
"Solvent sniffing. Physiologic effects and community control measures for intoxication from the intentional inhalation if organic solvents. I," by Press, E., et al. PEDIATRICS. 39:451-461, Mar, 1967.
--II, by Press, E., et al. PEDIATRICS. 39:611-622, Apr., 1967.
"Solvent systems for the identification of opiates in narcotic seizures by thin-layer chromatography," by Steele, J.A. JOURNAL OF CHROMATOGRAPHY. 19(2):300-303, 1965.
"Some analogs and drivatives of papaverine," by Lutz, W.B., et al. AMERICAN CHEMICAL SOCIETY, ABSTRACT PAPERS. 144: 9L, 1963.
"Some applications of paper chromatography in the detection of opium alkaloids," by Nakamura, G.R. BULLETIN ON NARCOTICS. 12(4):17-20, Oct.-Dec., 1960.
"Some aspects of the comparative pharmacology of morphine," by Maynert, E.W. FEDERATION PROCEEDINGS. 26(4):1111-1114, 1967.
"Some aspects of the fate and relationship of the N-methyl group of morphine to its pharmacological activity," by Elison, C., et al. JOURNAL OF MEDICINAL CHEMISTRY. 6: 237-246, 1963.
"Some central nervous properties of diethyldithiocarbamate," by Pfeifer, A.K., et al. JOURNAL OF PHARMACY AND PHARMACOLOGY. 18(4):254, 1966.
"Some changes in the peripheral blood of dogs after administration of certain tranquillizers and narcotics," by Collette, W.L., and Meriwether, W.F. VETERINARY MEDICINE-SMALL ANIMAL CLINICIAN. 60:1223-1226, 1965.
"Some effects of morphine and amphetamine on intellectual functions and mood," by Evans, W.O., and Smith, R.P. PSYCHOPHARMACOLOGIA. 6:49-56, 1964.
"Some effects of morphine and morphine antagonists on schedule-controlled behavior," by McMillan, D.E., et al.

JOURNAL OF PHARMACOLOGY AND EXPERIMENTAL THERAPEUTICS.
157:175-184, 1967.
"Some effects of morphine on respiration and metabolism of
rats," by Kokka, N., et al. JOURNAL OF PHARMACOLOGY AND
EXPERIMENTAL THERAPEUTICS. 148(3):386-392, 1965.
"Some human pharmacological studies of three psychotropic
drugs: thiothixine, molindone and w-1867," by Hollister,
L.E. JOURNAL OF CLINICAL PHARMACOLOGY AND THE JOURNAL OF
NEW DRUGS. 8(2):95-101, 1968.
"Some modern aspects of heroin analysis," by Lerner, M., and
Mills, A. BULLETIN ON NARCOTICS. 15(1):37-42, Jan.-
Mar., 1963.
"Some observations on the use of phenazocine (narphen) in
anaesthesia," by Macpherson, M. IRISH JOURNAL OF MEDICAL
SCIENCE. 450:289-293, 1963.
"Some pharmacological studies with 14-cinnamoyloxycodeine."
JOURNAL OF PHARMACY AND PHARMACOLOGY. 17(11):759-760,
1965.
"Some potent morphine antagonists possessing high analgesic
activity," by Gates, M., and Montzka, T.A. JOURNAL OF
MEDICINAL CHEMISTRY. 7(2):127-131, 1964.
"Some recent studies of the clinical pharmacology of local
anesthetics of practical significance," by Adriana, J.,
and Zepernick, R. ANNALS OF SURGERY. 158:666-671, 1963.
"Some relationships between catecholamines and morphine-
like drugs," by Smith, A.A., et al. RECENT ADVANCES IN
BIOLOGICAL PSYCHIATRY. 6:208-213, 1964.
"Species of fungi isolated from samples of opium from ten
different regions," by Eltutar, H., and Igneciler, M.
BULLETIN ON NARCOTICS. 15(1):35-36, Jan.-Mar., 1963.
"Specific and nonspecific antagonism of morphine-induced
respiratory depression," by Papadopoulos, C.N., and
Keats, A.S. ANESTHESIOLOGY. 23:86-91, 1962.
"Spontaneous opiate addiction in rhesus monkeys," by Clag-
horn, J.L., and Ordy, J.M. SCIENCE. 149:440-441, 1965.
"The stability of the drug metabolising enzymes of liver
microsomal preparations. BIOCHEMICAL PHARMACOLOGY. 13:
1607-1617, 1964.
"Standardization of scales wich evaluate subjective effects
of morphine, amphetamine, pentobarbital, alcohol, LSD-25,
pyrahexl and chlorpromazine." PSYCHOPHARMACOLOGIA. 4
(3):184-205, 1963.
"Staphylococcal endocarditis in heroin addicts," by Olsson,
R.A., and Romansky, M.J. ANTIMICROBIAL AGENTS AND CHEM-
OTHERAPY. pp. 121-126, 1961.
"Staphylacoccal tricuspid endocarditis in heroin addicts,"
by Olsson, R.A., and Romansky, M.J. ANNALS OF INTERNAL
MEDICINE. 57:755-762, 1962.
"Statistics of spontaneous electrical activity of suprs- and
ectosylvian gyri of the dog," by Tunturi, A.R. AMERICAN
JOURNAL OF PHYSIOLOGY. 204:51-59, 1963.
"Structures related to morphine," by Saito, S., and May, E.L.
JOURNAL OF ORGANIC CHEMISTRY. 27(3):948-951, 1962.
"Structures related to morphine. XXII. A benzomorphan con-

gener of meperidine," by Kugita, H., et al. JOURNAL OF
MEDICINAL AND PHARMACEUTICAL CHEMISTRY. 5(2):357-361,
1962.
--XXV. 5-propyl-and 5,9-depropyl-6,7-benzomorphans and a
pharmacologic summary," by Ager, J.H. JOURNAL OF MEDI-
CINAL AND PHARMACEUTICAL CHEMISTRY. 6(3):322-325, 1963.
--XXVI. Cyclization experiments with 2-benzyl-1,3,4-tri-
alkyl-1,2,5,6-tetrahydropyridines. Improved yields of
B-5,9-dialkyl-6,7-benzomorphans," by Ager, J.H., et al.
JOURNAL OF ORGANIC CHEMISTRY. 28(9):2470-2472, 1963.
--XXXI. 2'-substituted benzomorphans," by Jacobson, A.E.,
and May, E.L. JOURNAL OF MEDICINAL CHEMISTRY. 8(5):
563-566, 1965.
"Studies in detoxication by means of the isolated perfused
liver," by Evans, E.A., et al. TOXICOLOGY AND APPLIED
PHARMACOLOGY. 5:129-141, 1963.
"Studies in hyperkinetic behavior: II. Laboratory and clin-
ical evaluations of drug treatments," by Millichap, J.G.,
and Boldrey, E.E. NEUROLOGY. 17(5):467-471, 1967.
"Studies in mass spectrometry. IV. Steric direction of
fragmentation in cis- and trans-B: C ring-fused morphine
derivatives," by Mandelbaum, A., and Ginsburg, D. TETRA-
HEDRON LETTERS. 29:2479-2489, 1965.
"Studies of analgesic drugs. VIII. A narcotic antagonist
analgesic without psychotomimetic effects," by Keats, A.
S., and Telford, J. JOURNAL OF PHARMACOLOGY AND EXPERI-
MENTAL THERAPEUTICS. 143:157-164, 1964.
"Studies of analgesic drugs: respiratory effects of narcotic
antagonists," by Keats, A.S., and Telford, J. JOURNAL OF
PHARMACOLOGY AND EXPERIMENTAL THERAPEUTICS. 151:126-132,
1966.
"Studies of the dependence-producing potential of the nar-
cotic antagonist 2-cyclopropylmethyl-2'-hydroxy-5, 9-
dimethyl-6, 7-benzomorphan (cyclazocine, WIN-20, 740,
ARC II-c-3)," by Martin, W.R., et al. JOURNAL OF PHAR-
MACOLOGY AND EXPERIMENTAL THERAPEUTICS. 150:426-436,
Dec., 1965.
"Studies on antagonism of morphine miosis by nalorphine as
a diagnostic test for narcotic usage," by Chen, I.Y., et
al. BRITISH JOURNAL OF PHARMACOLOGY. 24:787-797, 1965.
"Studies on cellular adaptation to morphine and its reversal
by nolorphine in cerebral cortical slices of rats," by
Takemori, A.E. JOURNAL OF PHARMACOLOGY AND EXPERIMENTAL
THERAPEUTICS. 135:89-93, 1962.
"Studies on glucuronide synthesis in rats chronically treat-
ed with morphine and phenol," by Takemori, A.E., and Glo-
wacki, G.A. BIOCHEMICAL PHARMACOLOGY. 11:867-870, 1962.
"Studies on morphine alkaloids. II. Indolincodeine I. A
new skeletal rearrangement of 14-bromocodeine," by Okuda,
S., et al. CHEMICAL AND PHARMACEUTICAL BULLETIN. 13(9):
1092-1103, 1965.
"Studies on the enzymatic N- and O-demethylation of narcotic
analgesics and evidence for the formation of codeine from
morphine in rats and dogs," by Elison, C., and Elliott,

H.W. JOURNAL OF PHARMACOLOGY AND EXPERIMENTAL THERA-
PEUTICS. 144(2):265-275, 1964.
"Studies on the increased cerebral glucose utilization
caused by morphine," by Takemori, A.E. FEDERATION PRO-
CEEDINGS. 24(2, pt.1):548, 1965.
"Studies on the metabolic N-demethylation. IV. Effects
of phenobarbital and morphine on the oxidative demethyla-
tion in rat liver," by Kuroiwa, Y., et al. CHEMICAL AND
PHARMACEUTICAL BULLETIN. 13(6):731-734, 1965.
"Studies on the specificity of narcotic antagonists," by
Foldes, F.F., et al. ANESTHESIOLOGY. 26(3):320-328,
1965.
"Studies on the storage of norepinephrine and the effects
of drugs," by Potter, L.T., and Axelrod, J. JOURNAL OF
PHARMACOLOGY AND EXPERIMENTAL THERAPEUTICS. 140:199-206,
1963.
"Study of methadone as an adjunct in rehabilitation of her-
oin addicts," by Dole, V.P., and Nyswander, M. ILLINOIS
MEDICAL JOURNAL. 130:487-489, Oct., 1966.
"A study of some of the pharmacologic actions of fentanyl ci-
trate," by Gardocki, J.F., and Yelnosky, J. TOXICOLOGY
AND APPLIED PHARMACOLOGY. 6:48-62, 1964.
"A study of the interaction of nalorphine with fentanyl and
innovar," by Gardocki, J.F., et al. TOXICOLOGY AND AP-
PLIED PHARMACOLOGY. 6(5):593-601, 1964.
"Study of the narcotic antagonist," by Sadove, M.S., et al.
JOURNAL OF THE AMERICAN MEDICAL ASSOCIATION. 183:666-
668, 1963.
"A study on a colour reaction of morphine for the determin-
ation of the origin of opium and estimation of morphine,"
by Ramanathan, V.S. JOURNAL OF SCIENTIFIC AND INDUSTRIAL
RESEARCH. 21(12):449-460, 1962
"Study on the excitation induced by amphetamine, cocaine,
and -methyltryptamine," by Galambos, E., et al. PSYCHO-
PHARMACOLOGIA. 11(2):122-129, 1967.
"Study of the pharmacology of hasish," by Joachimoglu, G.,
and Miras, C. BULLETIN ON NARCOTICS. 15(3-4):7-8, 1963.
"Subjective drug effects: a factorial representation of sub-
jective drug effects on the Addiction Research Center In-
ventory," by Haertzen, C.A. JOURNAL OF NERVOUS AND MEN-
TAL DISEASE. 140(4):280-289, 1965.
"Subjective effects of heroin and morphine in normal sub-
jects," by Smith, G.M., and Beecher, H.K. JOURNAL OF
PHARMACOLOGY AND EXPERIMENTAL THERAPEUTICS. 136(1):47-
52, 1962.
"The sulphone analogue of d-methadone: assessment of antitussive activity in general practice," by Noel, P.R.
BRITISH JOURNAL OF DISEASES OF THE CHEST. 57(1):48-52,
1963.
"Suspected dependence on chlordiazepoxide hydrochloride
(librium)," by Slater, J. CANADIAN MEDICAL ASSOCIATION
Journal. 95:416, Aug. 27, 1966.
"Synthesis of a B/C trans-fused morphine structure," by Kugita, H., and Takeda, M. CHEMISTRY AND INDUSTRY. 51:
2099-2100, 1964.

"The synthesis of N-allylnorthebaine," by Bartels-Keith,
J.R. JOURNAL OF PHARMACY AND PHARMACOLOGY. 16:133-134,
1964.
"Synthesis of morphine-like structures. I. 9-hydroxmethyl-
2,5-dimethyl-6,7-benzomorphan," by Kugita, H., and Takeda, M. CHEMICAL AND PHARMACEUTICAL BULLETIN. 11(8):986-
989, 1963.
--II. 2'-methoxy-9-hydroxymethyl-2,5-dimethyl-6,7-benzo-
morphan." CHEMICAL AND PHARMACEUTICAL BULLETIN. 12(10):
1163-1166, 1964.
--III. Stereochemical control of addition of barane to 9-
methylenebenzomorphan." CHEMICAL AND PHARMACEUTICAL BUL-
LETIN. 12(10):1166-1171, 1964.
--IV. Further studies on addition of barane to 9-methylene-
benzomorphan." CHEMICAL AND PHARMACEUTICAL BULLETIN.
12(10):1172-1175, 1964.
"Tachyphylaxis to epinephrine and its modification by cocaine," by Perez-Reyes, M., and Lipton, M.A. PROCEEDINGS
OF THE SOCIETY FOR EXPERIMENTAL BIOLOGY AND MEDICINE.
112(1):181-186, 1963.
"Techniques utilized in the evaluation of psychotropic drugs
on animal activity," by Kinnard, W.J., Jr., and Watzman,
N. JOURNAL OF PHARMACEUTICAL SCIENCES. 55(10):995-1012,
1966.
"Temperature responses in the rat following intracerebral
microinjection of morphine." JOURNAL OF PHARMACOLOGY AND
EXPERIMENTAL THERAPEUTICS. 150(1):135-139, 1965.
"A theory of human pathologic pain and its measurement: the
analgesic activity of methotrimeprazine," by Kast, E.C.,
and Collins, V.J. JOURNAL OF NEW DRUGS. 6(3):142-148,
1966.
"Thyroxine and hypolipidaemic effect of clofibrate," by Dan-
owski, T.S., et al. LANCET. 1:854, Apr. 15, 1967.
"Time estimation, knowledge of results and drug effects," by
Rutschmann, J., and Rubinstein, L. JOURNAL OF PSYCHIATRIC
RESEARCH. 4(2):107-114, 1966.
"Titrium-labeled dihydromorphine: its metabolic fate and ex-
cretion in the rat," by Hug, C.C., Jr., and Mellett, L.B.
JOURNAL OF PHARMACOLOGY AND EXPERIMENTAL THERAPEUTICS.
149(3):446-453, 1965.
"Tolerance to and physical dependence on morphine in rats,"
by Martin, W.R., et al. PSYCHOPHARMACOLOGIA. 4(4):247-
260, 1963.
"Tolerance to morphine. I. Effects on catecholamines in
the brain and adrenal glands," by Maynert, E.W., and
Klingman, G.I. JOURNAL OF PHARMACOLOGY AND EXPERIMENTAL
THERAPEUTICS. 135:285-295, 1962
--II. Lack if effects on brain of 5-hydroxytryptamine and
y-aminobutytic acid," by Maynert, E.W., et al. JOURNAL
OF PHARMACOLOGY AND EXPERIMENTAL THERAPEUTICS. 135:296-
299, 1962.
--III. Effects on catecholamines in the heart, intestine
and spleen," by Klingman, G.I., and Maynert, E.W. JOURNAL
OF PHARMACOLOGY AND EXPERIMENTAL THERAPEUTICS. 135:300-

305, 1962.
"Tolerance to the lenticular effects of opiates," by Smith, A.A., et al. JOURNAL OF PHARMACOLOGY AND EXPERIMENTAL THERAPEUTICS. 156(1):85-91, 1967.
"Topical anesthesia for endoscopy," by Morse, H.R., and Hartman, M.M. PENNSYLVANIA MEDICAL JOURNAL. 68:39-42, 1965.
"Tourniquet pain: an experimental method sensitive to morphine," by Smith, G.M., et al. FEDERATION PROCEEDINGS. 24(2, pt.1):548, 1965.
"Trancylcypromine." LANCET. 1:388-389, 1963.
"Tranquillizing and related drugs: properties for their identification (part II)," by Rajeswaran, P., and Kirk, P.L. BULLETIN ON NARCOTICS. 13(4):21-32, Oct.-Dec., 1961.
"Transaminase activity after codeine administration," by Adams, P., et al. POSTGRADUATE MEDICAL JOURNAL. 38(440): 348-349, 1962.
"Transformation of codeine to an analog of the potent analgesic phenazocine," by Sargent, L.J., and Ager, J.H. JOURNAL OF MEDICINE AND PHARMACEUTICAL CHEMISTRY. 6(5): 569-572, 1963.
"Treatment of cardiac failure in infancy and childhood," by Kreidberg, M.B., et al. NEW ENGLAND JOURNAL OF MEDICINE. 268:23-30, 1963.
"Treatment of painful sickle cell crises with papaverine, preliminary report," by Diggs, L.W., and Williams, D.L. SOUTHERN MEDICAL JOURNAL. 56(5):472-474, 1963.
"The treatment of poor prognosis alcoholics by prolonged apomorphine aversion therapy," by Quinn, J.T., and Kerr, W.S. JOURNAL OF THE IRISH MEDICAL ASSOCIATION. 53:50-54, 1963.
"Treatment of respiratory insufficiency." MEDICAL LETTER ON DRUGS AND THERAPEUTICS. 8:63-64, 1966.
"Treatment of shock following myocardial infraction," by Goldberg, L.I., and Dorney, E.R. POSTGRADUATE MEDICINE. 37:52-57, 1965.
"Tritium-labeled dihydromorphine: an autoradiographic study of its tissue distribution in mice," by Hug, C.C., and Mellet, L.B. UNIVERSITY OF MICHIGAN MEDICAL BULLETIN. 29:165-174, 1963.
"An understanding of pain and its measurement," by Kast, E.C. MEDICAL TIMES. 94:1501-1553, 1966.
"The uptake and binding of circulating serotonin and the effect of drugs," by Axelrod, J., and Inscoe, J.K. JOURNAL OF PHARMACOLOGY AND EXPERIMENTAL THERAPEUTICS. 141: 161-165, 1963.
"Urine detection tests in the management of the narcotic addict," by Kurlan, A.A., et al. AMERICAN JOURNAL OF PSYCHIATRY. 122:737-742, 1966.
"Urine screening techniques employed in the detection of users of narcotics and their correlation with the nalorphine test," by Parker, K.D., et al. JOURNAL OF FORENSIC SCIENCES. 11:152-166, Apr., 1966.

"The use of alphaprodine (nisentil) for the production of
surgical anesthesia," by Hartman, M.M., and Schwab, J.M.
SURGICAL CLINICS OF NORTH AMERICA. 43:1229-1242, 1963.
"The use of codeine for the relief of pain in the recovery
room," by Sadove, M.S., et al. ILLINOIS MEDICAL JOURNAL.
125:151-153, 1964.
"The use of diamorphine (heroin) in therapeutics," by Vaille,
C. BULLETIN ON NARCOTICS. 15(3-4):1-5, July-Dec., 1963.
"The use of drugs in the management of drug dependence," by
Eddy, N.B. JOURNAL OF THE TENNESSEE MEDICAL ASSOCIATION.
60:269-273, 1967.
"The use of high dosage deprol in alcoholic and narcotic
withdrawal," by Snow, L., and Rickels, K. AMERICAN JOUR-
NAL OF PSYCHIATRY. 119(5):475, 1962.
"Use of hindlimb reflexes of the chronic spinal dog for com-
paring analgesics," by Martin, W.R., et al. JOURNAL OF
PHARMACOLOGY AND EXPERIMENTAL THERAPEUTICS. 144(1):8-11,
1964.
"The use of ion-exchange resin impregnated paper in the de-
tection of opiate alkaloids, amphetamines, phenothiazines
and barbiturates in urine," by Jaffe, J.H., and Kirkpa-
trick, D. PSYCHOPHARMACOLOGY BULLETIN; NATIONAL CLEARING-
HOUSE FOR MENTAL HEALTH INFORMATION. 3:49-52, 1966.
"Use of paper chromatographic technics on urine for evalu-
ating narcotic usage by the nalorphine pupil test," by
Lin, S.C., and Way, E.L. JOURNAL OF FORENSIC SCIENCES.
8:209-219, 1963.
"The use of potent analgesics," by Murphree, H.B. AMERICAN
JOURNAL OF NURSING. 63:104-109, 1963.
"The use of promazine, meperidine, and scopolamine in labor
and delivery," by Burgstiner, C.B. JOURNAL OF THE MEDICAL
ASSOCIATION OF GEORGIA. 52:101-103, 1963.
"Use of the new analgesic talwin in urology," by Anderson,
E.C., et al. JOURNAL OF UROLOGY. 96:584-585, 1966.
"Use of writhing test for evaluating analgesic activity of
narcotic antagonists," by Blumberg, H., et al. PROCEED-
INGS OF THE SOCIETY FOR EXPERIMENTAL BIOLOGY AND MEDICINE.
118(3):763-766, 1965.
"Uterine contractility in primates: a comparative study,"
by Scoggin, W.A., et al. SURGICAL FORUM; CLINICAL CON-
GRESS OF THE AMERICAN COLLEGE OF SURGEONS. 14:384-385,
1963.
"Variations in the strength of morphine induced analgesia
in relation to the autonomic nervous system," by Frommel,
E., et al. MEDICINA EXPERIMENTALIS. 8(3):171-175, 1963.
"Vegetable drugs and their derivatives," by Levine, J. JOUR-
NAL OF THE ASSOCIATION OF OFFICIAL AGRICULTURAL CHEMISTS.
46(1):20, 1963.
"Viral hepatitis associated with illicit parenteral use of
drugs," by Dismukes, W.E., et al. JOURNAL OF THE AMER-
ICAN MEDICAL ASSOCIATION. 206:1048-1052, Oct. 28, 1968.
"Viral hepatitis in narcotics users. An outbreak in Rhode
Island," by Rosenstein, B.J. JOURNAL OF THE AMERICAN
MEDICAL ASSOCIATION. 199(10):698-700, 1967.

"Von Recklinghausen's neurofibromatosis with long-standing
pelvic lesions, drug addiction, and mental sequelae," by
Sloan, W.R., and Nabney, J.B. JOURNAL OF OBSTETRICS AND
GYNAECOLOGY OF THE BRITISH COMMONWEALTH. 70:523-524,
1963.
"Withdrawal of ataractic medication in schizophrenic pa-
tients," by Garfield, S.L., et al. DISEASES OF THE NER-
VOUS SYSTEM. 27:321-325, May, 1966.
"Withdrawal symptoms after abrupt termination of imipramine,"
by Shatan, C. CANADIAN PSYCHIATRIC ASSOCIATION JOURNAL.
11 (suppl.):150-158, 1966.
"X-ray diffraction studies of cocaine and its substitutes,"
by Sullivan, R.C., and O'Brien, K.P. BULLETIN ON NAR-
COTICS. 20(3):31-40, July-Sept., 1968.

NARCOTICS CONTROL: Books and Essays

Agnew, Derek. UNDERCOVER AGENT: NARCOTICS; the dramatic
story of the world's secret war against drug racketeers.
London: Souvenir Press, 1960.
American Association for Health, Physical Education and Recreation. HOW CAN WE TEACH ADOLESCENTS ABOUT SMOKING,
DRINKING, AND DRUG ABUSE? Washington: National Education
Association, 1969.
Anslinger, Harry J. THE PROTECTORS; the heroic story of the
narcotic agents, citizens and officials and their unend-
ing, unsung battles against organized crime in America
and abroad. New York: Farrar and Strauss, 1964.
Anslinger, Harry Jacob, and Oursler, W. THE MURDERERS; the
story of the narcotic gangs. New York: Farrar, Strauss,
and Cudahy, 1961.
Bellizzi, John J. KEYNOTE ADDRESS. International Narcotic
Enforcement Officers Association, 8th Conference Report.
Louisville, Kentucky, 1967.
Blake, John B., editor. SAFEGUARDING THE PUBLIC: historical
aspects of medicinal drug control. Baltimore: Johns Hop-
kins Press, 1969.
Brill, Henry, et al. SECOND ON-SITE STUDY OF THE BRITISH
NARCOTIC SYSTEM. Albany: Narcotic Addiction Control Com-
mission, 1968.
Brotman, Richard, et al. A COMMUNITY APPROACH TO DRUG AD-
DICTION. Washington: Health, Education and Welfare, 1968.
Buckwalter, Jacob A. MERCHANT OF MISERY. Mountain View,
California: Pacific Press Pub. Association, 1961.
Buse, Renée. DEADLY SILENCE. Garden City, New York: Dou-
bleday, 1965.
Duster, Troy. THE LEGISLATION OF MORALITY; law, drugs, and
moral judgement. New York: Free Press, 1969.
Eldridge, W.B. NARCOTICS AND THE LAW: a critique of the
American experiment in narcotic drug control. New York:

New York University Press, 1962.
Felix, Robert H. "Demonstration of pilot programs to control narcotic addiction in the community," PROCEEDINGS: WHITE HOUSE CONFERENCE ON NARCOTIC AND DRUG ABUSE. Washington: Government Printing Office, 1962, pp. 80-84.
Fort, Joel. "Social and legal response to pleasure-giving drugs," UTOPIATES, by Richard Blum. New York: Atherton Press, 1964, pp. 203-223.
Gimlin, Joan S. LEGALIZATION OF MARIJUANA. Washington: Editorial Research Report, 1967 (2(6), Aug. 9).
Goodrich, Leland M. NEW TRENDS IN NARCOTICS CONTROL. New York: Carnegie Endowment for International Peace, 1960.
Harney, Malachi L., et al. NARCOTIC OFFICER'S NOTEBOOK. Springfield, Illinois: C.C. Thomas, 1961.
Hong Kong. Narcotics Advisory Committee. PROGRESS REPORT 1959/1960. Hong Kong: Government Printer, 1961.
Hong Kong. Secretary for Chinese Affairs. ANTI-NARCOTICS CAMPAIGN. S. C. A.'s Appeal to Every Government Servant for Help. Hong Kong, 1960.
Jeffee, Saul. NARCOTICS: AN AMERICAN PLAN. New York: Paul S. Eriksson, 1966.
Jones, T. DRUGS AND THE POLICE. London: Butterworth, 1968.
Louria, Donald B. DRUG SCENE. New York: McGraw-Hill, 1968.
Moore, Robin. FRENCH CONNECTION: the world's most crucial narcotics investigation. Boston: Little, Brown, 1969.
Moscow, Alvin. MERCHANTS OF HEROIN; an in-depth portrayal of business in the underworld. New York: Dial Press, 1968.
"Narcotics and drug abuse," THE CHALLENGE OF CRIME IN A FREE SOCIETY, by United States President's Commission on Law Enforcement and Adminstration of Justice. Washington: Government Printing Office, 1967.
New Jersey. Legislature. Narcotic Drug Study Commission. AN INTERIM REPORT: a study of the administration of narcotic control relating to the causes, prevention and control of drug addiction, constituted pursuant to Senate joint resolution no. 16, law of 1963. Trenton, 1964.
New York (City) Board of Education. PREVENTION OF NARCOTICS ADDICTION AND SUBSTANCE ABUSE. New York, 1966-1967 (Curriculum Bulletin, no. 16).
New York (State) Education Department. Curriculum Development Center. DRUG ABUSE; supplementary information for teachers on the use, misuse, and abuse of drugs. Albany, 1967.
New York (State). Investigation Commission. RECOMMENDATIONS OF THE NEW YORK STATE COMMISSION OF INVESTIGATION CONCERNING NARCOTICS ADDICTION IN THE STATE OF NEW YORK. New York, 1966.
New York (State) Narcotic Addiction Control Commission. THE STATE OF NEW YORK AND THE DRUG ADDICT. Albany, 1968.
O'Donnell, John. THE RELAPSE RATE IN NARCOTIC ADDICTION; a critique of follow-up studies. Albany: Narcotic Addiction Control Commission, 1968.
Saltman, Jules. WHAT WE CAN DO ABOUT DRUG ABUSE. New York:

Public Affairs Committee, Inc., 1966.

Schneider, George. DATA ON YOUTH 1967: A STATISTICAL DOC-
UMENT. Albany: New York State Division for Youth, 1967.

Siragusa, Charles. THE TRAIL OF THE POPPY: behind the mask
of the Mafia, as told to Robert Wiedrich. Englewood
Cliffs, New Jersey: Prentice-Hall, 1966.

Society for the Study of Addiction to Alcohol and other
drugs. PHARMACOLOGICAL AND EPIDEMIOLOGICAL ASPECTS OF
ADOLESCENT DRUG DEPENDENCE, ed Cedric W.M. Wilson. New
York: Pergamon Press, 1968.

United Arab Republic Committee for the investigation of
hashish consumption in the Egyptian region, Research in
progress: REPORT 1. The interviewing schedule: preparation, reliability, and validity. REPORT 2. Hashish consumption in Cairo City --- a pilot survey, by National
centre of Social and Criminological Research, Cairo, 1960
and 1963. Cairo: General Organization for Government
Printing Offices, 1963.

United Nations. ESTIMATED WORLD REQUIREMENTS OF NARCOTIC
DRUGS IN 1960. Statement issued by the Supervisory Body
under article 5 of the Convention of 13 July 1931 for limiting the manufacture and regulating the distribution
of narcotic drugs. New York, 1961.

--MULTILINGUAL LIST OF NARCOTIC DRUGS UNDER INTERNATIONAL
CONTROL, incorporating the names of narcotic drugs in alphabetical order - with proper cross-references - in the
working languages of the United Nations, and when possible in other languages: as far as possible the names of
drugs known to be used in the illicit traffic; the names
of known preparations which simply consist of the basic
drug in the form of tablets, solutions, or mixed only
with inactive ingredients; the names of the base-acid
combinations of narcotic substances known to be manufac-
tured; the structural formulae of the chemical substances.
New York, 1961.

--NARCOTIC DRUGS UNDER INTERNATIONAL CONTROL: MULTILINGUAL
LIST. New York: UN Document E-CN.7-436, 1963.

--Commission on Narcotic Drugs. SUMMARY OF ANNUAL REPORTS
OF GOVERNMENTS RELATING TO OPIUM AND OTHER NARCOTIC DRUGS
1957. This summary covers annual reports submitted by
governments in accordance with the treaties dealing with
the international control of narcotic drugs. New York,
1961.

United States. Bureau of Narcotics. CONTROL AND REHABILI-
TATION OF THE NARCOTIC ADDICT; a symposium. Washington:
Government Printing Office, 1961.

--PREVENTION AND CONTROL OF NARCOTIC ADDICTION. Washington: Government Printing Office, 1962.

--PREVENTION AND CONTROL OF NARCOTIC ADDICTION. Washington: Government Printing Office, 1964.

--PREVENTION AND CONTROL OF NARCOTIC ADDICTION. Washington: Government Printing Office, 1967.

United States. Congress. House of Representatives. Committee on Government Operations. Intergovernmental Re-

lations Subcommittee. DRUG SAFETY: HEARINGS. Mar. 24 -
June 18, 1964. Washington: Government Printing Office,
1964, 2 vols.
--Committee on Interstate and Foreign Commerce. DRUG ABUSE
CONTROL AMENDMENTS OF 1965: HEARINGS, Jan. 27-Feb. 10,
1965 (89th Congress, 1st session). Washington: Govern-
ment Printing Office, 1965.
--DRUG ABUSE CONTROL AMENDMENTS OF 1965: REPORT, Mar. 2,
1965, on H. R. 2, a bill to protect the public health
and safety by amending the Federal Food, Drug and Cos-
metic Act to establish special controls for depressant
and stimulant drugs and counterfeit drugs. Washington:
Government Printing Office, 1965.
United States. Congress. Senate. Committee on Government
Operations. ORGANIZED CRIME AND ILLICIT TRAFFIC IN NAR-
COTICS. Hearings before the Permanent Subcommittee on
Investigations of the Committee on Government Operations,
U.S. Senate, 88th Congress, 1st session pursuant to Senate resolution 17. Washington: Government Printing Office, 1963.
--ORGANIZED CRIME AND ILLICIT TRAFFIC IN NARCOTICS; REPORT,
together with additional combined views and individual
views. Washington: Government Printing Office, 1965.
--Subcommittee on Reorganization and International Organi-
zations. INTERAGENCY COORDINATION IN DRUG RESEARCH AND
REGULATION: HEARINGS, Agency coordination study (pursuant
to S. res. 27, 88th Congress, as amended): review of cooperation on drug policies among food and drug administration, National institutes of health and other agencies:
pt.5, June 19, 1963. Testimony and exhibits (including
subsequent 1963-1964 correspondence) on: (1) Commission
on drug safety; (2) Pharmaceutical manufacturers Association; (3) Medical education on drug safety and other drug
issues. Washington: Government Printing Office, 1964.
--Subcommittee on Executive Reorganization. ORGANIZATION
AND COORDINATION OF FEDERAL DRUG RESEARCH AND REGULATORY
PROGRAMS: LSD. HEARINGS, 89th Congress, 2nd session.
May 24-26, 1966. Washington: Government Printing Office,
1966.
United States. Congress. Senate. Committee on Labor and
Public Welfare. Subcommittee on Health. CONTROL OF PSY-
CHOTOXIC DRUGS: HEARING, Aug. 3, 1964, on S. 2628, a
bill to protect the public health by amending the Federal
Food, Drug and Cosmetic Act to regulate the manufacture,
compounding, processing, distribution, delivery and pos-
session of psychotoxic drugs. Washington: Government
Printing Office, 1964.
--PSYCHOTOXIC DRUG CONTROL ACT OF 1964; REPORT TO ACCOMPANY
S. 2628. Washington: Government Printing Office, 1964.
United States. Department of Health, Education and Welfare.
TASK FORCE ON PRESCRIPTION DRUGS, BACKGROUND PAPERS: cur-
rent American and foreign programs. Washington: Govern-
ment Printing Office, 1968.
--TASK FORCE ON PRESCRIPTION DRUGS, DRUG PRESCRIBERS [with

list of references]. Washington: Government Printing Office, 1968.
--TASK FORCE ON PRESCRIPTION DRUGS, DRUG USERS [with list of references]. Washington: Government Printing Office, 1968.
--TASK FORCE ON PRESCRIPTION DRUGS, 2ND INTERIM REPORT AND RECOMMENDATIONS. Washington: Government Printing Office, 1968.
United States. Food and Drug Administration. REQUIREMENTS OF THE UNITED STATES FOOD, DRUG, AND COSMETIC ACT. Revised. Washington: Government Printing Office, 1964.
United States Government. Executive Office. President's commission on law enforcement and the administration of justice: task force report, NARCOTICS AND DRUG ABUSE [annotations and consultants' papers]. Washington: Government Printing Office, 1967.
--REPORT OF THE PRESIDENT'S ADVISORY COMMISSION ON NARCOTIC DRUG ABUSE. Washington: Government Printing Office, 1963.
United States. Treasury Department. Federal Bureau of Narcotics. PREVENTION AND CONTROL OF NARCOTIC ADDICTION. Washington: Government Printing Office, 1962.
United States. Treatises, etc. NARCOTIC DRUGS: limitation and regulation of poppy plant cultivation and production of trade in, and use of opium; protocol between the U.S.A. and other governments. Washington: Government Printing Office, 1963.
Vermes, Hal G. HELPING YOUTH AVOID FOUR GREAT DANGERS: smoking, drinking, VD, narcotic addiction. New York: Association Press, 1965.
Washington (State) Laws, Statutes, etc. STATUTES, RULES AND REGULATIONS GOVERNING THE PRACTICE OF PHARMACY, THE SALE AND DISPENSING OF DRUGS, POISONS, NARCOTICS AND MEDICINES. Olympia, Washington: Board of Pharmacy, 1964.
Way, E.L. CONTROL AND TREATMENT OF DRUG ADDICTION IN HONG KONG. Paper presented at the Narcotics Conference held at the University of California at Los Angeles, Apr. 27-28, 1963.
Wighton, Charles. DOPE INTERNATIONAL. London: Muller, 1960.
Wilkins, L.T. SOCIAL DEVIANCE: social policy, action and research. Englewood Cliffs, New Jersey: Prentice-Hall, 1965.
Williams, J.B. NARCOTICS. Dubuque, Iowa: Wm. C. Brown, 1963.
Williams, J.B. NARCOTICS AND HALLUCINOGENICS; a handbook. Revised edition. New York: Glencoe Press, 1967.

NARCOTICS CONTROL: Periodical Literature

"Addiction to drug abuse control amendments." PUBLIC HEALTH REPORTS. 81:511, 1966.

"Addicts fear narcotics control by computer." AMERICAN PRO-
FESSIONAL PHARMACIST. 33:42-47, 1967.
"Adolescents, parents and education; recommendations that
public schools update anti-alcohol and anti-narcotics
education," by Brickman, W.W. SCHOOL AND SOCIETY. 93:
238, Apr. 17, 1965.
"The adverse drug reaction reporting a scheme and the Aus-
tralian drug evaluation committee," by Walshe, A.M. MED-
ICAL JOURNAL OF AUSTRALIA. 2:82-85, July 13, 1968.
"Air spotting and destruction of clandestine opium poppy in
Mexico." BULLETIN ON NARCOTICS. 20(3):18, July-Sept.,
1968.
"Alarming rise in dope traffic." U.S. NEWS AND WORLD RE-
PORT. 65:43-45, Sept. 2, 1968.
"Alcohol and other drug dependencies," by Birchard, Carl.
CANADA'S MENTAL HEALTH. 15(5-6):31-33, 1967.
"Another look at narcotics control in hospitals," by Debag-
gio, C. HOSPITALS. 37:76-81, 1963.
"Aspects of law enforcement in drug control," by Larkworth,
F.R. AMERICAN ASSOCIATION OF INDUSTRIAL NURSES JOURNAL.
15:7-9, Aug., 1967.
"Assessment of adverse reactions within a drug surveillance
program," by Borda, I.T., et al. JOURNAL OF THE AMERICAN
MEDICAL ASSOCIATION. 205:645-647, Aug. 26, 1968.
"Attack on dope." AMERICA. 108:251-252, Feb. 23, 1963.
"Authorities respond to growing drug use among high school
students." PHI DELTA KAPPAN. 50:213, Dec., 1968.
"Automated narcotic control system saves time for pharmacy
and nursing," by Case, R.W., et al. HOSPITALS. 41:97-
98, 1967.
"The barbiturates, tranquillizers, amphetamines, and hallucinogens, and their control in Switzerland," by Campan-
ini, N. BULLETIN ON NARCOTICS. 19(2):13-34, Apr.-June,
1967.
"Bill for control of drug addiction." NURSING TIMES. 63:
497, Apr. 14, 1967.
"A brief history of the narcotics control controversy," by
Zusman, J. MENTAL HYGIENE. 45(3):383-388, 1961.
"Bureaucracy and morality: an organizational perspective on
a moral crusade," by Dickson, D.T. SOCIAL PROBLEMS.
16:145-156, Fall, 1968.
"A bust at gunpoint and an armed search at sunset." LIFE.
67:32-33, Oct. 31, 1969.
"Buying off the farmers," by Ehrlich, D.A. SCIENCE NEWS.
93:15, Jan. 6, 1968.
"Campus drug abuse gets second look." THE ATTACK ON NARCOT-
IC ADDICTION AND DRUG ABUSE. 2(4):1, Nov., 1968.
"Canada and controlled drugs," by Curran, R.E. MEDICAL SER-
VICES JOURNAL. 18:415-430, 1962.
"A case study in narcotics control," by Davis, N.M. HOSPI-
TALS. 36:56-64, 1962.
"Centralized narcotic accounting improves income and saves
time," by Barth, A. MODERN HOSPITAL. 107:90, 1966.
"City courts urged to get tough with addict selling nar-

cotics," by Kahn, J. NEW YORK POST. April, 1965.
"College guidance on drugs; Columbia University." SCHOOL AND SOCIETY. 95:139, Mar. 4, 1967.
"Colleges act on drug problem." THE ATTACK ON NARCOTIC ADDICTION AND DRUG ABUSE. 2(4):12-13, Nov., 1968.
"Combatting drug abuse." CHILDREN. 16(5):208, Sept.-Oct., 1969.
"Combination narcotic form facilitates recording, charging," by Mead, W.B., and Brazill, G. HOSPITAL TOPICS. 45:91-93, 1967.
"Coming into force of the Single Convention on Narcotic Drugs, 1961." BULLETIN ON NARCOTICS. 17(1):1, Jan.-Mar., 1965.
"Comments on narcotics addiction," by Hoch, P.H. COMPREHENSIVE PSYCHIATRY. 4(3):140-144, 1963.
"Commission research uncovers needed dangerous drugs sata. Initial studies provide aid for N.A.C.C. drug abuse program." THE ATTACK ON NARCOTIC ADDICTION AND DRUG ABUSE. 3:1-2, Summer, 1969.
"Complying with the Drug Abuse Control Amendments of 1965." HOSPITALS. 40:75, 1966.
"A computerized system for restricted drug control and inventory," by Wirth, B.P. AMERICAN JOURNAL OF HOSPITAL PHARMACY. 24:556-560, Oct., 1967.
"Concerned communities approve drug councils. Training programs underway as local activity accelerates." THE ATTACK ON NARCOTIC ADDICTION AND DRUG ABUSE. 3:1-2, Winter, 1969.
"Control listings...narcotic and controlled drugs," by Burnie, C.F. CANADIAN HOSPITAL. 45:39-45, Mar., 1968.
"Control of addiction possible says Pierce." THE ATTACK ON NARCOTIC ADDICTION AND DRUG ABUSE. 3:1, Winter, 1969.
"Control of dangerous drugs on university campuses," by Bruyn, H.B. JOURNAL OF THE AMERICAN COLLEGE HEALTH ASSOCIATION. 16:13-19, Oct., 1967.
"Control of drug addiction and pharmaceutical preparations in the U. S." INTERNATIONAL DIGEST OF HEALTH LEGISLATION. 18(2):438-439, 1967.
"Control of drug addiction in Illinois." INTERNATIONAL DIGEST OF HEALTH LEGISLATION. 18(1):214-215, 1967.
"The control of drugs and therapeutic freedom," by Dunlop, D. PROCEEDINGS OF THE ROYAL SOCIETY OF MEDICINE. 61: 841-846, Aug., 1968.
"The control of narcotic drugs." WHO CHRONICLE. 14:309-311, 1960.
"Control of pharmaceutical samples." JOURNAL OF THE LOUISIANA STATE MEDICAL SOCIETY. 120:36-37, Jan., 1968.
"Control of psychotropic substances - Resolution of the Twenty-first World Health Assembly." BULLETIN ON NARCOTICS. 20(4):1, Oct.-Dec., 1968.
"Control of restricted drugs by automatic data processing," by Richards, C.F. AMERICAN JOURNAL OF HOSPITAL PHARMACY. 21:377-379, 1964.
"Control of some chemicals used in the manufacture of nar-

cotics." BULLETIN ON NARCOTICS. 21(1):46, Jan.-Mar., 1969.
"Controls on narcotics should keep them from getting out of hand," by Bowles, G. MODERN HOSPITAL. 95:98-100, 1960.
"Controlling the addict - British system," by Brill, Henry. NEWSWEEK. 55:80, Jan., 1960.
"Crackdown on bootleg drugs; campaign to end traffic in counterfeit drugs," by Irwin, T. TODAY'S HEALTH. 45: 18-19 passim, Jan., 1967.
"Criminal justice notes: drug abuse up 1500 per cent." NCCD NEWS. 48(4):10, Sept.-Oct., 1969.
"Criteria for exemption of combination products from provisions of the drug abuse control amendments," by Spratto, G.R. AMERICAN JOURNAL OF HOSPITAL PHARMACY. 25:532-534, Sept., 1968.
"Curbing the drug traffic in Britain; plans to change prescription system," by Wenham, B. NEW REPUBLIC. 156: 9-10, Mar. 18, 1967.
"The dangerous drug problem," by Louria, D.B., et al. NEW YORK MEDICINE. 22:241-246, 1966.
"Dangerous Drugs Act 1967. Restrictions on the prescribing of heroin or cocaine to addicts." NURSING TIMES. 64: 486, Apr. 12, 1968.
"Data on the illicit traffic in cocaine and coca leaves in South America with an annex on narcotics control in Brazil by Parreiras, D. BULLETIN ON NARCOTICS. 13(H):33-36, Oct., Dec., 1961.
"Dependence on alcohol and other drugs." WHO CHRONICAL. 21:219-226, June, 1967.
"Diagnosis and management of depressant drug dependence," by Ewing, J.A., and Bakewell, W.E. AMERICAN JOURNAL OF PSYCHIATRY. 123(8):909-917, 1967.
"Dope control." U.S. NEWS AND WORLD REPORT. 67:108, Oct. 20, 1969.
"Does your school board have a policy on drug abuse?" TEXAS OUTLOOK. 53:52, Mar., 1969.
"Dope control," by Berrellez, R. U.S. NEWS AND WORLD REPORT. 65:84, Aug. 26, 1968.
"Dream farm; field of marijuana destroyed by narcotic agents." TIME. 90:17-18, Sept. 8, 1967.
"Drug abuse and addiction; reporting in a general hospital," by Schremly, J.A., and Solomon, P. JOURNAL OF THE AMERICAN MEDICAL ASSOCIATION. 189:512-514, 1964.
"Drug abuse and control," by Smythe, H.A. CANADIAN HOSPITAL. 45:41-42, Apr., 1968.
"Drug abuse and social policy." CANADA'S MENTAL HEALTH. 17:26-32, Jan.-Feb., 1969.
"The Drug Abuse Control Amendments of 1965." RHODE ISLAND MEDICAL JOURNAL. 49:189, 1966.
"Drug control in Sweden," by Goldberg, L., and Lindgren, C. BULLETIN ON NARCOTICS. 13(4):7-15, Oct.-Dec., 1961.
"Drug regulation and the public health," by Austern, T. NEW YORK UNIVERSITY LAW REVIEW. 39:771-784, Nov., 1964.
"Drug trafficking," by Armstrong, G. JOURNAL OF THE FOREN-

SIC SCIENCE SOCIETY. 7:2-11, Jan., 1967.
"Drug usage: a two-way attack." U.S. NEWS AND WORLD REPORT.
67:9, Nov. 3, 1969.
"Drug usage and the law: the adolescent and an archaic con-
cept," by Barton, W. CLINICAL PROCEEDINGS OF THE CHILD-
REN'S HOSPITAL OF WASHINGTON, D.C. 24:180-184, 1968.
"Drugmakers and the government, who makes the decisions?" by
Lear, J. SATURDAY REVIEW. 43:37-42, July 2, 1960.
"Drugs and drug addiction: opinions on the taking of 'soft'
drugs." MEDICINE, SCIENCE AND THE LAW. 6:167-168, 1966.
"Drugs and drug addiction: unjust operation of the dangerous
drugs act." MEDICINE, SCIENCE AND THE LAW. 6:168, 1966.
"Drugs and public opinion: New York State residents speak
out on drug abuse." THE ATTACK ON NARCOTIC ADDICTION AND
DRUG ABUSE. 3(4):305, Fall, 1969.
"Drugs and regulations," by Russo, R.H. AMERICAN ASSOCIA-
TION OF INDUSTRIAL NURSES JOURNAL. 16:12-14, Oct., 1968.
"Drugs and teenagers," by Jones, A. JOURNAL OF THE FOREN-
SIC SCIENCE SOCIETY. 7:12-16, Jan., 1967.
"Drugs; new move for reform." TIME. 94:26, Oct. 24, 1969.
"Drugs on campus; undercover agents at Cornell and Fairleigh
Dickinson Universities." TIME. 89:36 passim, Mar. 24,
1967.
"Drugs out of control." JOURNAL OF THE IRISH MEDICAL ASSOC-
IATION. 61:217-218, June, 1968.
"Drugs: the new prohibition." NEWSWEEK. Feb. 7, 1966, p.
21.
"Education: drug misuse weapon." THE ATTACK ON NARCOTIC AD-
DICTION AND DRUG ABUSE. 3:13, Winter, 1969.
"An effective narcotic control system using electronic data
processing," by Eckel, F., and Latiolais, C.J. AMERICAN
JOURNAL OF HOSPITAL PHARMACY. 22:519-523, 1965.
"Eighteenth session of the Commission on Narcotic Drugs, and
Thirty-sixth session of the Economic and Social Council."
BULLETIN ON NARCOTICS. 15(3-4):39-42, 1963.
"The epidemiology of drug addiction and reflections on the
problem and policy in the U. S.," by Mattick, H.W. ILLI-
NOIS MEDICAL JOURNAL. 130:436-447, 1966.
"Establishment of a new drug addiction program," by McIsaac,
W.M. PSYCHOPHARMACOLOGY BULLETIN; NATIONAL CLEARINGHOUSE
FOR MENTAL HEALTH INFORMATION. 3:40-44, Dec., 1966.
"Estimated world requirements of narcotic drugs in 1960-[an-
nual]. BULLETIN ON NARCOTICS. 12(1):39-40, Jan.-Mar., 1960.
"The evolving role of the Canadian government in assessing
drug safety," by Hapmen, R.A. CANADIAN MEDICAL ASSOCIA-
TION JOURNAL. 98:294-300, Feb. 10, 1968.
"Failure of permissiveness; addiction increasing in Great
Britain." TIME. 89:76, Feb. 17, 1967.
"Federal control of narcotics and dangerous drugs," by Vin-
son, F.M., Jr. JOURNAL OF THE AMERICAN PHARMACEUTICAL
ASSOCIATION. 8:437-438 passim, Aug., 1968.
"Federal drug controls," by McKim, T.R. CANADIAN HOSPITAL.
45:46-47 passim, May, 1968.
"Federal Food and Drug Administration. Revised New-Drug

Regulation. Title 21--Food and Drugs." JOURNAL OF ORAL
THERAPEUTICS AND PHARMACOLOGY. 4:148-164, Sept., 1967.
"The fight against narcotics," by Mabileau, J.F. UNITED
NATIONS REVIEW. 11:29-34, Feb., 1964.
"First report of the International Narcotics Control Board."
BULLETIN ON NARCOTICS. 21(3):33-38, July-Sept., 1969.
"Forecast for back-to-school!" THE ATTACK ON NARCOTIC AD-
DICTION AND DRUG ABUSE. 3:9, Spring, 1969.
"A forty-years' chronicle of international narcotics con-
trol - the work of the Permanent Central Narcotics Board
1928-1968 and of the Drug Supervisory Body 1933-1968,"
by Greenfield, H. BULLETIN ON NARCOTICS. 20(2):1-4,
Apr.-June, 1968.
"Forty years of the campaign against narcotic drugs in the
United Arab Republic," by El Hadka, A.A. BULLETIN ON NAR-
COTICS. 17(4):1-12, Oct.-Dec., 1965.
"Four record forms plus vigilance help to safeguard narcot-
ics," by Stephens, W.L. AMERICAN PROFESSIONAL PHARMACIST.
29(12):23-26, 1963.
"General assembly, 32nd session, 21-26 Aug., 1963." INTER-
NATIONAL CRIMINAL POLICE REVIEW. 18(173):305-314 passim,
1963.
"Give drugs to addicts so we can be safe," by Goldstein,
J.J. SATURDAY EVENING POST. pp. 12 passim, July 30,
1966.
"Government and the dangerous drugs," by Joffe, M.H. CLIN-
ICAL PROCEEDINGS OF THE CHILDREN'S HOSPITAL OF DC. 24:
190-193, May, 1968.
"The Grand Old Men of the League of Nations," by Renborg,
B.A. BULLETIN ON NARCOTICS. 16:1-11, Oct.-Dec., 1964.
"Growing drive against drugs." U.S. NEWS AND WORLD REPORT.
67(24):38-40, Dec. 15, 1969.
"Guidance councils set throughout [New York] State." THE
ATTACK ON NARCOTIC ADDICTION AND DRUG ABUSE. 3:1-2,
Spring, 1969.
"Hallucinogens: the drugs and their effects on the user;
the present legal response to the new drug problem and
suggested alternate means of control. COLUMBIA LAW RE-
VIEW. 68:521-560, Mar., 1968.
"Haverford policy on drug use," by Borton, H. SCHOOL AND
SOCIETY. 95:250 passim, Apr. 15, 1967.
"The hazards of drugs and their control in Ireland," by
Boles, W.E. JOURNAL OF THE IRISH MEDICAL ASSOCIATION.
61:213-216, June, 1968.
"Herbert L. May," by Anslinger, H.J. BULLETIN ON NARCOTICS.
15(2):1-7, Apr.-June, 1963.
"Here and there " CANADA'S MENTAL HEALTH. 17:32, Jan.-
Feb., 1969.
"Hide and seek; conflict between the Mexican government and
Mexican poppy growers." NEWSWEEK. 67:60, Mar. 14, 1966.
"History of legal and medical roles in narcotic abuse in the
U.S.," by Simrell, E.V. PUBLIC HEALTH REPORTS. 83:587-
593, July, 1968.
"House votes controls on barbiturates, amphetamines [admin-

istration-backed bill (HR 2), expanding federal controls over depressant and stimulant drugs]." CONGRESSIONAL QUARTERLY WEEKLY REPORT. 23:373-375, Mar. 12, 1965.

"How new drugs are brought under international narcotics control by the procedure of the Single Convention on Narcotics Drugs, 1961 - the case of etorphine and acetorphine," BULLETIN ON NARCOTICS. 20(2):51-52, Apr.-June, 1968.

"How one district combats the drug problem," by Birnbach, S. SCHOOL MANAGEMENT. 10:102-106, June, 1966.

"How to cope with drug addiction in hospitals," by Krantz, J.C. MODERN HOSPITAL. 94:66-68, Feb., 1960.

"The identification of amphetamine type drugs," by Clarke, E.G.C. JOURNAL OF THE FORENSIC SCIENCE SOCIETY. 7(1): 31-36, Jan., 1967.

"The identification of some proscribed psychedelic drugs," by Clarke, E.G.C. JOURNAL OF THE FORENSIC SCIENCE SOCIETY. 7:46-50, Jan., 1967.

"Inn of synthetic dreams," by Jacob, A. ATLAS. 16:35-38, Nov., 1968.

"Innovations in drug education." JOURNAL OF SCHOOL HEALTH. 39:236-239, Apr., 1969.

"International control of narcotic drugs; administrative arrangements." UN MONTHLY CHRONICLE. 4:71-72, June, 1967.

"International control of narcotics," by Kusevic, V. UNESCO COURIER. 21:6-8, May, 1968.

"International drug conference." THE ATTACK ON NARCOTIC ADDICTION AND DRUG ABUSE. 3:4, Spring, 1969.

"The International Narcotics Control Board enters upon its functions. BULLETIN ON NARCOTICS. 20(2):49-50, Apr.-June, 1968.

"The international system of narcotics control," by Steinig, L. BULLETIN ON NARCOTICS. 20(3):1-6, July-Sept., 1968.

"Interpol fights the narcotic traffic." LISTEN. 16(5): Sept.-Oct., 1963.

"Interpol versus the underworld of narcotics," by Nepote, J. UNESCO COURIER. 21:24-29 passim, May, 1968.

"The Ithaca College program for the control of illegal drug usage," by Hammond, J.D. JOURNAL OF THE AMERICAN COLLEGE HEALTH ASSOCIATION. 16:35-37, Oct., 1967.

"Kick; government agencies efforts to stamp out drugs." NEW REPUBLIC. 154:10, Apr. 16, 1966.

"LBJ's Narco plan: lining up the big guns; crackdown on the way?" by McNeil, D. VILLAGE VOICE. pp. 11ff, Mar. 11, 1968.

"LSD: control, not prohibition." LIFE. 60:4, Apr. 29, 1966.

"LSD is no problem for us, public schoolmen report; school administration poll." NATION'S SCHOOLS. 78:55, Aug., 1966.

"Laboratory experience in drug abuse control," by Davidow, B. PSYCHOPHARMACOLOGY BULLETIN; NATIONAL CLEARINGHOUSE FOR MENTAL HEALTH INFORMATION. 3:30-33, Dec., 1966.

"Law enforcement and drug abuse," by Cowden, J., and Horan,
R. CLINICAL PROCEEDINGS OF THE CHILDREN'S HOSPITAL OF
DC. 24:161-180, 1968.
"Law-medicine notes: law, medicine, and LSD," by Chayet,
N.L. NEW ENGLAND JOURNAL OF MEDICINE. 277(5):253-254,
1967.
"The legal aspects of narcotic control in New York State,"
by Bellezzi, J.J. HEALTH NEWS. 37:4-9+, Aug., 1960.
"Let's think twice about 'free' narcotics," by Bloomquist,
E.R. GP. 21:156-162, 1960.
"Limitation and control of natural narcotics raw materials:
scheme of the League of Nations and the United Nations,"
by Renborg, B. BULLETIN ON NARCOTICS. 15(2):13-26, 1963.
"List of drugs under international narcotics control." WHO
TECHNICAL REPORT SERIES. 229:13-16, 1962.
"Local drug council formed." THE ATTACK ON NARCOTIC ADDIC-
TION AND DRUG ABUSE. 2(4):1, Nov., 1968.
"Logistics of junk," by Lyle, D. ESQUIRE. 65:59-67 passim,
Mar., 1966.
"Major effort to halt drug abuse." NEW YORK STATE EDUCATION.
56:32-33, Dec., 1968.
"Marijuana control: a perspective," by McGlothlin, W.H.
JOURNAL OF SECONDARY EDUCATION. 43:223-227, May, 1968.
"Medical profession seen as leader in combating narcotics
addiction," by Holmes, S.J. PAPERS ON DRUGS -- ADDIC-
TIONS, ALCOHOLISM AND DRUG ADDICTION RESEARCH FOUNDATION,
TORONTO, 1965, pp. 45-53.
"The meeting of the interamerican consultative group on nar-
cotics control: Rio de Janeiro, 27 Nov.-7 Dec., 1961,"
by Parreiras, D. BULLETIN ON NARCOTICS. 15(2):47-53,
1963.
"Merchants of heroin; condensation," by Moscow, A. READER'S
DIGEST. 93:203-228, Aug., 1968;
--93:199-207 passim, Sept., 1968.
"A model continuum for a community-based programme for the
prevention and treatment of narcotic addiction," by Freed-
man, A.M., et al. AMERICAN JOURNAL OF PUBLIC HEALTH.
54:791-802, 1964.
"More on lithium carbonate," by Reagan, J.J. AMERICAN JOUR-
NAL OF PSYCHIATRY. 124:1267-1268, Mar., 1968.
"N.A.C.C. (New York State Narcotic Addiction Control Commis-
sion) mobile unit." THE ATTACK ON NARCOTIC ADDICTION AND
DRUG ABUSE. 3:10, Spring, 1969.
"Nalorphine testing for illegal narcotic use in California:
methods and limitations," by Terry, J.G., and Teixeira,
T.C. JOURNAL OF NEW DRUGS. 2:206-210, 1962.
"Narcotic policy: the British example," by Schur, E.M. CON-
TEMPORARY ISSUES. pp. 18-21, June-July, 1963.
"Narcotic prevention and early treatment," by McGee, R.A.
CALIFORNIA YOUTH AUTHORITY QUARTERLY. 17(4):3-11, 1964.
"The narcotic problem," by Schwartz, G. WESTERN MEDICINE.
6:335-338, 1965.
"Narcotics addiction and the physician," by Miller, D.E.
JOURNAL OF THE AMERICAN OSTEOPATHIC ASSOCIATION. 66:

1232-1236, July, 1967.
"Narcotics and drug abuse: the federal response." SCIENCE. 162:1254, Dec. 13, 1968.
"Narcotics and medical practice - medical use of morphine and morphine-like drugs and management of persons dependent on them." JOURNAL OF THE AMERICAN MEDICAL ASSOCIATION. 202(3):209-212, 1967.
"Narcotics and their regulation - lawyer's view," by Acheson, D.C. ILLINOIS MEDICAL JOURNAL. 130:432-326, 1966.
"Narcotics control act decreases addiction." THE UNION SIGNAL. 87:116, Oct. 28, 1961.
"Narcotics control in Ghana - a case study," by Sagoe, T.E.C. BULLETIN ON NARCOTICS. 18(2):5-13, Apr.-June, 1966.
"Narcotics control in Switzerland," by Bertschinger, J.P., et al. BULLETIN ON NARCOTICS. 16:1-16, Apr.-June, 1964.
"Narcotics control in the Republic of Togo," by Johnson-Romuald, F. BULLETIN ON NARCOTICS. 21(1):41-45, Jan.-Mar., 1969.
"Narcotics control seen." SCIENCE NEWS LETTER. 81:198, Mar. 31, 1962.
"Narcotics control: WHO's share in the International System," by Halback, H. UNITED NATIONS REVIEW. 8:26-27, Sept., 1961.
"Narcotics - the semantics and control of addiction." MEDICAL TRIBUNE. pp. 2-3, Oct., 1965.
"New approaches to the narcotic problem. New approaches at the national level," by Javits, J.K. BULLETIN OF THE NEW YORK ACADEMY OF MEDICINE. 40:292-298, 1964.
--New approaches at the New York City level," by Rosenthal, T. BULLETIN OF THE NEW YORK ACADEMY OF MEDICINE. 40: 304-313, 1964.
--New approaches at the state level," by Hoch, P.H. BULLETIN OF THE NEW YORK ACADEMY OF MEDICINE. 40:299-303, 1964.
--Summary and discussion," by Wortis, S.B. BULLETIN OF THE NEW YORK ACADEMY OF MEDICINE. 40:314-318, 1964.
"New control on drugs?" BUSINESS WEEK. p. 44, Sept. 14, 1968.
"New trends in narcotic addiction control," by Hess, C.B. PUBLIC HEALTH REPORTS. 81:277-281, 1966.
"New trends in narcotic control," by Goodrich, L. INTERNATIONAL CONCILIATION. 530:214, 1960.
"New views on the narcotic problem." by Kirkpatrick, A.M. CANADIAN MEDICAL ASSOCIATION JOURNAL. 82:1317-1322, 1960,
"New York hospitals join addiction fight," by Vandow, E.S., and Knapp, S.E. MODERN HOSPITAL. 101:115-116, 1963.
"New York's narcotic addiction program," by Meislas, H. PSYCHIATRIC QUARTERLY. 37:203-209, 1963.
"XIXth session of the Commission on Narcotic Drugs, 37th session of the Economic and Social Council." BULLETIN ON NARCOTICS. 16:41-45, Oct.-Dec., 1964.
"Note - changes in the scope of control." BULLETIN ON NARCOTICS. 12(2):51, Apr.-June, 1960; 15(2):55, Apr.-June, 1963; 16:56, Apr.-June, 1964; 17(4):47, Oct.-Dec., 1965;

18(4):47-48, Oct.-Dec., 1966.

"The obligations of states under the Single Convention on Narcotic Drugs, 1961," by Reuter, P. BULLETIN ON NAR-COTICS. 20(4):3-7, Oct.-Dec., 1968.

"Official control of the administration of drugs. Historical notes on early attempts at regulation," by Stevenson, L.G. EXPERIMENTAL MEDICINE AND SURGERY. 22:147-154, June-Sept., 1964.

"Olfactronic detection of narcotics and other controlled drugs," by Kroloszynski, B.K., et al. POLICE. 13(3): 20-25, Jan.-Feb., 1969.

"One possible approach to the control of drug addiction in Delaware," by Vandervort, W.J. DELAWARE MEDICAL JOURNAL. 38:172, 1966.

"One way or the other it all goes up in smoke." LIFE. 67: 29, Oct. 31, 1969.

"Organization of an admistrative organ for the control of narcotic drugs," by Lobato, J.B. BULLETIN ON NARCOTICS. 18(2):1-4, Apr.-June, 1966.

"Our new narcotic law. JOURNAL OF THE MEDICAL SOCIETY OF NEW JERSEY. 65:78-79, Feb., 1968.

"Patterns of change. Federal Drug Agency responsible for both safety and effectiveness," by Goddard, J.L. RHODE ISLAND MEDICAL JOURNAL. 51:448-452, July, 1968.

"Permanent central narcotics board; final session at Geneva." UN MONTHLY CHRONICLE. 4:95-96, Dec., 1967.

"The physician's role in abating drug addiction," by Myers, I.L. JOURNAL OF THE MEDICAL ASSOCIATION OF ALABAMA. 36: 565 passim, Nov., 1966.

"The position of the Bureau of Narcotics," by Gaffney, G.H. ILLINOIS MEDICAL JOURNAL. 130:516-520, Oct., 1966.

"Preventing drug abuse: a graduate narcotics institute for teachers: Queens College," by Mackell, T.J. JOURNAL OF SCHOOL HEALTH. 39:113-115, Feb., 1969.

"Prevention and control of narcotic addiction." THE UNION SIGNAL. 87:6-7, Oct. 28, 1961.

"The prevention of drug abuse," by Giordana, H. HUMANIST. 28:20-23, 1968.

"Problems in prescribing and dispensing narcotics," by Herron, J.T. JOURNAL OF THE ARKANSAS MEDICAL SOCIETY. 56: 499-501, 1960.

"Professor Joachimoglu retires from international narcotics control organs." BULLETIN ON NARCOTICS. 20(2):43-44, 1968.

"Progress on Iran: the struggle against the evil of narcotics up to 1960," by Wright, A.W. BULLETIN ON NARCOTICS. 12 (3):1-4, July-Sept., 1960.

"Psychedelics and the law: a prelude in question marks," by Bates, R. PSYCHEDELIC REVIEW. no. 4, 1964.

"Psychotomimetic agents," by Scigliano, J.A. JOURNAL OF THE AMERICAN PHARMACEUTICAL ASSOCIATION. 8:28-29, Jan., 1968.

"Public health and drug safety," by Ingraham, H.S. VITAL SPEECHES. 32:231-234, Feb. 1, 1966.

"Punishment of a narcotic addict for crime of possession.

Eighth amendment implications. VALPARAISO LAW REVIEW. 2(2), 1968.
"Putting the brakes on speed; government to restrict the flow of illegal drugs." BUSINESS WEEK. p. 92 passim, Oct. 28, 1967.
"The rapid screening test for potential addiction liability of new analgesic agents," by Shemano, I., and Vendel, H. TOXICOLOGY AND APPLIED PHARMACOLOGY. 6:334-339, 1964.
"Recommended future international action against abuses of alcohol and other drugs," by Fort, J. BRITISH JOURNAL OF ADDICTION. 62:129-146, Mar., 1967.
"Reformation, not legislation," by Campbell, N.A. AMERICAN JOURNAL OF PHARMACY AND THE SCIENCES SUPPORTING PUBLIC HEALTH. 139:200-204, Sept.-Oct., 1967.
"Regional conferences on the illicit traffic in drugs," by United Nations Department of Social Affairs. BULLETIN ON NARCOTICS. 12(4):29-36, 1960.
"Regulations to curb illicit drug traffic," by Stetler, C.J. MEDICAL ANNALS OF THE DISTRICT OF COLUMBIA. 35:149, 1966.
"Resolution of the United Nations General Assembly." BULLETIN ON NARCOTICS. 21(3):1-2, July-Sept., 1969.
"A review of drug abuse and counter measures in Japan since World War II," by Nagahama, M. BULLETIN ON NARCOTICS. 20(3):19-24, July-Sept., 1968.
"Review of the twentieth session of the commission on narcotic drugs, and the fortieth session of the economic and social council." BULLETIN ON NARCOTICS. 18(1):63-67, 1966.
"Review of the twenty-second session of the commission on narcotic drugs and the forty-fourth session of the economic and social council." BULLETIN ON NARCOTICS. 20 (2):37-41, 1968.
"Review of the twenty-third session of the commission on narcotic drugs and the forty-sixth session of the economic and social council." BULLETIN ON NARCOTICS. 21 (3):23-31, July-Sept., 1969.
"Rockefeller and the drug plan," by Buckley, W.F., Jr. NATIONAL REVIEW. 18:257, Mar. 22, 1966.
"The road to controls: barbiturates, amphetamines, tranquilizers and hallucinogens. BULLETIN ON NARCOTICS. 19 (1):15-19, Jan.-Mar., 1967.
"STP under abuse control: that's a proposal of FDA." OIL, PAINT AND DRUG REPORT. 192:7 passim, Nov. 27, 1967.
"Safety of drugs." BRITISH MEDICAL JOURNAL. 3:758, Sept. 28, 1968.
"Seizures in the Federal Republic of Germany." BULLETIN ON NARCOTICS. 20(3):6, July-Sept., 1968.
"Services for the prevention and treatment of dependence on alcohol and other drugs. Fourteenth report of the WHO Expert Committee on Mental Health. WHO TECHNICAL REPORT SERIES. 363:1-45, 1967.
"Silver snuffbox; Dr. Leary and daughter Susan." TIME. 87:

85, Mar. 18, 1966.
"A simplified narcotic distribution system," by Austin, L.H.
AMERICAN JOURNAL OF HOSPITAL PHARMACY. 24:561-565, Oct.,
1967.
"Simplified systems for control of narcotics on nursing
floors," by Crider, H.F. HOSPITAL TOPICS. 43:87-91,
1965.
"Single convention on narcotic drugs, 1961," by Lande, A.
INTERNATIONAL ORGANIZATION. 16:776-797, 1962.
"Solvent sniffing. Physiologic effects and community con-
trol measures for intoxication from the intentional in-
halation of organic solvents. I.," by Press, E., and
Done, A.K. PEDIATRICS. 39(3):451-461, 1967.
--II. PEDIATRICS. 39(4):611-622, 1967.
"Some aspects of narcotics control in Mexico," by Barona, J.
BULLETIN ON NARCOTICS. 16:1-5, July-Sept., 1964.
"Some aspects of the production, turnover and control of
narcotic drugs in Poland," by Egierszdorff, I., and De-
long, T. BULLETIN ON NARCOTICS. 19(3):1-6, July-Sept.,
1967.
"Some chemical aspects of drug legislation," by Phillips,
G.F. JOURNAL OF THE FORENSIC SCIENCE SOCIETY. 7:17-30,
Jan., 1967.
"The South-East Asia Consultative Group on Narcotics Control,
Bangkok, Dec., 1960." BULLETIN ON NARCOTICS. 13(4):
37-38, Oct.-Dec., 1961.
"A Soviet law (USSR Ministry of Public Health, Order no.
530, 5 July 1967)." BULLETIN ON NARCOTICS. 20(2):52,
1968.
"The special contributions of a hospital halfway house," by
Wayne, G.J. MENTAL HOSPITALS. 14:440-442, 1963.
"Spies, J.G.; campus-spy game." NEWSWEEK. 69:112, Mar. 27,
1967.
"State-level liaison in narcotics control: a report." AR-
CHIVES OF GENERAL PSYCHIATRY (Chicago). 18:513-517,
May, 1968.
"The statutory presumption in federal narcotics prosecu-
tions," by Sandler, G. JOURNAL OF CRIMINAL LAW, CRIM-
INOLOGY AND POLICE SCIENCE. 57:7-16, 1966.
"Stimulant and depressant dependence: drug abuse control
amendments," by Dobbs, D.S., et al. MEDICAL ANNALS OF
THE DISTRICT OF COLUMBIA. 36:425-427, July, 1967.
"The story of narcotics control in India (opium)," by Kohli,
D.N. BULLETIN ON NARCOTICS. 18(3):3-12, July-Sept.,
1966.
"Strip packaging and simplified records bring new efficiency
in narcotics distribution," by Kenna, F.R. HOSPITALS.
39:107-113, 1965.
"The struggle for control of drug prescriptions," by Lear,
J. SATURDAY REVIEW. 45:35-39, Mar. 3, 1962.
"A study of illicit amphetamine drug traffic in Oklahoma
City," by Griffith, J. AMERICAN JOURNAL OF PSYCHIATRY.
123:560-569, 1966.
"Substances not under international control [note by the

editor⌋." BULLETIN ON NARCOTICS. 18(4):iv, Oct.-Dec.,
1966.
"The Supreme Court narcotics decision: implications for alcohol," by Deitrick, I.G. QUARTERLY JOURNAL OF STUDIES
ON ALCOHOL. 24:122-127, 1963.
"A survey of narcotic control in hospitals," by Gautreaux,
R., et al. AMERICAN JOURNAL OF HOSPITAL PHARMACY. 24:
566-573, Oct., 1967.
"Symposium on drug safety. The role of regulatory agencies
and industry in assessment of the safety of drugs for
use in man. The situation in the United Kingdom," by Ca-
hal, D.A. CANADIAN MEDICAL ASSOCIATION JOURNAL. 98:
271-275, Feb. 10, 1968.
"Temper rise over search for drugs." U.S. NEWS AND WORLD
REPORT. 67:16, Oct. 13, 1969.
"Testimony concerning the Bureau of Narcotics before House
of Representatives." THE UNION SIGNAL. 87:10-11, Oct.
28, 1961.
"Three years of nalline," by Brown, T. POLICE. 5:49-52,
Mar.-Apr., 1961.
"Time for decision on narcotics addiction," by Javits, J.K.
COMPREHENSIVE PSYCHIATRY. 4:137-139, June, 1963.
"To drug or not to drug: Britain." NATIONAL REVIEW. 20:
536, June 4, 1968.
"To seal a border." TIME. 94:p. 70, Sept. 26, 1969.
"Toughness to the task; Federal bureau of narcotics and the
bureau of drug abuse control combined." NEW REPUBLIC.
159:10-11, Nov. 2, 1968.
"Towards a solution of regional narcotics problems: recent
projects of UN technical assistance." BULLETIN ON NAR-
COTICS. 20(1):41-49, Jan.-Mar., 1968.
"Toxicity of new drugs," by Lowinger, P. SCIENCE. 161:
632, Aug. 16, 1968.
"Twenty-first session of the commission on narcotic drugs -
forty-second session of the economic and social council."
BULLETIN ON NARCOTICS. 19(2):59-61, Apr.-June, 1967.
"Twenty-four hour narcotic disposition recording system,"
by Zellers, D.D., et al. AMERICAN JOURNAL OF HOSPITAL
PHARMACY. 24:550-555, Oct., 1967.
"Twenty years of narcotics control under the United Nations.
Review of the work of the commission of narcotic drugs
from its 1st to its 20th session." BULLETIN ON NARCOTICS.
18(1):1-60, Jan.-Mar., 1966.
"Two new laws relating to psychedelics: 1. Federal law. 2.
New York State law," by Metzner, R. PSYCHEDELIC REVIEW.
no. 7:3-10, 1966.
"Uniform state regulation of narcotics - a national need."
JOURNAL OF THE AMERICAN MEDICAL ASSOCIATION. 194(5):
352-353, 1965.
"The United Nations and the illicit traffic in narcotic
drugs." BULLETIN ON NARCOTICS. 12(4):21-27, Oct.-Dec.,
1960.
"The United Nations and the opium problem," by Gregg, R.W.
INTERNATIONAL AND COMPARATIVE LAW QUARTERLY. 13:96-115,

Jan., 1964.
"United Nations consultative group on narcotic problems in Asia and the Far East." BULLETIN ON NARCOTICS. 17(2): 39-46, 1965.
"United Nations consultative group on opium problems, New Delhi, 1967." BULLETIN ON NARCOTICS. 20(4):15-19, Oct.-Dec., 1968.
"The United Nations narcotics laboratory." BULLETIN ON NARCOTICS. 19(3):7-15, July-Sept., 1967.
"United Nations plans soft drug misuse drive." THE ATTACK ON NARCOTIC ADDICTION AND DRUG ABUSE. 3:10, Spring, 1969.
"United States and Mexico discuss illicit traffic in narcotic drugs." DEPARTMENT OF STATE BULLETIN. 55:968, Dec.26, 1966.
"United States: re-organization of narcotics control." BULLETIN ON NARCOTICS. 20(3):30, July-Sept., 1968.
"The United States views on the single convention on narcotic drugs." BULLETIN ON NARCOTICS. 15(2):9-11, Apr.-June, 1963.
"Unusual aspects of narcotics control," by Durant, W.J. HOSPITALS. 36:82-88, 1962.
"Use and control of hazardous drugs," by Gimlin, J.S. EDITORIAL RESEARCH REPORT. 2:586-589, Aug. 9, 1967.
"Use and misuse of drugs." NURSING TIMES. 63:1612-1613, Dec. 1, 1967.
"Waging a war on drug abuse." BUSINESS WEEK. pp. 106-107, Jan. 20, 1968.
"War on addiction," by Campion, D.R. AMERICA. 112:356-359, Mar. 13, 1965.
"War on narcotics; illegal fields of marijuana and amapola in Mexico," by Bell, J.N. TODAY'S HEALTH. 45:48-62, July, 1967.
"We're winning the war against dope," by Anslinger, H.J. THE UNION SIGNAL. 87:8-9, Oct. 28, 1961.
"We stopped giving our narcotics away," by De Caprariis, H.V., and Minahan, J.R. AMERICAN JOURNAL OF HOSPITAL PHARMACY. 21:366-371, 1964.
"What to tell young people about alcohol and narcotics," by Northup, D.W. WEST VIRGINIA MEDICAL JOURNAL. 59: 374-377, 1963.
"Wheeling and dealing with tragedy," by Shepherd, J. LOOK. 32:56-59, Mar. 5, 1968.
"Where we stand on drug abuse," by Watts, M.S., et al. CALIFORNIA MEDICINE. 107:357-358, Oct., 1967.
"While you weren't looking; Senate ratifies a new international treaty." NEW REPUBLIC. 157:7, July 8, 1967.
"Whips or scorpions?" LANCET. 1:1241, June 8, 1968.
"The work of the Permanent Central Opium Board in 1959." BULLETIN ON NARCOTICS. 12(1):37-38, Jan.-Mar., 1960; 13(2):39-41, 1961; 15(1):45-49, Jan.-Mar., 1963; 16:45-50, Jan.-Mar., 1964; 17(1):45-50, Jan.-Mar., 1965; 18 (2):43-48, Apr.-June, 1966; 19(1):23-28, Jan.-Mar., 1967.
"Workshop on the detection and control of abuse of narcotics, barbiturates and amphetamines, San Juan, Puerto Rico,

Dec. 13-15, 1965," by Leonard, F. PSYCHOPHARMACOLOGY
BULLETIN; NATIONAL CLEARINGHOUSE FOR MENTAL HEALTH IN-
FORMATION. 3:21-26, Dec., 1966.

NARCOTICS LAWS AND LEGISLATION: Books and Essays

Blum, Richard H. "Legislators and drugs," SOCIETY AND DRUGS.
San Francisco: Jossey-Bass, 1969, pp. 293-320.
California. Department of Justice. Bureau of Criminal
Statistics. NARCOTIC ARRESTS AND THEIR DISPOSITIONS IN
CALIFORNIA, 1960. Sacramento, 1961 - [yearly].
Duster, Troy. THE LEGISLATION OF MORALITY; law, drugs, and
moral judgment. New York: Free Press, 1969.
Eldridge, W.B. NARCOTICS AND THE LAW: a critique of the
American experiment in narcotic drug control. Chicago:
American Bar Foundation, 1962.
Goodrich, Leland M. NEW TRENDS IN NARCOTICS CONTROL. New
York: Carnegie Endowment for International Peace, 1960.
India (Republic) Laws, statutes, etc. LAW AND PRACTICE RE-
LATING TO THE OPIUM ACT, 1878 along with the rules, cen-
tral and states, and allied laws and dangerous drugs act,
193, by J.P. Bhatnager. Allahabad: Central Law Agency,
1963.
Jeffee, Saul. NARCOTICS: an American plan. New York: Paul
S. Eriksson, 1966.
Kavaler, Franklin. OUTLINE OF PHARMACEUTICAL LAW: New York
City, New York State, Federal. New York, 1960.
Kennedy, Harold W. THE LOS ANGELES COUNTY NARCOTIC DRUG
LAW PROGRAMS. Los Angeles, 1960.
Lindesmith, Alfred R. THE ADDICT AND THE LAW. Bloomington:
Indiana University Press, 1965.
Louria, Donald B. DRUG SCENE. New York: McGraw-Hill, 1968.
National Council on Crime and Delinquency. NARCOTICS LAW
VIOLATIONS; a policy statement (of the) Advisory Council
of Judges. New York, 1964.
New Jersey. Legislature. Narcotic Drug Study Commission.
AN INTERIM REPORT: a study of the administration of nar-
cotic control relating to the causes, prevention and con-
trol of drug addiction, constituted pursuant to Senate
joint resolution No. 16, Laws of 1963. Trenton, 1964.
--PUBLIC HEARING. April 16, 1964. Trenton, 1964.
Smith, Kline and French Laboratories. DRUG ABUSE; a manual
for law enforcement officers. Philadelphia, 1965.
Sonnenreich, Michael R., et al. HANDBOOK OF FEDERAL NARCOTIC
AND DANGEROUS DRUG LAWS. Washington: Government Printing
Office, 1969.
Toulmin, A.A. A TREATISE ON THE LAW OF FOODS, DRUGS, AND
COSMETICS, 2nd edition. Cincinnati: Anderson Publishing,
1963.
Udell, Gilman G. OPIUM AND NARCOTIC LAWS (Feb. 9, 1909 -

Oct. 24, 1968). Washington: Government Printing Office, 1968.

United Nations. LAWS AND REGULATIONS PROMULGATED TO GIVE EFFECT TO THE PROVISIONS OF THE CONVENTION OF 13 July 1931 FOR LIMITING THE MANUFACTURE AND REGULATING THE DISTRIBUTION OF NARCOTIC DRUGS. New York, 1961.

--NARCOTIC DRUGS UNDER INTERNATIONAL CONTROL. New York, 1963.

--Commission on Narcotic Drugs. NATIONAL LAWS AND REGULATIONS RELATING TO THE CONTROL OF NARCOTIC DRUGS. New York, 1947/56+; CUMULATIVE INDEX, 1947-1964. New York, 1965 (UN Document E/NL. 1964).

--Conference for the Adoption of a Single Convention on Narcotic Drugs, 1961. OFFICIAL RECORDS. New York, 1964 (UN Document E/C^N 7/Ac3/1-2).

--SINGLE CONVENTION ON NARCOTIC DRUGS. New York, 1961(UN Document E/CONF34/22).

United States. Bureau of Narcotics. REGULATIONS NO. 1, RELATING TO THE IMPORTATION, MANUFACTURE, PRODUCTION COMPOUNDING, SALE, DEALING IN, DISPENSING, PRESCRIBING, ADMINISTERING, AND GIVING AWAY OF MARIHUANA, under the act of Aug. 2, 1937, Public no. 238, 75th Congress; joint marihuana regulations made by the Commissioner of Narcotics and the Commissioner of Internal Revenue with the approval of the Secretary of Treasury; effective date, July 2, 1964. Washington: Government Printing Office, 1964.

--President's Commission on Law Enforcement and Administration of Justice. TASK FORCE REPORT: NARCOTIC AND DRUG ABUSE. Washington: Government Printing Office, 1967.

NARCOTICS LAWS AND LEGISLATION: Periodical Literature

"The addict and the law," by Schur, E.M. DISSENT. 8:43-52, Winter, 1961.

"Addiction: beginning of wisdom," by Lindesmith, A.R. NATION. 196:49-52, Jan. 19, 1963.

"America's social frontiers: why not smoke pot?" by Etzioni, A. CURRENT. 95:38-41, May, 1968.

"Aspects of law enforcement in drug control," by Larkworth, F.R. AMERICAN ASSOCIATION OF INDUSTRIAL NURSES JOURNAL. 15:7-9, Aug., 1967.

"Barbiturate curbs to go into effect; producers and distributors of barbiturates, amphetamines and drugs must keep records." OIL, PAINT AND DRUG REPORT. 188: 7 passim, Dec. 27, 1965.

"Benevolent coercion: New York's dope nostrum; Nelson Rockefeller's program," by Prisendorf, A. NATION. 204:486-489, Apr. 17, 1967.

"Bill for control of drug addiction." NURSING TIMES. 63:497, 1967.

"A brief history of the narcotics control controversy," by Zusmann, J. MENTAL HYGIENE. 45:383-388, July, 1961.
"British narcotics policies," by Schur, E.M. JOURNAL OF CRIMINAL LAW, CRIMINOLOGY AND POLICE SCIENCE. 51:619-629, Mar.-Apr., 1961.
"The British narcotic system," by Larimore, G.W., and Brill, H. NEW YORK STATE JOURNAL OF MEDICINE. 60:107, 1960.
"British system," by Schur, E.M. NEW MEDICAL MATERIAL. pp. 16-17, Dec., 1962.
"British way with the junkie," by Samuels, G. NEW YORK TIMES MAGAZINE. p. 37+, Oct. 18, 1964.
"Can we punish for the acts of addiction?" by McMorris, S.C. AMERICAN BAR ASSOCIATION JOURNAL. 54:1081-1085, Nov., 1968.
"Canadian narcotics legislation, 1908-1923: a conflict model interpretation," by Cook, S.J. CANADIAN REVIEW OF SOCIOLOGY AND ANTHROPOLOGY. 6(1):36-46, Feb., 1969.
"Conference on narcotics studies liaison of medicine law." JOURNAL OF THE MEDICAL ASSOCIATION OF THE STATE OF ALABAMA. 36:1156-1157, Mar., 1967.
"Congress: a new option for addicts; a look at LSD," by Walsh, J. SCIENCE. 152:1728-1729, June 24, 1966.
"Controlling narcotic drug addiction in Canada: recent developments," by Macdonald, R. St. J. CURRENT LAW AND SOCIAL PROBLEMS. pp. 243-261, 1961.
"Controversial issues in the management of drug addiction: legalization, ambulatory treatment and the British system," by Ausubul, D.P. MENTAL HYGIENE. 44:535-544, Oct., 1960.
"Criminal law and the narcotics problem," by Canton, D.J. JOURNAL OF CRIMINAL LAW. 51(5):512-527, Jan.-Feb, 1961.
"Dangerous drugs act 1967. Restrictions on the prescribing of heroin or cocaine to addicts." NURSING TIMES. 64: 486, Apr. 12, 1968.
"Dangerous law?" COMMONWEAL. 86:76, Apr. 7, 1967.
"Dihydrocodeinone drugs; first narcotics casualties." OIL, PAINT AND DRUG REPORT. 179:5 passim, Jan. 12, 1961.
"Dilemma for drug addicts; current laws," by Murtagh, J.M. AMERICA. 108:740-742, May 25, 1963.
"Don't dodge the drug questions," by Hawkins, M.E. SCIENCE TEACHER. 33:32-35, Nov., 1966.
"Drug abuse in the eyes of the law," by Ledger, L. THE TEXAS OUTLOOK. 51:37-39, Nov., 1967.
"Drug abuse law; over-the-counter barbiturates given more time." OIL, PAINT AND DRUG REPORT. 189:4, Jan. 17, 1966.
"Drug addiction; a pharmacist's viewpoint," by Kesling, J.H. JOURNAL OF SCHOOL HEALTH. 39:174-179, Mar., 1969.
"Drug addiction and the law: N.Y. academy of medicine calls for a new approach." WALL STREET JOURNAL. 161:18, Apr. 24, 1963.
"Drug is a drink is a smoke," by Plumb, J.H. SATURDAY REVIEW. 50:25-26, May 27, 1967.
"Drug regulation and the public health," by Austern, T. NEW YORK UNIVERSITY LAW REVIEW. 39:771-784, Nov., 1964.

"Drug usage: a two-way attack." U.S. NEWS AND WORLD REPORT. 67:9, Nov. 3, 1969.
"Drug usage and the law: the adolescent and an archaic concept," by Barton, W. CLINICAL PROCEEDINGS OF THE CHILD-REN'S HOSPITAL, DC. 24:180-184, 1968.
"Drugs and regulations," by Russo, R.H. AMERICAN ASSOCIATION OF INDUSTRIAL NURSES JOURNAL. 16:12-14, Oct., 1968.
"Drugs and the law." NEW REPUBLIC. 159:11, Nov. 30, 1968.
"Drugs and the young law-breaker," by Gibbens, P.C. MENTAL HEALTH. 25(3):36-37, 1966.
"Drugs cases; philosophy of punishment." ECONOMIST. 224: 476-477, Aug. 5, 1967.
"Drugs on the market; steps to remove ineffective remedies from the market." NEWSWEEK. 71:56-57, Feb. 5, 1968.
"Drugs subject to federal narcotics lawa." WISCONSIN MEDICAL JOURNAL. 62:43-47, 1963.
"Effect of Mapp versus Ohio on police search-and-seizure practices in narcotics cases [Police practices in misdemeanor narcotics cases in New York City before and after the Supreme Court's decision in Mapp versus Ohio in 1961]. COLUMBIA JOURNAL OF LAW AND SOCIAL PROBLEMS. 4:87-104, Mar., 1968.
"Federal Food and Drug Administration. Revised New-drug regulation. Title 21--Food and Drugs." JOURNAL OF ORAL THERAPEUTICS AND PHARMACOLOGY. 4:148-164, Sept., 1967.
"Federal narcotics czar," by Meisler, S. NATION. 190:159-163, Feb. 20, 1960.
"First facts about drugs," by Kelsey, F.O. JOURNAL OF HEALTH, PHYSICAL EDUCATION AND RECREATION. 36:26-27, Feb., 1965.
"Food and Drug Administration tightens regulations on drugs." SCIENCE. 132:456, Aug. 19, 1960.
"For the long distance runner who got caught a twenty-year sentence," by Howard, J. LIFE. 67:30-31, Oct. 31, 1969.
"Freedom to be unfit," by Gould, D. NEW STATESMAN. 74: 254, Sept. 1, 1967.
"GH poll: should marijuana laws be changed?" GOOD HOUSE-KEEPING. 167: 10 passim, July, 1968.
"Goddard reluctantly supports strong law on hallucinogens." AMERICAN DRUGGIST. 157:18, Mar. 11, 1968.
"Hallucinogens: the drugs and their effects on the user; the present legal response to the new drug problem and suggested alternate means of control." COLUMBIA LAW RE-VIEW. 68:521-560, Mar., 1968.
"Hard pill for drug makers to down: FDA is extending insistence on proof of therapeutic equivalence as well as effectiveness of new versions of products it has already approved." BUSINESS WEEK. 2032:59-60, Aug. 10, 1968.
"The Harrison act and drug addiction: scientific treatment of this disease, not criminal prosecution, is the answer," by Gassman, B. BAR BULLETIN. 22(1):22-27, 1964.
"History of legal and medical roles in narcotic abuse in the U.S.," by Simrell, E.V. PUBLIC HEALTH REPORTS. 83: 587-593, July, 1968.
"History of the opium and narcotic drug legislation of Can-

ada," by Trasov, G.E. CRIMINAL LAW QUARTERLY. 4:274,
  1962.
"How hazardous are drugs from abroad " U.S. NEWS AND WORLD
  REPORT. 53:4, Dec. 17, 1962.
"How to deal with drugs." NEWSWEEK. 71:85-86, Mar. 11,
  1968.
"Imprisonment for the 'crime' of narcotics addiction held
  unconstitutional as cruel and unusual punishment." UNI-
  VERSITY OF PENNSYLVANIA LAW REVIEW. 111:122-136, Nov.,
  1962.
"International control of narcotic drugs." INTERNATIONAL
  ORGANIZATION. 14:200-201, Winter, 1960.
"Interpretations of Miranda rules governing interrogations
  and confessions," by Greenwald, R.L., and Vogelman, R.P.
  JOURNAL OF CRIMINAL LAW, CRIMINOLOGY AND POLICE SCIENCE.
  60:369-372, Sept., 1969.
"A judge looks at LSD," by Oliver, J.W. FEDERAL PROBATION.
  32(5):11, Mar., 1968.
"Keep off the grass?" NEW REPUBLIC. 156:5-6, June 17, 1967.
"LBJ and drug traffic; narcotics message." NEW REPUBLIC.
  158:11, Feb. 17, 1968.
"LSD crackdown," by Sanford, D. NEW REPUBLIC. 158:11-12,
  Mar. 16, 1968.
"LSD is seen needing no new control laws." OIL, PAINT AND
  DRUG REPORT. 189:4 passim, May 30, 1966.
"LSD, law and society," by Leary, T. THE REALIST. 69,
  Sept., 1966.
"LSD may become legal if it gets religion." SCIENCE NEWS.
  90:22, July 9, 1966.
"LSD tough laws: move is on in Congress." OIL, PAINT AND
  DRUG REPORT. 192:7 passim, Nov. 27, 1967.
"Law and LSD." TIME. 87:34, June 10, 1966.
"Law and the nurse," by Hershey, N. AMERICAN JOURNAL OF
  NURSING. 64:111-112, 1964.
"Law enforcement and drug abuse," by Cowden, J., and Horan,
  R. CLINICAL PROCEEDINGS OF THE CHILDREN'S HOSPITAL, DC.
  24:161-180, May, 1968.
"Law-medicine notes: law, medicine, and LSD," by Chayet, N.L.
  NEW ENGLAND JOURNAL OF MEDICINE. 277(5):253-254, 1967.
"The law of entrapment in narcotics arrest," by Gallick, L.J.
  NOTRE DAME LAWYER. 38(6):741-750, 1963.
"Law said too easy on deadly goofballs, pep pill pushers,"
  by Sims, P. NEW ORLEANS STATES AND ITEM. Oct., 1965.
"The legal aspect of narcotics control in N.Y. State," by
  Bellizzi, J.J. HEALTH NEWS. 37:4-9+, Aug., 1960.
"Legalization of marijuana," by Gimlin, J.S. EDITORIAL RE-
  SEARCH REPORT. 2(6), Aug. 9, 1967.
"Legislation to control addiction," by Reid, R.F. ADDIC-
  TIONS. 13(4):36-48, 1966.
"The legislator looks at addiction," by Moran, J.B. ILL-
  INOIS MEDICAL JOURNAL. 130:524-529, Oct., 1966.
"Legislators on social scientists and a social issue: a re-
  port and commentary on some discussions with lawmakers
  about drug abuse," by Blum, R.H., and Funkhouser, M.L.

JOURNAL OF APPLIED BEHAVIORAL SCIENCE. 1(1):84-112, 1965.

"Limitation and control of natural narcotics raw materials: schemes of the League of Nations and the United Nations," by Renborg, B.A. BULLETIN ON NARCOTICS. 15:13-26, Apr.-June, 1963.

"A lobby for people?" by Blum, R.H., and Funkhouser, M.L. AMERICAN PSYCHOLOGIST. 20(3):208-210, 1965.

"Madness to relax cannabis law." PHARMACEUTICAL JOURNAL. 199:122-123, 1967.

"Marihuana and the law." CANADIAN MEDICAL ASSOCIATION JOURNAL. 97:1359-1362, 1967.

"Marihuana and the new American hedonism," by Bleibtreu, J.N. PSYCHEDELIC REVIEW. no. 9:72-79, 1967.

"Marijuana before the bench." TIME. 90:77 passim, Sept. 29, 1967.

"Marijuana control: a perspective," by McGlothlin, W.H. JOURNAL OF SECONDARY EDUCATION. 43:223-227, May, 1968.

"Marijuana is still illegal: Massachusetts ruling," by Oteri, J. TIME. 90:38 passim, Dec. 29, 1967.

"Marijuana law," by Shane, J. NEW REPUBLIC. 158:9-10, Mar. 23, 1968.

"Marijuana madness," by Der Marderosian, A.H. JOURNAL OF SECONDARY EDUCATION. 43:200-205, May, 1968.

"Marijuana: the law vs. twelve million people." LIFE. 67:27-28, Oct. 31, 1969.

"Medicine and the law in the treatment of drug addiction," by Lowry, J.V., and Simrell, E.V. BULLETIN ON NARCOTICS. 15(3-4):9-16, July-Dec., 1963.

"The medico-legal conflict," by Ostrow, S. AMERICAN JOURNAL OF NURSING. 63:67-71, July, 1963.

"Medico-legal conflict in drug usage," by Bowen, O.R. JOURNAL OF SCHOOL HEALTH. 39:165-172, Mar., 1969.

"Menace of drug abuse," by Goddard, J.L. AMERICAN EDUCATION. 2:4-7, May, 1966.

"A model law for the application of the single convention on narcotic drugs, 1961," by Vaille, C. BULLETIN ON NARCOTICS. 21(2):1-12, Apr.-June, 1969.

"More drugs included under drug abuse law." SCIENCE NEWS. 89:235, Apr. 9, 1966.

"More taking pep pills: drugs bill (prevention of misuse)." TIMES (London) EDUCATIONAL SUPPLEMENT. 2555:1265, May 8, 1964.

"Narcotic and dangerous drug problems. Current status of legislation, control and rehabilitation," by Quinn, W.F. CALIFORNIA MEDICINE. 106(2):108-111, 1967.

"Narcotic and drug abuse: report of Advisory Commission prescribes for old problems new dangers," by Walsh, J. SCIENCE. 143:662-666, Feb. 14, 1964.

"Narcotic drug addiction: some legal aspects," by Debaggio, C. JOURNAL OF THE MISSISSIPPI STATE MEDICAL ASSOCIATION. 6:6-10, 1965.

"Narcotic drug labels must now be in metric units." OIL, PAINT AND DRUG REPORT. 180:7 passim, July 24, 1961.

"Narcotic law enforcement and false propaganda," by Giordano, H.L. POLICE. 10(4):22-25, 1966.
"Narcotics and crime; why our cities are taking a new look." SENIOR SCHOLASTIC. 81:16-19, Nov. 14, 1962.
"Narcotics and the law," by Sparks, W. COMMONWEAL. 74: 467-469, Aug. 25, 1961.
"Narcotics and the law: a critique of the American experiment in narcotic drug control by W.B. Eldridge. A review," by J. Fort. SATURDAY REVIEW. 45:30-31, Aug. 18, 1962.
"Narcotics and their regulation--a lawyer's view," by Acheson, D.C. ILLINOIS MEDICAL JOURNAL. 130:432-436, Oct., 1966.
"Narcotics dilemma: crime or disease?" by Kobler, J. SATURDAY EVENING POST. 235:64-66+, Sept. 8, 1962.
"Narcotics, drug abuse bureaus: Congress favoring Johnson plan to put them in Justice Dept." OIL, PAINT AND DRUG REPORT. 193:7 passim, Mar. 25, 1968.
"Narcotics legislation." JOURNAL OF THE AMERICAN MEDICAL ASSOCIATION. 194(1):25-26, 1965.
"Nature of the mind and the effect of drugs upon it," by Wilms, J.H. NATIONAL ASSOCIATION OF WOMEN DEANS AND COUNSELORS JOURNAL. 31:24-30, Fall, 1967.
"New control on drugs?" BUSINESS WEEK. p. 44, Sept. 14, 1968.
"New legislation in Spain: driving under the influence of narcotics." BULLETIN ON NARCOTICS. 21(1):40, Jan.-Mar., 1969.
"The new narcotics law in Iran," by Radji, A.H. BULLETIN ON NARCOTICS. 12(2):1-3, Apr.-June, 1960.
"New prohibition? intensified federal drugs crackdown." NEWSWEEK. 67:21-22, Feb. 7, 1966.
"New trends in narcotics control," by Goodrich, L.M. INTERNATIONAL CONCILIATION. 530:181-242, Nov., 1960.
"New York's narcotic addiction program." by Meiselas, H. PSYCHIATRIC QUARTERLY. 37(2):203-209, 1963.
"1969 drug legislation." THE ATTACK ON NARCOTIC ADDICTION AND DRUG ABUSE. 3:5, Summer, 1969.
"The Nixon drug law: a crucial fault." LIFE. 67:32, Sept. 5, 1969.
"Nixon's new plan to deal with the marijuana problem." U.S. NEWS AND WORLD REPORT. 67(17):14, Oct. 27, 1969.
"Now, tighter rules for some old remedies." U.S. NEWS AND WORLD REPORT. 64:12, Feb. 5, 1968.
"The obligations of states under the single convention on narcotic drugs, 1961," by Reuter, P. BULLETIN ON NARCOTICS. 20(4):3-7, 1968.
"Our new narcotic law." JOURNAL OF THE MEDICAL SOCIETY OF NEW JERSEY. 65:78-79, Feb., 1968.
"Penalties for LSD." TIME. 91:53, Mar. 8, 1968.
"The physician and state narcotic laws." ILLINOIS MEDICAL JOURNAL. 124:332-333, 1963.
"The physician and the drug abuse laws." JOURNAL OF THE AMERICAN MEDICAL ASSOCIATION. 205(11):788-789, 1968.

"Pills bill passes Senate, some ironing-out needed. (Controls over production and marketing of barbiturates, amphetamines, etc.)." OIL, PAINT AND DRUG REPORT. 187: 3 passim, June 28, 1965.

"Pot penalties too severe," by McBroom, P. SCIENCE NEWS. 90:270, Oct. 8, 1966.

"Pot's luck; Massachusetts ban." NEWSWEEK. 71:14, Jan. 1, 1968.

"Potty laws [in the U.S.]." ECONOMIST. 225:160, Oct. 14, 1967.

"Problems of competence in international law with regard to the punishment of narcotic drug offences and the extradition of narcotics offenders," by Henrichs, W. BULLETIN ON NARCOTICS. 12(1):1-7, Jan.-Mar., 1960.

"Psychedelics and the law: a prelude in question marks," by Bates, R.C. PSYCHEDELIC REVIEW. no. 1:379-393, 1964.

"Public Law 89-74 (H. R. 2). Drug Abuse Control Amendments of 1965 as applicable to hospitals and nursing homes," by Archambault, G.F. AMERICAN JOURNAL OF HOSPITAL NURSING. 22:674-675, Dec., 1965.

"Questions and answers; concerning laws," by Mead, M. REDBOOK. 120:28, Mar., 1963.

"Recommended future international action against abuses of alcohol and other drugs," by Fort, J. BRITISH JOURNAL OF ADDICTION. 62:129-146, 1967.

"Reflections on narcotic addiction," by Hoffman, M. YALE REVIEW. 54:17-30, Oct., 1964.

"The regulation of psychedelic drugs," by Barrigar, R.H. PSYCHEDELIC REVIEW. 1:394-441, 1964.

"Rehabilitative effectiveness of a community correctional residence for narcotic users," by Fisher, S. JOURNAL OF CRIMINAL LAW, CRIMINOLOGY AND POLICE SCIENCE. 56:190-196, June, 1965.

"Responsibility and addiction: the law in Canada," by Alexander, E.R. ADDICTIONS. 13(4):11-35, 1966.

"Should it be legalized? Soon we will know," by Goddard, J.L. LIFE. 67:34-35, Oct. 31, 1969; also READER'S DIGEST. 96(573):70, Jan., 1970.

"Single convention on narcotic drugs adopted." UNITED NATIONS REVIEW. 8:28-29, May, 1961.

"Some chemical aspects of drug legislation," by Phillips, G.F. JOURNAL OF THE FORENSIC SCIENCE SOCIETY. 7:17-30, Jan., 1967.

"A Soviet law." BULLETIN ON NARCOTICS. 20(2):52, Apr.-June, 1968.

"Speaking out; give drugs to addicts," by Straus, N. SATURDAY EVENING POST. 237:6+, Aug. 8, 1964.

"Stimulant and depressant dependence: drug abuse control amendments," by Dobbs, D.S., and Peele, R. MEDICAL ANNALS OF THE DISTRICT OF COLUMBIA. 36:425-427, July, 1967.

"Three years of nalline," by Brown, T. POLICE. 5:49-50+, Mar.-Apr., 1961.

"Time for decision on narcotics addiction," by Javits, J.K. COMPREHENSIVE PSYCHIATRY. 4(3):137-139, 1963.

"Treating addicts humanely." CHRISTIAN CENTURY. 83:131-132,
    Feb. 2, 1966.
"Two new laws relating to psychedelics." PSYCHEDELIC REVIEW.
    no. 7:3-10. 1966.
"Uniform state regulation of narcotics - a national need."
    JOURNAL OF THE AMERICAN MEDICAL ASSOCIATION. 194(5):
    552-553, 1965.
"Volstead exhumed? Dangerous drug penalty amendments of
    1968," by Shoben, E.J., Jr. NATION. 207:306-308, Sept.
    30, 1968.
"War on addiction," by Campion, D.R. AMERICA. 112:356-359,
    Mar. 13, 1965.
"What every chief should know about narcotics," by Skousen,
    W.C. LAW AND ORDER. 12(2):10-12, 1964.
"What price euphoria? The case against marijuana," by Mc-
    Morris, S.C. MEDICO-LEGAL JOURNAL. 34:74-79, 1966;
    also BRITISH JOURNAL OF ADDICTION. 62:203-208, Mar.,
    1967.
"What's wrong with pot?" NEWSWEEK. 70:30, Oct. 2, 1967.

NARCOTICS AND CRIME: Books and Essays

Anslinger, Harry J. THE PROTECTORS; the heroic story of the
    narcotic agents, citizens and officials and their unend-
    ing, unsung battles against organized crime in America
    and abroad. New York: Farrar Strauss, 1964.
  --and Oursler, W. THE MURDERERS; the story of the narcotic
    gangs. New York: Farrar, Strauss and Cudahy, 1961.
Blum, Richard H. "Drugs, behavior and crime," SOCIETY AND
    DRUGS. San Francisco: Jossey-Bass, 1969, pp. 277-291.
California. Department of Justice. Bureau of Criminal Sta-
    tistics. DRUG ARREST AND DISPOSITIONS IN CALIFORNIA.
    Sacramento, 1962.
Chein, Isador, et al. THE ROAD TO H; narcotics, delinquency
    and social policy. New York: Basic Books, 1964.
Cloward, Richard A., and Ohlin, L. DELINQUENCY AND OPPOR-
    TUNITY: a theory of delinquent gangs. New York: Free
    Press of Glencoe, 1960.
Eysenck, H.J. CRIME AND PERSONALITY. Boston: Houghton Mif-
    flin, 1964.
McGrath, John H. "A comparative study of adolescent drug
    users, assaulters, and auto thieves" (Thesis, unpublished,
    Rutgers State University). DISSERTATION ABSTRACTS. 28
    (10-A):4290, 1968.
Rubin, S. CRIME AND JUVENILE DELINQUENCY. 2nd edition.
    New York: Oceana, 1961.
Steiner, L.R. UNDERSTANDING JUVENILE DELINQUENCY. New Jer-
    sey: Chilton and Company, 1960.
Tunley, Paul. KIDS, CRIME AND CHAOS; a world report on juv-
    enile delinquency. New York: Harper, 1962.

United States. Congress. Senate. Committee on Government
Operations. ORGANIZED CRIME AND ILLICIT TRAFFIC IN NAR-
COTICS. Hearings before the Permanent Subcommittee on
Investigations of the Committee on Government Operations,
U.S. Senate, 88th Congress, 1st session, pursuant to Sen-
ate resolution 17, 88th Congress. Washington: Government
Printing Office, 1963-.
--Permanent Subcommittee on Investigations. ORGANIZED
CRIME AND ILLICIT TRAFFIC IN NARCOTICS; report, together
with additional combined views and individual views.
Washington: Government Printing Office, 1965.
--Committee on the Judiciary. JUVENILE DELINQUENCY: TREAT-
MENT AND REHABILITATION OF JUVENILE DRUG ADDICTS. Wash-
ington: Government Printing Office, 1968.
--JUVENILE DELINQUENCY: HEARINGS PURSUANT TO S. RES. 240,
pt. 19, March 4-6, 1968, LSD and marijuana among young
people. Washington: Government Printing Office, 1968.
--91st Congress. 1st session. DRUG ABUSE IN WASHINGTON
AREA. Springfield, Virginia. For sale by Clearinghouse,
1969.
Yolles, Stanley F. RECENT RESEARCH ON LSD, MARIJUANA, AND
OTHER DANGEROUS DRUGS. Statement before the Subcommittee
on Juvenile Delinquency of the Committee on the Judiciary, U.S. Senate, Mar. 6, 1968. Washington: Government
Printing Office, 1968.

NARCOTICS AND CRIME: Periodical Literature

"Addiction and criminal responsibility," by Caplan, L. MED-
ICO-LEGAL JOURNAL. 30:85-97, 1962.
"Addicts turn to property theft to support habit." THE AT-
TACK ON NARCOTIC ADDICTION AND DRUG ABUSE. 3(2):1-2,
Spring, 1969.
"Amphetamine and delinquency," by Scott, P.D. LANCET. 2:
534-535, 1964.
"Behavioral science and criminal law," by Sachas, E.J. SCI-
ENTIFIC AMERICAN. 209:39-45, 1963.
"Bennies + gasoline + death," by Drzazga, J. POLICE MAGA-
ZINE. 6:66-68, Mar.-Apr., 1962.
"Cannabis and violence." BULLETIN ON NARCOTICS. 20(2):44,
Apr.-June, 1968.
"Case of the hypnotic hippie." NEWSWEEK. 74(24):30-37,
Dec. 15, 1969.
"Cops in the world of junk: narcotic squad, New York City,"
by Lipsyte, R.M. NEW YORK TIMES MAGAZINE. p. 63, Oct.
14, 1962.
"A correctional dilemma: the narcotics addict," by Nahren-
dorf, R.O. SOCIOLOGY AND SOCIAL RESEARCH. 53:21-33,
Oct., 1968.
"Correctional problems the court can help," by Bennett, J.V.

CRIME AND DELINQUENCY. 7:1-8, Jan., 1961.
"Criminal justice notes: juvenile drug data; Arizona."
NCCD NEWS. 48(4):7, Sept.-Oct., 1969.
"Criminal justice notes: juveniles jailed for first mari-
juana offenses." NCCD NEWS. 48(4):11, Sept.-Oct., 1969.
"The criminal law and the narcotics problem," by Cantor,
D.J. JOURNAL OF CRIMINAL LAW, CRIMINOLOGY AND POLICE
SCIENCE. 51(5), Jan.-Feb., 1961.
"Criminological problems in the sixties," by Huffman, A.V.
AMERICAN JOURNAL OF CORRECTION. 28(1):4-6, 1966.
"Current aspects of delinquency and addiction," by Cooley,
A.E. ARCHIVES OF GENERAL PSYCHIATRY. June, 1961.
"The decriminalization of narcotics addiction," by McMorris,
S.C. AMERICAN CRIMINAL LAW QUARTERLY. 3(2):84-88, 1965.
"Delinquency and the amphetamines," by Scott, P.D., and Will-
cox, D.R.C. BRITISH JOURNAL OF PSYCHIATRY. 111(478):
865-876, 1965.
"Doctor's conviction for unlawful possession of narcotics
upheld." JOURNAL OF THE INDIANA STATE MEDICAL ASSOCIA-
TION. 56(12):1536, 1963.
"Drug addiction and crime," by Winick, C. CURRENT HISTORY.
52:349-353 passim, June, 1967.
"Drugs and delinquency," by Stewart, H., et al. MEDICO-
LEGAL JOURNAL. 33(2):56-71, 1965.
"Drugs and public opinion: New York State residents speak
out on drug abuse." THE ATTACK ON NARCOTIC ADDICTION
AND DRUG ABUSE. 3(4):3-5, Fall, 1969.
"Drugs and the young law-breaker," by Gibbens, T.C. MENTAL
HEALTH. 25(3):36-37, 1966.
"Drugs, behavior, and crime," by Blum, R.H. ANNALS OF THE
AMERICAN ACADEMY OF POLITICAL AND SOCIAL SCIENCE. 374:
135-146, Nov., 1967.
"Epidemiology of criminal narcotic addiction in Canada," by
Richman, A., and Humphrey, B. BULLETIN ON NARCOTICS.
20(1):31-39, Jan.-Mar., 1969.
"From hard to soft drugs: temporal and substantive changes
in drug usage among gangs in a working class community,"
by Klein, J., and Phillips, D.L. JOURNAL OF HEALTH AND
SOCIAL BEHAVIOR. 9:139-145, June, 1968.
"The great narcotics muddle," by DeMott, B. HARPER'S MAG-
AZINE. 224:46-54, Mar., 1962.
"Halfway houses for delinquent youth," by Carpenter, K.S.
CHILDREN. 10:224-229, 1963.
"Hong Kong's prison for drug addicts." BULLETIN ON NARCOT-
ICS. 13:13-20, Jan.-Mar., 1961.
"Marihuana and crime," by Munch, J.C. BULLETIN ON NARCOT-
ICS. 18(2):15-22, Apr.-June, 1966.
"Marijuana smoking and the onset of heroin use," by Ball,
J.C. BRITISH JOURNAL OF CRIMINOLOGY. 7(4):408-413,
1967; also BULLETIN ON NARCOTICS. 20(3):29, July-Sept.,
1968.
"Narcotic addiction and crime," by O'Donnall, J. SOCIAL
PROBLEMS. 13:374-385, Spring, 1966.
"The negro addict as an offender type," by Roebuck, J.B.

JOURNAL OF CRIMINAL LAW, CRIMINOLOGY AND POLICE SCIENCE. 53(1):36-43, 1962.
"The negro numbers man as a criminal type: the construction and application of a typology," by Roebuck, J.B. JOURNAL OF CRIMINAL LAW, CRIMINOLOGY AND POLICE SCIENCE. 54(1): 48-60, 1963.
"Prevention of narcotic offenses (part two)," by Talukdar, A.R. THE DETECTIVE. 8(10):27-29, 1964.
--Part four. THE DETECTIVE. 8(13):12-14, 1964.
--Part five. THE DETECTIVE. 8(14):6-7, 1964.
--Part six. THE DETECTIVE. 8(15):6-7, 1964.
--Part seven. THE DETECTIVE. 8(16):13-14, 1964.
--Part nine. THE DETECTIVE. 8(18):10-11, 1964.
"A psychopharmacologic experiment in a training school for delinquent boys: methods, problems, findings," by Eisenberg, L., et al. AMERICAN JOURNAL OF ORTHOPSYCHIATRY. 33(3):431-447, 1963.
"Psychosis, psychoneurosis, mental deficiency, and personality type in criminal drug addicts," by Messinger, E., and Zitrin, A. QUADERNI DI CRIMINOLOGIA CLINICA. 7(2): 137-154, 1965.
"The rehabilitative effectiveness of a community correctional residence for narcotic users," by Fisher, S. JOURNAL OF CRIMINAL LAW, CRIMINOLOGY AND POLICE SCIENCE. 56(2): 190-196, 1965
"The scent of danger," by Macmillan, W.L., Jr. POLICE CHIEF. 20(5):42-44, 1963.
"Statistical study of criminal drug addicts," by Messinger, E., and Zitrin, A. CRIME AND DELINQUENCY. 11(3):283-292, 1965.
"Stealing and addiction are linked problems." SCIENCE NEWS LETTER. 84:3, July 6, 1963.
"Teen-age drinking and drug addiction," by Pollack, J.H. NEA JOURNAL. 55:8-12, May, 1966.
"These fighters against youth crime need your help," by Hoover, J.E. READER'S DIGEST. 78:145-152, Apr., 1961.
"Thieves, convicts and the inmate culture," by Cressey, D., and Irwin, J. SOCIAL PROBLEMS. 10:45, 1962.
"Two patterns of narcotic addiction in the United States," by Ball, J.C. JOURNAL OF CRIMINAL LAW, CRIMINOLOGY AND POLICE SCIENCE. 56(2):203-211, 1965.
"What psychiatry can do for criminology," by Frym, M. BULLETIN OF THE MENNINGER CLINIC. 25(4), July, 1961.
"The world of the righteous dope fiend," by Sutter, A.G. ISSUES IN CRIMINOLOGY. 2:177-222, Fall, 1966.

NARCOTICS BIBLIOGRAPHY

"Abstract of articles and papers on narcotic habit." THE ANNOTATED BIBLIOGRAPHY. 2(6):1-11, 1964

"Bibliography on drugs," by Israelstam, D. CALIFORNIA LAW
    REVIEW. Jan., 1968.
"Bibliography: scientific publication on narcotic drugs in
    1959." BULLETIN ON NARCOTICS. 12(3):35-53, July-Sept.,
    1960.
THE DRUG SCENE: printed materials on drugs and addiction,
    rev. Marjorie Christman. Northbrook, Illinois: Public
    Library, 1969.
Hollander, C. "Selected bibliography," BACKGROUND PAPERS
    ON STUDENT DRUG INVOLVEMENT, ed C. Hollander. Washington:
    United States National Student Association, 1967, pp.
    159-162.
Kalant, Oriana Josseau. AN INTERIM GUIDE TO THE CANNABIS
    (MARIJUANA) LITERATURE. Toronto: Addiction Research
    Foundation, 1968.
"A marijuana bibliography," by Bruin Humanist Forum (Issues
    Study Committee). NEW WEST. 2:16, 1967.
Moore, Laurence A., Jr. MARIJUANA (CANNABIS) BIBLIOGRAPHY,
    1960-1968. Los Angeles: Bruin Humanist Forum, 1969.
New York (State). Narcotic Addiction Control Commission.
    ANNOTATED BIBLIOGRAPHY OF LITERATURE ON NARCOTIC ADDIC-
    TION. Compiled by the Narcotic Addiction Control Com-
    mission in cooperation with the United States Department
    of Justice, Federal Bureau of Prisons. Albany, 1968.
Pearlman, Samuel, editor. DRUGS ON CAMPUS: an annotated
    guide to the literature. Brooklyn College, 1968.
--"A selected bibliography on drug usage in colleges and
    universities." COLLEGE STUDENT SURVEY: AN INTERDISCI-
    PLINARY JOURNAL OF ATTITUDE RESEARCH. 2:5-7, Spring,
    1968.
"Selected bibliography on narcotic addiction treatment,
    1960-1966. Reports of treatment programs," by Dole, V.P.,
    et al. AMERICAN JOURNAL OF PUBLIC HEALTH. 57:2005-2008,
    Nov., 1967.
Sells, Helen F. A BIBLIOGRAPHY ON DRUG DEPENDENCE. Fort
    Worth, Texas: Texas Christian University Press, 1967.
United States. National Clearinghouse for Mental Health
    Information. BIBLIOGRAPHY ON DRUG DEPENDENCE AND ABUSE,
    1928-1966. Chevy Chase, Maryland, 1969.
--National Library of Medicine. DRUG LITERATURE; a fact-
    ual survey on 'the nature and magnitude of drug litera-
    ture'. Report prepared for the study of 'Interagency
    coordination in drug research and regu0ation', by the
    Subcommittee on Reorganization and International Organi-
    zations of the Senate Committee on Government Operations.
    Washington: Government Printing Office, 1963.
--NARCOTICS ADDICTION; a selected list of references in
    English. Washington: Reference Division, National Library
    of Medicine, 1960.
Washington (State) State Library. DRUG ABUSE. Olympia, 1968.

AUTHOR INDEX

Aaron, H., 103
Aaronson, B.S., 52
Abeles, H., 55, 140, 146
Abelson, P.H., 51, 52, 89
Abély, P., 7
Abenson, M.H., 11
Aberfeld, D.C., 157
Aberle, D.F., 76
Abrams, S., 40, 77, 93
Abramson, H.A., 53, 69, 70
Abramson, M., 135, 137
Abreu, L., 81
Abse, D.W., 233
Abt, L.E., 192
Accardo, N., 164
Acheson, D.C., 209, 269, 281
Achte, K.A., 133
Adams, B.G., 27
Adams, H.J., 35
Adams, P., 255
Adams, R., 77
Adams, S., 103
Adams, W.T., 6
Adawi, A., 30
Adey, W.R., 67, 72
Adler, T.K., 221
Adriana, J., 157, 220, 221, 251
Adshead, S.A.M., 192
Africa, T.W., 144
Ager, J.H., 252, 255
Aghajanian, G.K., 62, 71
Agnew, D., 257
Agnew, N.M., 9
Ahmed, S.N., 114
Aitken, D., 77
Akera, T., 214
Akers, R.L., 144
Alamel, P., 188
Alaxandris, A., 15
Alden, J.D., 144
Aldrich, M., 77, 89, 91, 192
Alexander, E.J., 51
Alexander, E.R., 282
Alexander, G., 69
Alexander, L., 156
Alexander, M., 15, 40
Alexander, S., 85
Alha, A., 38

Alksne, H., 178
Allen, E.J., 189
Allen, J.R., 49, 87, 133
Allen, S.M., 6, 9
Allison, G.E., 120
Allsop, K., 148
Alpert, R., 40, 58, 72, 81
Amaral Vieira, F.J., 98
Amarel, M., 58, 74
Amias, A.G., 233
Anand, R.D., 235
Anant, S.S., 151, 186
Anderson, C., 185
Anderson, E.C., 256
Anderson, H., 121
Anderson, J., 120
Anderson, R.C., 239
Anderson, S.M., 38
Andrade, O.M., 85
Andrec, A., 97
Andrews, G., 40, 61, 77
Andry, A.C., 104
Angers, P., 133
Ankermann, H., 242
Anslinger, H.J., 77, 104, 257, 266, 274, 283
Antell, M.J., 141, 180
Aoki, Y., 165
Appel, J.B., 23, 54, 57, 62, 7
Apter, J.T., 74
Archambault, G.F., 282
Archer, S., 208, 240
Arena, J.M., 248
Arieff, A.J., 153
Armitage, G.H., 25
Armstrong, A., 67
Armstrong, G., 191, 264
Armstrong, J.C., 186
Armstrong, J.D., 148
Arndt, R.R., 234
Arneson, G.A., 56
Arthur, R.J., 8, 181
Asatoor, A.M., 233
Ashcroft, G.W., 9
Asher, H., 59
Askew, B.M., 19
Astin, A.W., 120, 137, 155
Aston, R., 34, 235
Asuni, T., 94

288

Atal, C., 99
Atkinson, B.L., 2
Audier, H., 238
Auerbach, R., 69
Augenstein, L., 52
Austern, T., 264, 277
Austin, C.G., 90
Austin, L.H., 272
Ausubel, D.P., 104, 121, 123, 149, 153, 277
Avico, U., 203
Axelrod, J., 243, 255
Ayd, F.J., 223
Azelrod, J., 232
Baarschers, W.H., 234
Bach, G.R., 179
Bacharuch, A.L., 108
Bachrich, P.R., 209
Baekeland, F., 20, 36
Baerheim-Svendsen, A., 247
Baganz, P.C., 133, 176
Bagdon, W.J., 233
Bain, G., 240
Bair, J.R., 238
Baker, A.A., 121
Baker, E.F.W., 76
Baker, R.S., 145
Bakewell, W.E., 143, 166, 264
Balagot, R.C., 241
Balduzzi, E., 167
Baldrey, E.C., 38
Baldrighi, G., 32
Baldwin, B.A., 32
Ball, J., 84, 118, 121, 122, 139, 140, 147, 152, 171, 285, 286
Ballante, A., 91
Ballard, B.E., 244
Balster, R.L., 13
Ban, T.A., 193
Banerjee, R., 8, 231
Banic, B., 231
Baptisti, A., 232
Barber, B., 193
Barber, C.G., 92
Barber, G.O., 205
Barbero, A., 86
Barish, H., 104
Barker, G.H., 6
Barman, M.L., 10
Barnard, G.W., 165
Barnard, M., 49, 87
Barnes, C.D., 19
Barnes, H.E., 145

Barona, J., 272
Barowsky, J., 239
Barr, H.L., 70
Barr, M., 126, 175
Barrett-Connor, E., 69
Barrigar, R., 57, 282
Barron, F., 40, 49
Barry, H., 12, 31, 32, 222
Bartels-Keith, J.R., 254
Barth, A., 262
Bartholomew, A.A., 134, 146, 152
Bartlett, S., 6
Barton, D.H.R., 237
Barton, W., 131, 265, 278
Basham, A., 77
Bass, P., 230
Bastron, R., 231
Bate, L.C., 217
Bateman, K., 60, 63
Bates, R., 57, 270, 282
Bates, W.M., 143, 182, 186, 209
Battegay, R., 152, 157, 187
Batterman, R.C., 220
Battersby, A.R., 242
Battista, O., 77, 193
Baudelaire, C.P., 45, 77
Bay, R., 127
Baytop, T., 77
Beale, M.A., 193
Beall, L.L., 143, 209
Beamish, P., 8
Beavan, K.A., 85
Beaver, W.T., 35, 174, 222
Beazley, J.M., 248
Bechard, A.J., 121
Becker, A.H., 61
Becker, D.I., 74
Becker, H.G., 173
Becker, H.K., 203
Becker, H.S., 50, 77, 104, 124, 131, 136
Beckett, A.H., 6, 12, 22, 23, 29
Beckett, H.D., 150
Beckman, H., 1
Beecher, H.K., 13, 19, 148, 253
Beechey, N.R., 230
Behrendt, H., 125
Bejarano, J., 145
Belden, E., 69
Beliaev, N.V., 98

Harris, M., 93, 245
Harris, R., 13, 74, 189
Harris, W.D., 165
Harrold, T., 243
Harry, J., 214
Hart, R., 8
Harthoorn, A.M., 221
Hartley, E., 28
Hartley, W., 28
Hartman, M.A., 70
Hartman, M.M., 256
Hartmann, E., 32, 65
Harui, T., 30
Hausman, R., 142
Hausner, M., 71, 72
Havens, J., 54
Havlena, J., 36
Hawkins, M.E., 6, 26, 47, 277
Hat, R.K., 238
Hayter, A., 195
Heard, G., 46
Hearst, E., 18
Heaton, J., 80
Heaysman, L., 61
Hebbard, F.W., 66
Heimstra, N.W., 16, 17, 21, 22, 71
Hekimiam, L.J., 155
Helpern, M., 124, 195, 204
Hemmi, T., 141
Henderson, A., 96
Henley, W.L., 162
Henrichs, W., 282
Henshaw, J.R., 210
Hensala, J.D., 52, 69
Hensiak, J.F., 240
Hentoff, N., 107, 130
Herich, R., 99
Herisset, A., 103
Herman, M., 143
Hermon, H., 57
Herron, J.T., 270
Herrick, A.D., 196
Hershey, N., 279
Heslop-Harrison, J., 97, 102
Hess, A.G., 107
Hess, C.B., 269
Hess, J.W., 29
Hewetson, J., 187
Hayman, J.J., 162
Hibbeln, P., 34, 235
Hicks, J.T., 84
Hidalgo, J., 217
Higgins, L., 208

Hill, G.B., 39
Hill, H., 117, 149, 155, 160, 163, 179
Hill, P.J., 108, 196
Hill, R.M., 160
Hill, W.T., 88
Hillman, H.H., 238
Himwich, H.E., 16, 38
Hirsch, R., 177
Hobson, J.A., 66
Hoch, P.H., 122, 263, 269
Hochbaum, G.M., 136
Hockman, W.S., 177
Hodos, W., 12, 30
Hoff, H.R., 216
Hoffer, A., 1, 41, 64
Hoffman, F., 157, 196
Hoffman, M., 128, 147, 282
Hoffman, R., 57
Hofling, C., 107
Hofman, A., 61, 62
Hofmann, H., 235
Holden, H.M., 147, 149
Holfeld, H., 73
Hollander, C., 80, 108, 196, 287
Holliday, A.R., 67
Hollifield, H.C., 244
Hollister, L.E., 37, 48, 63, 67, 76, 167, 203, 231, 251
Hollister, W.G., 131
Holmberg, M.B., 159
Holmes, S.J., 141, 180, 268
Holmstedt, B., 196
Holt, R.R., 73
Holzinger, R., 61, 185
Honigfeld, G., 65, 75, 227, 242
Hoover, J.E., 286
Honn, F.R., 153
Hopkins, J., 42
Hopkins, S.I., 196
Horan, R., 268, 279
Hordern, A., 196
Hornick, N., 48
Horovitz, Z., 22
Horowitz, M., 150, 160
Hoskin, H.F., 173
Houde, R.W., 248
Houston, J., 43, 57, 82
Houston, K., 73
Howard, A.H., 237
Howard, J., 87, 278
Howe, H.S., 108

Kamano, D.K., 16, 29
Kamm, G., 38
Kane, A.A., 243
Kane, F.J., 160, 238
Kane, J.J., 60, 68, 108, 152
Kaplan, K., 156
Kapoor, L.D., 250
Karamustafaoglu, V., 36
Kareva, G.F., 227
Karlsberg, P., 229
Karnow, S., 192
Kasanen, A., 164
Kase, Y., 245
Kast, E., 52, 61, 62, 69, 75,
    238, 254, 255
Kato, R., 35
Kato, T., 69
Katsiafics, M.D., 61
Katz, M.M., 62
Katz, S., 50
Kaufman, J., 93
Kavaler, F., 275
Keane, C.B., 196
Keats, A.S., 38, 252
Keele, C.A., 210
Keeler, M., 8, 15, 57, 60, 63,
    69, 84, 87, 90, 92, 94, 98
Keeler, O., 172
Kelman, H., 117, 162, 181, 241
Kelsey, F.O., 206, 278
Keniston, K., 81, 108, 206
Kenna, F.R., 272
Kennedy, H.W., 275
Kennedy, J.D., 129
Kennedy, R.F., 120
Kent, L.R., 39
Kerr, W.S., 255
Kesling, J.H., 128, 277
Keup, W., 214
Key, B.J., 66, 67
Khalefa, A.M., 211
Khan, N.H., 245
Khandelwal, I.C., 189
Khazan, N., 14, 31, 65
Kieffer, S.N., 181
Kielholz, P., 152, 187
Kiernan, C.C., 20
Kihm, J.J., 112
Killam, K.F., 235
Kiloh, L.G., 7, 8
King, F.W., 54, 89
King, W., 213
Kingston, C., 101, 212
Kinnard, W.J., 254

Kinne, S., 46
Kiplinger, G.F., 244, 245
Kirk, P., 101, 255
Kirkham, J.E., 18, 33
Kirkpatrick, A.M., 269
Kirkpatrick, D., 256
Kirpekar, S.M., 227
Kissin, B., 92, 225
Kistner, J.M., 2
Kitzinger, A., 108, 196
Klare, H.S., 112
Klaveter, R.E., 71
Kleber, H.D., 56, 59, 72, 164
Kleckner, J.H., 56
Klee, G.D., 70
Klein, J., 87, 285
Klein, M., 133
Kleinman, K.M., 32
Klinger, W., 27
Klingman, G.I., 254
Klonsky, G., 169
Kluever, H., 42, 81
Knapp, S.E., 269
Kneebone, G.M., 9
Knight, D.A., 21, 247
Knotts, G.R., 203
Knox, J.W., 243
Knox, S.C., 155
Kobayasshi, T., 31, 225
Kobler, J., 47, 120, 143, 209,
    281
Koch, B., 165
Kochi, H., 96
Koella, W.P., 42
Koestner, A., 239
Koff, R.S., 167
Kohlan, R.G., 59
Kohli, D.N., 272
Kohn, B., 66
Kokka, N., 251
Kokoski, R.J., 245
Kolb, L., 108, 127
Kolodny, A.L., 235
Konietzko, K.C., 182
Konsky, G., 177
Kook, C.C., 243
Kopell, B.S., 16
Koppanyi, T., 249
Kornetsky, C., 240, 245
Korngold, M., 52
Korte, F., 81, 92, 101, 103
Koslin, A.J., 225
Kosman, M., 16
Koutsky, C.D., 116

301

Lee, H.A., 39
Lee, W.J., 232
Lee Peng, C.H., 230
Leech, K., 81, 197
Leeds, D.P., 109, 115
Leffler, L., 52
Lefkowitz, B., 211
Lehman, D.J., 127
Lehmann, H.E., 21, 163, 247
Lehmann, J., 36
Leibowitz, M., 115
Leighton, F.S., 151
Lemere, F., 6
Lendon, N., 86, 132
Lennard, H.L., 211
Leonard, B.E., 31
Leonard, F., 23, 39
Lerner, A.M., 155, 219
Lerner, M., 51, 53, 61, 81,
    92, 97, 100, 240, 251
Lerner, P., 101
Lesser, E., 172
Lettvin, J., 61, 154
Leuner, H., 73
Levi, M., 197
Levine, E.E., 115
Levine, J., 52, 56, 61, 63, 64,
    68, 125, 141, 175, 248, 256
Levitt, L.I., 150, 184, 185
Levy, A., 182
Levy, N.J., 152
Levy, S., 19
Lewin, L., 81, 197
Lewis, B., 81
Lewis, D.C., 162, 206, 240, 241
Lewis, J.J., 231
Liberman, R., 172
Lieberman, D., 159
Lieberman, L., 123, 183
Liebert, R., 86, 97, 158, 204
Lienert, G.A., 54, 70
Lin, R.K.S., 243
Lin, S.C., 256
Lindesmith, A.R., 81, 109,
    116, 149, 276
Lindgren, C., 264
Lindmann, E., 86
Ling, T.M., 43, 76
Lingeman, R.R., 55, 197
Lingh, S.D., 32
Lingl, F.A., 160, 237
Linton, H.B., 59, 68, 72, 73
Lionel, P. 60
Lipinski, E., 55

Lippincott, W.T., 45, 116
Lipsyte, R.M., 123, 284
Lipton, L., 81
Lipton, M.A., 254
Lister, R.E., 38, 213
Little, J.C., 30
Little, R.B., 152, 160, 179,
    187
Litwin, E.M., 176
Litwin, G., 48, 56
Livingston, R.B., 109, 142
Lobato, J.B., 270
Lobb, H., 10
Loiselle, R., 22
Lombardi, D.N., 133, 157
Long, J.P., 245
Long, R.H., 26
Loranger, A.W., 223
Lorr, M., 35
Lotti, V.J., 214, 216
Loughman, W.D., 70
Louria, D.B., 46, 47, 53, 81,
    85, 86, 109, 160, 197, 203,
    208, 258, 264, 275
Louroc, N.C., 214
Lovingood, B.W., 3, 16
Lowinger, P., 273
Lowry, J.T., 163
Lowry, J.V., 139, 179, 280
Luby, E., 67
Luce, C.B., 119
Luce, J., 132
Lucena, J., 81
Luckin, W., 138
Ludlow, F., 82
Ludlow, P. 88
Ludvigson, H.W., 11
Ludwig, A., 52, 56, 61, 63, 64,
    68, 75, 159, 177
Lundberg, G.D., 23
Lundell, F.W., 15
Lundquist, G., 249
Lundy, J.S., 117
Luther, B.R., 3, 202
Lutz, W.B., 250
Lyerly, S.B., 14
Lyle, D., 139, 268
Mabileau, J.F., 206, 266
McBay, A.J., 25
McBroom, P., 28, 52, 54, 93,
    116, 282
McCann, H.W., 140
McCarrick, H., 128, 175
McClane, T.K., 230

Plass, H.F., 37, 248
Pletscher, A., 46
Plotnikoff, N., 18, 21
Plumb, J.H., 277
Poe, R.H., 10
Pollack, J.H., 151, 286
Pollard, J.C., 43, 58, 151
Polsky, N., 82, 153, 198
Pond, T.A., 150
Popham, R.E., 198
Portoghese, P.S., 241
Poschel, B.P.H., 17
Poser, M., 198
Post, B., 23
Potter, H.P., 160
Potter, L.T., 253
Potthoff, C.J., 26
Poulton, E.C., 235
Powars, D., 11
Powelson, H., 48
Poze, R.S., 163
Preble, E., 149
Prescott, L.F., 216
Presnell, M., 46
Press, E., 250, 272
Price, A.C., 119
Prichard, E.N., 26
Priest, R.G., 26
Prince, A.M., 51
Prisendorf, A., 120, 143, 276
Prout, C.T., 9
Pruden, E., 138
Publey, H.C., 127
Puro, H.E., 159, 233
Purtell, D.J., 206
Purtell, T.C., 111
Putnam, P.L., 141
Quarton, G.C., 20
Quastel, J.H., 230
Quinn, J.T., 255
Quinn, W., 54, 91, 141, 142, 147, 180, 280
Radecka, C., 65
Radin, S.S., 146
Radji, A.H., 281
Rado, S., 111, 159, 177, 233
Radosevic, A., 95
Raevskaia, V.V., 39
Rajeswaran, P., 255
Ram, H., 100
Ramanathan, V.S., 209, 211, 253
Ramirez, E., 135, 158, 178
Rand, M.E., 150
Randrup, A., 22

Rao, D.A., 235
Rapp, M.S., 152, 213
Rappaport, M., 12, 30
Raskin, H.A., 116, 171, 184
Rasor, R.W., 137, 178
Ratcliffe, S.G., 239
Rathbone, J.L., 198
Rathod, N.H., 148, 164
Rausch, J., 242
Ray, M.B., 175
Ray, O.S., 20, 56, 163, 228, 243
Raybin, H.W., 25
Raymond, M.J., 186
Raz, M.B., 123
Read, D., 198
Reagan, J.J., 268
Rechtschaffen, A., 14
Rector, M.G., 86
Redlich, F.C., 111
Redmond, N., 238
Reed, F.S., 5
Rees, W.L., 127
Regal, L.H., 163
Regardie, I., 83
Reice, S., 84
Reich, G., 54
Reichert, H., 35
Reichle, C.W., 221
Reid, R.F., 279
Reifler, C.B., 59, 98
Reinke, D., 18
Reivich, M., 73
Relin, L., 111
Remington, F.B., 39
Remmer, H., 25, 30
Renborg, B., 208, 266, 268, 280
Resnick, O., 61, 69
Retterstol, N., 111, 157
Retting, S., 166
Reuben, D., 89
Reuter, P., 270, 281
Reves, S., 173
Revzin, A.M., 67
Reynolds, H.H., 73
Riccio, V., 140
Rice, J., 142, 162, 180
Rich, L., 51
Rich, R.H., 10, 11
Richards, C.F., 263
Richards, L.G., 126
Richards, W.A., 51
Richman, A., 159, 285

308

Richman, S., 116, 171
Rickels, K., 156, 188, 256
Rigby, W., 97
Riding, J.E., 220
Rinkel, M., 57
Riva, H.L., 232
Rizy, E.F., 17, 32
Robbins, E., 68
Roberts, A.H., 73
Roberts, H.J., 4
Roberts, M., 55, 75, 166
Robertson, J.P.S., 111
Robin, A.A., 206
Robins, L., 131, 204
Robinson, D.W., 210
Robinson, J.L., 7
Robinson, J.T., 121
Robinson, L., 130
Rockwell, D.A., 4, 5
Roddick, J.W., 223
Rodin, E., 67
Rodman, M.J., 198
Rodriguez, A.A., 211, 245
Roe, B.B., 218
Roebuck, J.B., 143, 285, 286
Rogers, L.A., 231
Rogers, P.G., 126
Rogg, S.G., 60
Rohde, I.M., 116, 129, 176
Rohr, J.H., 241
Rollins, R.L., 187
Rolo, A., 69, 72, 176, 226
Romansky, M.J., 251
Romauld, F., 269
Ronney, E.A., 149
Roper, P., 176
Roper, W.L., 202
Rose, A., 162
Rose, P., 83
Roseman, B., 44
Rosen, A.J., 32
Rosenberg, C.M., 53, 154
Rosenberg, D.E., 35, 38, 71
Rosenfeld, A., 6, 59, 91, 132, 206
Rosenfeld, H., 144
Rosenstein, B.J., 167, 256
Rosenthal, S.H., 71
Rosenthal, T., 122, 164, 269
Rosevear, J., 83
Ross, G.S., 33
Ross, I., 136
Ross, J., 182
Ross, S., 14, 18, 226

Rossi, A., 20
Rossi, G., 140, 183, 208
Rossides, E.T., 192
Roszak, T., 123
Roth, W.T., 15
Rothmann, K., 214
Rothstein, E., 239
Rothwell, N.D., 178
Roubicek, 61
Rowe, D.H., 233
Rowland, M., 23
Roy, A.T., 190
Royfe, E.H., 159
Rubin, A., 236
Rubin, D.R., 47
Rubin, M.M., 141, 180
Rubin, R.T., 24
Rubin, S., 283
Rubington, E., 128, 152
Rubinstein, L., 23, 38, 254
Rumelhart, D.E., 18
Runk, B., 88
Rushton, R., 13, 15
Russo, J.R., 2
Russo, R.H., 265, 278
Rutschmann, J., 23, 38, 254
Sabath, G., 149, 152, 184, 187
Sachas, E.J., 284
Sadove, M.S., 241, 244, 253, 256
Sadusk, F.J., 144
Sadusk, J.F., Jr., 8
Sadusk, J.R., 150
Sagehorn, R., 56
Sagoe, T.E.C., 269
Saihoo, P., 136
Sainsbury, M.J., 130
St. Angelo, A., 99
St. Charles, A.J., 111
St. Pierre, C.A., 188
Saito, S., 251
Saker, J., 8
Sallee, S.J., 17
Salsbury, C.A., 10
Saltman, J., 83, 111, 258
Salustiano, J., 97
Sampaio, C., 99
Sampurnanand, 55
Samuels, G., 111, 120, 145, 189, 277
Sand, W.T., 115
Sanders, K., 129
Sanders, M.K., 152
Sandison, R.A., 50

309

314